LEAD
versus
HEALTH
**Sources and Effects
of Low Level Lead
Exposure**

LEAD
versus
HEALTH
Sources and Effects of Low Level Lead Exposure

edited by

Michael Rutter
Professor of Child Psychiatry
Institute of Psychiatry
De Crespigny Park
Denmark Hill
London SE5

Robin Russell Jones
Deputy Chairman
CLEAR
2 Northdown Street
London N1

A Wiley Medical Publication

JOHN WILEY & SONS
Chichester · New York · Brisbane · Toronto · Singapore

RA
1231
L4
L44

Copyright © 1983 by John Wiley & Sons Ltd.

Library of Congress Cataloging in Publication Data:

International Symposium on Low Level Lead Exposure and
    Its Effects on Human Beings (1982: London, England)
    Lead versus health.
    (A Wiley medical publication)
    Includes bibliographical references and index.
    1. Lead-poisoning—Congresses.   2. Lead—
    Environmental aspects—Congresses.   I. Rutter,
    Michael.   II. Russell Jones, Robin.   III. Title.
    IV. Series. [DNLM: 1. Lead poisoning—Congresses.
    QV 164L 1982]
    RA1231.L41545 1982   363.1'79   82-16020
    ISBN 0 471 90028 1

British Library Cataloguing in Publication Data:

International Symposium on Low Level Lead Exposure and
    its Effects on Human Beings *(1982: London)*
    Lead versus health.
    1. Lead—Physiological effects—Congresses
    I. Title   II. Rutter, Michael
    III. Russell Jones, Robin
    612'.01524   RA1231.L4

    ISBN 0 471 90028 1

Printed in Great Britain

LIST OF CONTRIBUTORS

Augustinos Anagnostopoulos,   Professor of Inorganic Chemistry,
Aristotlian University of
Thessaloniki,
School of Chemical Engineering,
Thessaloniki,
Greece.

Joseph L. Annest,   Geneticist and Statistician,
National Center for Health Statistics,
3700 East West Highway,
Hyattsville,
Maryland 20782,
U.S.A.

Curtis Barton,   Graduate Student in Psychometrics,
Department of Psychology,
University of North Carolina,
Chapel Hill,
NC 27514
U.S.A.

Vernon Benignus,   Physiological Psychologist,
Environmental Protection Agency,
Research Triangle Park,
NC 27711,
U.S.A.

Irwin H. Billick,   Program Manager,
Lead Poisoning Research,
Environmental Research Group,
Department of Housing and Urban
Development,
Washington DC,
U.S.A.

Julian Clark,   Psychiatrist,
Department of Psychiatry,
State University of New York,
Downstate Medical Center,
Brooklyn NY 11203,
U.S.A.

Oliver David,   Associate Professor of Psychiatry,
State University of New York,
Downstate Medical Center,
Brooklyn NY 11203,
U.S.A.

Michael J. Duggan,

Scientific Officer,
Greater London Council,
County Hall,
London SE1.

Gary Grad,

Psychiatrist,
Department of Psychiatry,
Downstate Medical Center,
Brooklyn NY 11203,
U.S.A.

Philippe Grandjean,

Director,
Department of Occupational Medicine,
Danish National Institute of
Occupational Health,
Baunegaardsvej 73,
DK - 2900 Hellerup,
Denmark.

Stanley Hoffman,

Research Psychologist,
Department of Psychiatry,
State University of New York,
Downstate Medical Center,
Brooklyn NY 11203,
U.S.A.

Richard Lansdown,

Principal Psychologist,
Department of Psychological
Medicine,
The Hospital for Sick Children,
Great Ormond Street,
LONDON WC1.

Ian B. Millar,

District Community Physician,
Greenwich Health District,
London.

Michael R. Moore,

Senior Lecturer in Medicine,
University of Glasgow,
Department of Medicine,
Western Infirmary,
Glasgow G11 6NT.

Keith Muller,

Psychometrician,
Department of Epidemiology,
University of North Carolina,
Chapel Hill,
North Carolina 27514,
U.S.A.

Herbert L. Needleman,

Associate Professor of Child
Psychiatry and Paediatrics,
Children's Hospital of Pittsburgh,
125 De Soto Street
Pittsburgh PA 15213,
U.S.A.

David Otto,

Research Psychologist,
United States Environmental
Protection Agency,
Research Triangle Park,
North Carolina 27711,
U.S.A.

Clair C. Patterson,

Geochemist,
California Institute of Technology,
Pasadena,
California 91125,
U.S.A.

Robin Russell Jones,

Deputy Chairman,
CLEAR,
2 Northdown Street,
LONDON N1.

Michael Rutter,

Professor of Child Psychiatry,
Institute of Psychiatry,
De Crespigny Park,
London SE5 8AF.

Ellen K. Silbergeld,

Chief Toxics Scientist,
Environmental Defense Fund,
1525 18th Street NW,
Washington DC 20036,
U.S.A.

Robert S. Stephens,

Reader in Chemistry,
Department of Chemistry,
University of Birmingham,
PO. Box 363,
Birmingham B15 2TT.

Jeffrey Sverd,

Child Psychologist,
Department of Psychiatry,
State University of New York,
Downstate Medical Center,
Brooklyn NY,
U.S.A.

Marie-Ann Urbanowicz,

Research Psychologist,
Department of Psychology,
University of London,
Institute of Psychiatry,
De Crespigny Park,
London SE5 8AF.

Gerhard Winneke,

Director,
Psychophysiology Section,
Medical Institute of Environmental
Hygiene,
University of Dusseldorf,
Gurlittstrasse 53,
D 4000 Dusseldorf,
Germany.

William Yule,

Reader in Applied Psychology,
Institute of Psychiatry,
De Crespigny Park,
London SE5 8AF.

PREFACE

This volume represents the edited proceedings of an international symposium on 'Low Level Lead Exposure and Its Effects on Human Beings' that took place in London at the Institute of British Architects from May 10-12th, 1982. The symposium was organized by the CLEAR Charitable Trust and was sponsored by Pura Foods Ltd; we express our appreciation to both organizations.

The prime purpose of the symposium was to allow a rigorous, critical and thoughtful reappraisal of the evidence on the effects of low level lead exposure. The speakers were chosen on the basis of their active current research involvement in the topic, with special reference to those new investigations claimed to be throwing new light on the subject. The meeting was widely advertised and open to all who wished to attend, but special invitations were extended to many of the key figures in the controversies surrounding the question of whether low levels of exposure can be damaging to health. The discussion periods following each paper were designed to allow full opportunities for participants to raise conceptual and methodological concerns over the evidence and the inferences based on it. Equally, they gave speakers the occasion to consider criticisms and to put such counter-arguments as might be appropriate. Because these discussions served both to clarify some of the research findings and to highlight some of the crucial points of difficulties or disagreements over the interpretations of the findings, we have retained them in the volume. Whether or not the evidence allows consensus on the conclusions to be drawn must be left to readers to decide for themselves. However, certainly our hope is that the volume might provide a considered "state of the art" appraisal of what we know and what we do not know, together with the implications that stem from that appraisal.

All but two of the papers given at the symposium have been included. The first omission was a preliminary report on lead levels and abnormal births that the author wished to hold until the study was complete. As the topic is an important one, Dr Ellen Silbergeld was asked to prepare a chapter on the experimental studies of the effects of lead on reproduction. We are most grateful to her for producing an authoritative review with the necessary speed to meet publication deadlines. The second omission, Dr Philip Day's review of research into environmental sources of lead exposure, stemmed from his inability to produce a paper in time for publication. Again, as the material covered was crucial to this volume, one of us (R.R.J.) joined with Dr Robert Stephens to prepare a review of the topic. During the course of the meeting it became clear that lead-contaminated dust might constitute an important source of lead exposure for children; accordingly, we are very pleased to include Dr Michael Duggan's appraisal of that issue as a further additional chapter beyond those given at the symposium. Also, we are glad to be able to include a chapter by Dr David Otto who was invited to the meeting but who was unable to attend.

The book is divided into five parts. In the first chapter, Rutter introduces the topic with an outline of the scientific concerns and a brief review of the main evidence prior to 1980 on the psychological sequelae of lead exposure in children. The second section is concerned with the sources of lead in the environment. Patterson compares natural levels of lead with those that are found in our present-day environment, whilst the chapters by Annest and Billick focus on recent trends in lead levels in the U.S.A. Moore describes his findings on lead in drinking water, and both Anagnostopoulos and Duggan focus on the role of lead in dust. Finally, Russell Jones and Stephens provide an extensive review of the evidence that identifies lead in petrol as a significant contributor to human lead intake.

The third section deals with the toxicology of lead. Grandjean discussed what is known about organolead compounds and Silbergeld devotes two chapters to the findings from animal research. The first discusses experimental studies of lead neurotoxicity and the second considers the effects of lead on reproduction. These chapters are included because any understanding of the mechanisms and processes underlying lead effects must rely on experimental studies.

The fourth section is concerned with the effects of lead on children's behaviour and intellectual functioning. Needleman describes his American epidemiological study based on dentine lead; Winneke provides the findings from his two studies in Germany using tooth lead; Lansdown et al report a British study based on blood levels; David et al give an account of the use of chelation to study the behavioural effects of lead in hyperactive American children with moderately elevated lead levels; and Otto et al report on the relationships between electrophysiological measures and blood lead levels in early childhood. In the final chapter, Rutter seeks to draw together these (and other) findings in an overall appraisal of the sources and effects of low level lead exposure, this is followed by a discussion of the policy implications that stem from the scientific evidence.

Numerous people have provided generous help in the preparation of this volume. While we cannot record them all, we would like to express a particular note of appreciation to the chapter authors who willingly and cheerfully met very tight deadlines in order to bring the volume to completion as swiftly as possible. Also we owe a deep debt of gratitude to the secretaries who coped admirably with a tremendous load of work. Particular thanks are due to Joy Maxwell and Jenny Smith at the Institute of Psychiatry, to Sue Dibb and Patricia Simms at CLEAR, to Anita Salvador for her help with the typing, and to Sylvia Holmes who assisted with the illustrations. Finally, we are most indebted of all to Des Wilson of CLEAR without whom the symposium would not have taken place at all.

Michael Rutter and Robin Russell Jones

PART 1
Introduction

Lead Versus Health
Edited by M. Rutter and R. Russell Jones
© 1983 John Wiley & Sons Ltd.

SCIENTIFIC ISSUES AND STATE OF THE ART IN 1980

Michael Rutter

Department of Child and Adolescent Psychiatry
Institute Of Pyschiatry
De Crespigny Park
Denmark Hill
London SE5.

INTRODUCTION

The topic of low level lead exposure constitutes a difficult area for research with many technical problems in measurement and even greater difficulties in statistical analysis that stem from the multitude of interacting variables. As various reviews of the evidence have emphasised (see Rutter, 1980; U.S. Environmental Protection Agency, 1977; U.S. Committee on Lead in the Human Environment, 1980), it has been no easy or straightforward matter to separate out the psychological effects of lead exposure per se from the manifold adverse social influences with which it tends to be associated. Nevertheless, that is what must be done if we are to understand how lead affects human functioning.

The papers included in this volume aim to summarise the scientific issues and findings, and to assess the quality and strength of the evidence on the sources of lead on the environment and on the possible effects of that lead on children's development and neuropsychological functioning. Inevitably with a topic of this kind, policy issues intertwine with scientific considerations. This occurs not only because the health of the nation's children and the future of the next generation is an emotive subject, but also because there is a general awareness that almost all research findings in this field have potential policy implications. Nevertheless, as Rein and White (1977) have argued, research and policy making constitute rather different fields of actions. They suggest that the 'game' of science lies in the determination of value-neutral facts, whereas the 'game' of politics involves the design of value-expressive action. Of course, in the real world, facts are never truly value-neutral. Even so, the strength of science lies in its ability to devise means of testing ideas and of finding answers to questions. It is the responsibility of the researcher to undertake this task with rigour, with dispassionate care to test the validity of one hypothesis against the claims of other competing hypotheses, and with the creative imagination to see how studies may be planned for this purpose. Science does not comprise a body of knowledge; rather it involves a process of enquiry - a means of finding out about how things work. As

1

Medawar (1969) put it: "The purpose of scientific enquiry is not to compile an inventory of factual information.. (instead) It begins as a story about a Possible World - a story which we invent and criticise and modify as we go along, so that it ends by being, as nearly as we can make it, a story about real life". It is that aspect of science with which this volume is concerned.

Politicians need to understand the factual evidence on levels of risk and on mechanisms of action that is relevant to their decision--making and, in particular, need to know which actions are likely to be most effective in meeting their value determined aims. Hopefully, the subject matter of this book will help to provide that evidence. However, the development of policies necessarily also involves decisions on values and on political aims and objectives, as well as analyses of financial implications. All those matters are outside the scope of this volume.

The symposium on which it is based was not designed to provide the forum for political debate, or for the accusations and counter-accusations on personalities and values that that so often involves. It is profoundly to be regretted that, in some quarters, the scientific discussion on lead has degenerated into heated exchanges of ex cathedra assertions that this person's work is 'not to be trusted' because he has taken some supposed political stand, or signed some official report, or accepted Government or Industry funds for research. Rather than cast aspersions on the scientific probity of our colleagues we need to look at the quality of their work. It is on that basis that they should be judged.

Scientists are also citizens and it is their responsibility to come to such conclusions on policy matters as may be possible, and to act accordingly. The fact that we have not all chosen to act in precisely the same way is a reflection of the lack of certainty in the empirical evidence. Of course, science does not deal in certainties; rather, it provides evidence on probabilities and it is on those probabilities that political decisions have to be taken. The responsibility of participants in this symposium was to weigh the empirical research findings in order to come to the best judgement possible on the likely effects of low level lead exposure.

But, if our concern is to foster normal development and to reduce the risks of damage to children and adults in our society (and that must be the concern of all of us), perhaps we should pause to question whether there was a need for this symposium at all. After all, it is only two years since a Department of Health and Social Security Working Party (1980), the Lawther Committee, produced their report on exactly these issues. Did we need to go over the same ground yet again? I think we did. That report has not been free from criticism and the symposium provided the opportunity for a fresh look. But, more especially, new evidence had become available during that two years and we needed to consider whether that strengthened or weakened the case that there were significant ill-effects from low lead level exposure. After all, the Lawther

Committee was quite explicit that further research was required in order to provide a satisfactory estimate of the level of risk at low levels of lead. Did the new evidence allow that estimate to be made?

Of course, some may feel that that gets us unnecessarily involved in scientific niceties. Researchers may quibble on whether or not there is a 'safe' limit of lead exposure and, if there is, what that limit may be. But do we need to bother with that? After all, it is well established that lead is a serious toxin with potentially damaging effects on the nervous system. Moreover, lead has no known physiological benefits. As everyone is agreed that lead could do harm and definitely does not do good, is that not enough to get on with the urgent business of getting lead out of the environment? Undoubtedly, that is enough for some public health actions and those should be implemented without further delay. It should always be remembered that no decision to act is a decision 'not to act'. Even so, we cannot leave the matter there for two rather different reasons.

Firstly, although some public health actions are inexpensive and without risks, others are costly and carry risks of their own. Thus, some 'experts' advocate treating people exposed to lead by chelation - a chemical treatment designed to eliminate lead from the body. That treatment is not free from risks and before we embark on any policy of widespread chelation we need to be sure that the cure is not worse that the disease. Or, again, some argue that we should cease using lead for any purposes at all. That may be right but there are many instances in which lead seems to be the best substance for the purpose (Lin-Fu, 1973) and before we advocate changing everything, we need to know that it is necessary. Another example is provided by lead-emitting ore smelters. Should the evidence that they have seriously contaminated the environment with toxic lead mean that the area should be evacuated? Perhaps, but it is not a neutral action to remove people from their homes or deprive them of their jobs. That circumstance requires rather a high level of probability on the risks.

The second reason why we need to be able to assess the level of risk from particular levels of lead exposure concerns actions on 'non-lead' factors in the environment. Over the years enthusiastic claims have been made that lead toxicity constitutes one of the main causes of criminality and educational difficulties. Indeed, British newspapers in 1981 reported one claim that lead pollution played a dominant role in the riots in Brixton and Toxteth! If that were so, it would constitute a very considerable cause for relief among politicians. The saving in money would be enormous. After all, some would feel that it relieved them from having to bother further about social disadvantage or racial discrimination or even patterns of policing! But before we give up attempts at social reform we need to be sure that lead really is responsible for most of the ills of society. Of course, such extreme claims are wholly inconsistent with the empirical evidence and do not warrant serious discussion.

Nevertheless, the issues they raise are serious, for our conclusions on the extent of damage from low levels of lead exposure do have implications for our actions on <u>other</u> health hazards. It is for these reasons that we need to consider the evidence carefully. Our understanding of the effects of low level lead exposure involves a serious scientific purpose but, also, that purpose has crucial implications for policy.

Because the chapters that follow are largely concerned with very recent research findings, we need first to consider briefly the state of play before those investigations were undertaken. What had been shown by the earlier research, and what scientific issues had it raised?

RESEARCH PRIOR TO 1980

The story of the concern over the possibly adverse effects of (relatively) low levels of exposure to lead had its origins in the general recognition in the early years of this century that high doses of lead could cause encephalopathy, with convulsions and coma often followed by death (e.g. Thomas and Blackfan, 1914). It was found, too, that many children who recovered from encephalopathy were left with permanent neurological sequelae. Then, some years later, there came the first reports that there could be persistent neurotoxic impairment following milder episodes of lead poisoning that fell short of overt encephalopathy (Byers and Lord, 1943; Perlstein and Attala, 1966). However, until the 1970's there was a general assumption that increased lead levels were of little clinical importance if there were no recognisable symptoms of poisoning (in terms of anaemia, peripheral neuropathy, renal damage, or neurological dysfunction) and if blood lead levels were below about 50 or 60 µg/dl. During the last dozen years or so, that assumption has been called in questions increasingly and it has been argued that there may be adverse effects of lead on behaviour and cognition even at levels hitherto regarded as safe or acceptable (Bryce-Smith and Waldron, 1974; Conservation Society, 1978; Repko and Corum, 1976). The empirical evidence underpinning those arguments derived from studies using a variety of different research strategies.

<u>Clinic-Type Studies with High Lead Levels</u>   Perhaps the most commonly used approach was the comparison of clinic children with high lead levels and controls known or supposed to have low levels. For example, De la Burde and Choate (1972; 1975) compared 70 four-year-old children with pica and blood lead levels of at least 40 µg/dl (or at least 30 µg/dl in association with X-ray lead line findings), and 72 controls who were reasonably well matched over a good range of appropriate background variables, including maternal IQ. Comparisons both at 4 and 7 years showed the high lead children to have intellectual scores of some 3 to 5 points below the controls and to include a higher proportion with behavioural difficulties. The study was a generally satisfactory one but details were lacking on some important issues and the groups were not

equated for pica (so that there was the possibility that the group differences reflected the lower IQ and greater behavioural deviance of children with pica, rather than an effect of high lead levels per se).

Similarly, Perino and Ernhart (1974) contrasted 30 black preschool children with blood lead levels in the 40 to 70 µg/dl range, with 50 whose levels were in the 10 to 30 range. Inadequate details were given on sampling and matching but there seemed to be sound blood lead assessments. The high lead group had a mean McCarthy scale IQ 10 points below the controls (80 vs. 90); also, the parent-child IQ correlation was significantly lower in the high lead group (0.10 vs. 0.52) - suggesting that lead toxicity had attenuated the usual parental effect on child IQ.

Most other studies of this type produced broadly comparable results but some gave rise to essentially negative findings (e.g. Baloh et al., 1975). However, the general indication from the better investigations was that lead levels persistently raised above 60 tend to be associated, on average, with a 3 to 4 point reduction in IQ, even among asymptomatic children. Conclusions were much less certain with respect to levels in the 40 to 60 range but there were pointers to the possibility of adverse sequelae in some instances. The main limitations lay in the paucity of data on the effects of lead levels below 40 µg/dl and the often rather weak statistical controls for the confounding effects of pica and of social background.

Studies of Mentally Retarded or Behaviourally Deviant Children
David and his colleagues (1972; 1976; 1977) conducted several studies of the relationships between lead levels and mental retardation or hyperkinesis in clinic children. The usual design involved a comparison of the blood lead levels of a psychiatric clinic group and a paediatric clinic control group; together with a further subcomparison within the clinic group of those children for whom there was a known non-lead aetiology and those with an unknown aetiology. The general finding was that lead levels were higher in the psychiatric group than in paediatric controls, and higher in those with an unknown aetiology than in those where the cause of the disorder was thought to have been established. All these studies have numerous weaknesses including a paucity of data on relevant background variables, arbitrary and uncertain designations of 'cause', and missing data. In view of these limitations (with David's and with other studies, such as those by Beattie et al, 1975 and Moore et al, 1977), no firm conclusions are possible from this research strategy. The consistent finding of higher lead levels in deviant groups is provocative but it is uncertain whether they represent a cause, or an effect, or a mixture of the two.

Chelation Studies   Chelation studies in which chemical means are used to eliminate lead from children with high lead levels approximate to the experimental model, in that if it could be shown that a reduction in body lead was followed by intellectual gains or behavioural improvement this would provide powerful evidence for a

causal link. However, for this strategy to be valid it is essential:
a) to employ contrasting interventions in order to determine
whether the gains are specifically due to the fall in lead levels; and
b) to use control groups or baseline periods to check whether the
alterations in IQ or behaviour exceed those due to random
fluctuations or to maturational changes. Unfortunately, none of the
published studies (e.g., Pueschel et al, 1972; David et al, 1976;
Sachs et al, 1978) adequately met these minimal criteria and no
worthwhile conclusions were possible.

Smelter Studies   One of the major difficulties in the interpretation
of most studies showing an association between raised lead levels
and impaired intelligence or disturbed behaviour was the question of
which led to which. Were less intelligent, behaviourally deviant
children more likely to exhibit pica and hence absorb excessive lead
as a result of their behaviour, or did an increased burden of body
lead cause a lowering IQ and an increase in abnormal behaviour?
The only really satisfactory means of avoiding this dilemma is to
study children whose exposure to lead is extrinsic to and
independant of their own behaviour. In theory, investigations of
children living near a lead smelter should provide this opportunity.
Unfortunately, in practice such studies have been bedevilled by the
possibility that families living near a smelter differ in social or
other characteristics from those living further away (homes are not
allocated randomly!). Also, many of the investigations have
suffered from a weak or unknown relationship between blood levels
and proximity to the smelter (e.g. Hebel et al., 1976; Lansdown et
al., 1974; Landrigan et al., 1975a and b), from small sample size
(Ratcliffe, 1977), from subject loss (Gregory et al, 1976) or from
problems in the presentation of findings (McNeil et al, 1975).
These methodological difficulties severely limit the conclusions that
can be drawn from smelter sites; nevertheless, it may be noted that
four of the six studies were consistent with a small (1 to 5 points)
intellectual deficit associated with raised lead levels in the 40 to
80 µg/dl range (see Rutter, 1980).

General Population Studies   It was clear during the 1970s that
epidemiological enquiries were likely to be required in order to deal
with methodological defects in the studies using other research
strategies. Needleman et al's (1979) investigation in Massachusetts
which sought to relate dentine lead levels and measures of neuropsychological functioning provided the first well planned large scale
enquiry of that kind. There were some important questions and
reservations about the study as reported in 1979 (but see also
chapter 12) but none were sufficient to invalidate the findings and,
in 1980, I concluded that it provided: "the most impressive evidence
to date on the possibly damaging effects of raised lead levels in the
range usually previously considered harmless" (p.19).

Overview to Studies Prior to 1980   With respect to the subject of
this volume, the most obvious feature of the pre-1980 studies is
that scarcely any, with the possible exception of Needleman's, dealt
at all systematically with blood lead levels below 35 µg/dl. In view

of the <u>absence</u> of empirical evidence on the effects of low level lead exposure below that cut-off, <u>no conclusions were possible on the consequences of lead levels below 35</u>. Accordingly, the first need was to undertake enquiries with a specific focus on that group. Later chapters in this volume do just that.

In addition, however, these earlier investigations highlighted several crucial methodological considerations that needed to be dealt with if more firmly based conclusions were to be drawn. First, there was the problem of selection bias stemming from a) the use of clinic sample, or b) the use of volunteer subjects, or c) the differential loss of subjects and the failure to obtain systematic data on all individuals in the study. The implication was that epidemiological studies of the general population or of high risk groups were desirable.

Second, many studies used weak and insensitive measures of neuropsychological functioning - often with screening questionnaires or poorly validated tests only. In that the empirical evidence was entirely consistent in showing that the effects of low level lead exposure were <u>small</u>, it was imperative to use sensitive, well validated, broad range measures of cognitive performance and of behaviour.

Third, for the same reason, it was essential to study quite large samples. If the effects are small, it follows that large groups will be needed to produce statistically significant results.

Fourth, there were the problems stemming from inadequate markers of exposure to lead. Most early studies relied on single blood lead levels, often with measures obtained several years prior to the psychological assessment of the children. Because blood lead levels reflect only very <u>recent</u> ingestion of lead, they provide an unsatisfactory guide to the overall lead burden (especially when there is an acute source of high lead exposure), they fail to give information on <u>past</u> exposure or on the <u>duration</u> of exposure, and they cannot differentiate between short-term and long-term lead intoxication. Moreover, many of the published reports were unclear as to whether the measures referred to peak blood levels, to average levels during the main period of lead exposure, or to the levels found <u>after</u> removal of the lead source. This problem seemed to point to the need to use indices, such as tooth or dentine lead, that did reflect the long-term overall body lead burden.

Fifth, although some studies suffered from the use of a single weak psychological outcome measure, others suffered from the problems that derive from the use of a large number of measures. The difficulty in the latter situation is that many univariate statistical comparisons are bound to produce a few differences that are simply the result of chance. There are several available means of dealing with this problem, however. These include the use of multivariate statistics, determination of whether the significant differences always fell in the same direction (chance differences should favour

all groups equally), and determination of whether the same differ
ences (on the same tests) are replicated in different investigations
(see Rutter, 1980).

Finally, there was the need to provide adequate statistical controls
for possible confounding variables - especially pica and psychosocial
background. As this is such a crucial issue, and as it has been so
widely misunderstood by those concerned about lead pollution, it
warrants more detailed discussion.

CONFOUNDING VARIABLES

The need to control for confounding variables arises when the
groups (e.g. high lead and low lead) to be compared with respect
to some dependent variable (e.g. IQ), differ in terms of some third
variable (e.g. social class or maternal IQ) which also correlates
with the dependent measure. In this situation all three variables
inter-correlate with one another and the question is: Which is
causing which? Thus, in some studies it has been found that the
IQ of the high lead children is, on average, lower than that of the
low lead children - suggesting a neurotoxic effect by which lead
lowers IQ levels. However, when maternal IQ and social class are
'controlled', by entering them into the multivariate analysis before
lead, the high lead and low lead groups no longer differ in IQ.
The inference that stems from that analysis is that there was no
'true' lead effect on IQ; rather, it resulted from the prior association between social background and lead exposure. Somehow,
especially if one is personally committed to the need to get lead out
of the environment, that seems a bit of unacceptable statistical
jiggery-pokery that has misleadingly succeeded in 'explaining away'
a real effect of lead. Surely, if the high lead and low lead groups
initially differed in IQ (before statistical controls for confounding
variables were introduced) there must be some sort of real effect of
lead on IQ? How could it just disappear in the statistical analysis?

Perhaps the point is illustrated most easily by means of an analogy.
If the total population of England was studied systematically, a
highly significant correlation would be found between baldness and
height. It might, therefore, be inferred that baldness caused
tallness (or, if you prefer, that tallness caused baldness). But,
the careful investigator would also have observed that both
baldness and tallness themselves correlated with age and sex.
Statistical controls would then be introduced for age, with the
result that the correlation between baldness and height would drop
markedly. This reduction in the association, of course, would have
arisen because scarcely any children are bald and it would not be
sensible to examine the links between baldness and height without
first taking that into account (either through statistical manipulation
or through a restriction of the sample to adults). Then, further
statistical controls would need to be added in order to deal with sex
differences. At that point the correlation between baldness and
height would disappear altogether. The original correlation arose
only because, on average, men are taller than women and because

although some men are bald, scarcely any women lose much of their hair. Within a sample of men, baldness is unassociated with height. The initial correlation carried with it no causal implications; it was just an artefact of the fact that baldness is largely restricted to adult males.

Interestingly, if the study had been restricted to adult men the correlation would have been the other way round - i.e. between baldness and shortness! In that case, the association (once again artefactual) would have arisen simply because old men (who are more likely to be bald) tend to be shorter - both because of shrinking with age and because less well nourished past generations tended to be shorter than the young adults of today.

Not only is it apparent that the introduction of appropriate controls for confounding variables can correctly cause a correlation to 'disappear' completely, but also it can reverse a correlation. That is not statistical juggling but, rather, a means of better representing the true state of affairs. The example of baldness serves to illustrate why that is necessary if totally false inferences are not to be drawn. The same need arises with respect to lead, social background and psychological functioning.

The main facts here are reasonably straightforward, although their interpretation is not. That is to say, it is well established that there is a very substantial overlap between social disadvantage and high level exposure. It is apparent in terms of the general population studies (see chapters 3, 4, 12, 13 and 14) and also it has been evident in more detailed studies of the home environment of children known to have raised lead levels. For example, Milar et al (1980) studied 52 asymptomatic children, aged 10 to 73 months, who had been referred to a lead screening programme. The families of children with lead levels above 30 μg/dl were systematically compared with those whose lead levels were below that cut-off - using, amongst other things, measures of maternal IQ and the Caldwell HOME inventory, which provides an assessment of the quality of the caregiving environment. The findings showed that in the younger age group of children (below 30 months of age) the maternal IQ in the high lead group was significantly lower (75.0 vs. 85.1) and the HOME inventory scores were also lower (i.e. 'worse'). The differences were less marked in the older age group of children.

The importance of this finding (and others of a similar kind) is that is it well known that, for reasons unconnected with lead, maternal IQ and the quality of caregiving have an influence on children's psychological development (see Rutter, 1983a; Rutter and Madge, 1976). In part, that causal influence reflects genetic factors and, in part, environmental effects. However, there are several reasons why we know that the associations are not explicable in terms of lead exposure. Most obviously, lead cannot account for the correlations between the maternal IQ of biological mothers and the IQ of their children who have been adopted by other parents and hence who have not shared the same environment; nor can it account for the associations between the quality of institutional environments and the development of children reared in them. Accordingly, it is clear that children's social background has an independent effect (partly genetic and partly environmental) on their psychological functioning. Moreover, it is apparent from the strength of these associations that these independent effects of the social environment are substantially greater than the effects of low level lead exposure. It is obvious that it is essential to control for the confounding effects of social background factors if we are to assess whether lead, too, has a causal effect on psychological functioning.

However, in undertaking the necessary multivariate statistical analyses to control for confounding variables it is important to bear in mind the various alternative hypotheses to be considered. First, there are the two extremes. That is it could be that the only true effect is that due to social background - lead only seems to have an effect because high lead levels are more commonly found in children from socially disadvantaged homes. In the studies undertaken prior to 1980, this did not seem to be the case but there were doubts because most studies had rather weak measures of social variables. Alternatively, it could be that the only true effect is that due to lead. As already noted, we can rule out that hypothesis completely because we know that there are effects of the social environment that have nothing to do with lead.

Secondly, there are various 'intermediate' hypotheses. The simplest is that the effects are a bit of both - that is that both lead and the social background have effects on psychological functioning but that these are separate and unconnected. That remains a real possibility. But, also, there are more complicated (but still highly plausible) ways in which the causal processes might work. For example, it could be that an adverse social environment (living in an old house with lead plumbing, or living near a lead smelter, or living adjacent to a motorway with high lead pollution of the air) serves to increase the likelihood of high lead exposure which then, in turn, has an adverse effect on children's psychological functioning. In that case the effects of the social environment and of lead exposure would be inter-linked in that the former predisposed to the latter.

Thirdly, various different types of interaction may be postulated. For example, on the basis of what is known about the effects of other biological hazards, it reasonably could be proposed that the adverse effects of lead might be greater in the case of children who, for other reasons, already have a lower IQ or some behavioural disturbance or who come from a socially disadvantaged background. In other words, the presence of one type of disadvantage potentiates or increases the effect of another type. If that were so, we might expect to see greater effects of lead among children from a poor background than among those living in more affluent circumstances. This is more than a remote theoretical possibility in that there is good evidence for other biological hazards (such as malnutrition or perinatal complications) that this sort of potentiation does indeed occur. Statistical means are available to test for these (or other) interaction effects but it is important to recognise that there are many different forms of interaction and that considerable care is needed in the choice of statistical tests if they are to be detected (see Rutter, 1983b).

Of course, too, it is apparent that from a public policy point of view it is not enough to consider the links between lead exposure and social adversity only in terms of the possible implications for an understanding of the mechanisms underlying the associations with some dependent variable with respect to children's psychological development. Also, we have to ask why social adversity and lead exposure are linked in the first place, and what implications the answer to that question may have for policies of prevention. The chapter by Dr. Moore later in this volume deals quite explicitly with that issue in terms of the means by which water can become lead-polluted. However, the point is a general one that applies to all routes by which lead may enter the body.

BIOLOGICAL MECHANISMS

One further issue with respect to the state of play prior to 1980 on the research into the possible adverse effects of low level lead exposure concerns the need to identify the biological mechanisms involved. Quite rightly, there is always a good deal of scepticism regarding causal inferences based on weak statistical associations (as is the case with lead) so long as the biological mechanisms remain unknown. Of course, it could be argued that the mechanism is likely to involve small degrees of brain damage, on the grounds that if high levels of lead exposure lead to severe damage (which, it is known that they do) then low levels should cause slight damage. However, that is a weak and unsatisfactory argument for several different reasons. In the first place, the general concept of 'minimal brain dysfunction' remains both controversial and poorly supported (see Rutter, 1983c). It is not that anyone doubts that minor degrees of damage can occur - obviously they can and do take place. Rather, the problem lies in doubts as to whether such minor damage has any functional consequences, and in the lack of convincing evidence that there is any coherence to the syndromes supposedly associated with minor damage to the brain. Secondly, because high levels of lead exposure lead to severe brain damage it does not follow that lower levels will have similar, but lesser, effects. There are numerous examples of biological agents that have different effects at different levels (thus, many elements are beneficial, and indeed necessary for life, at low levels but toxic at high levels), and of agents that cause damage only above some threshold. It is not acceptable to argue downwards by extrapolation from what is known about the effects of high lead exposure. Instead, the need is for direct studies of the biological effects of low level exposure.

Prior to 1980, there were few satisfactory studies of that kind. In humans, research had been limited by the lack of satisfactory tools with which to assess brain functioning. It was known that the ordinary EEG was useless for that purpose and at that time little use had been made of computer assisted EEG analyses with lead exposed children. In contrast, there had been many animal studies but these had other limitations of a serious kind (U.S. Environmental Protection Agency, 1977). Firstly, there were problems of species differences. For example, in rats lead intoxication commonly leads to paraplegia and serious growth retardation whereas this is unusual in humans. Secondly, the great majority of experimental studies had failed to take account of undernutrition. This was a major shortcoming because high lead exposure in animals was usually accompanied by serious undernutrition and because undernutrition is known to have effects on brain structure and functioning. Thirdly, many investigations had rather unsatisfactory measures of the level of body lead being studied. Insofar as such measures were available it was evident that, almost always, rather high levels of lead exposure were involved. In particular, the animal research threw little light on the mechanisms involved in effects occurring with blood lead levels below 35 µg/dl. Fourthly, the animal models of human behavioural syndromes tended to rely on weak and inappropriate analogies as well as on unsatisfactory behavioural measures (especially assessments of overall activity level). Thus, the use of animal studies to investigate the role of lead intoxication in the hyperkinetic syndrome (e.g. Silbergeld and Goldberg, 1973; 1974), which at one time seemed so hopeful, have not stood the test of time. Not only were the results seriously confounded by undernutrition, but also it has become apparent that the behavioural measures used had serious limitations. As a consequence, subsequent studies have produced discrepant findings that allow of no overall conclusion.

Nevertheless, during the 1970s, researchers were becoming aware of these methodological problems and were taking steps to remedy the deficiencies of the earlier research. By the late 1970s it was already apparent that the better recent research was beginning to provide useful insights into the biological mechanisms that might underlie the effects of low level lead exposure. Some of that research is succinctly summarized in Dr. Silbergeld's two chapters on animal studies in this volume.

CONCLUSIONS

The research prior to 1980 had been important in showing that lead had important effects on neuropsychological functioning even when there had been no overt encephalopathy. As a result, it had become generally accepted that there were important adverse sequelae with blood lead levels above 60 µg/dl; and that, probably, there might also be sequelae with levels in the 40 to 60 µg/dl range. However, little was known on the effects of lead when blood lead levels remained below 40. As I concluded in 1980,....
"The more difficult issue is how far there may be cognitive

impairment with blood lead levels in the 20 to 40 µg/dl range....
The Needleman et al study ... suggests a threshold for toxicity far
below that suggested by most other investigations... (but) there
are reasons for considering that caution is needed before too much
is built into this one study. Nevertheless, a good case has been
made which cannot so far be disproven and it is essential to
conduct further studies which could settle the matter one way or
the other" (pp. 19-20). During the last two years there has been
substantial further research into the effects of low level lead
exposure; the chapters that follow outline what has been done and
what has been found. The discussion sections following each
chapter report the debate that took place during the CLEAR
symposium on just what inferences could be drawn from these
findings.

REFERENCES

Baloh, R., Sturn, R., Green, and Gleser, B., (1975), Neuro-
    psychological effects of chronic asymptomatic increased lead
    absorption. Arch. Neurol., 32, 326-330.
Beattie, A.D., Moore, M.R., Goldberg, A., Finlayson, M.J.W.,
    Graham, J.F., Mackie, E.M., Main, J.C., McLaren, D.A.,
    Murdoch, R.M. and Stewart, G.T., (1975), Role of chronic low-
    level lead exposure in the aetiology of mental retardation.
    Lancet, 1, 589-592.
Bryce-Smith, D. and Waldron, H.A., (1974), Lead, behaviour and
    criminality. Ecologist, 4, 367-377.
Byers, R.K. and Lord, E.E., (1943), Late effects of lead poisoning
    on mental development. Amer. J. Dis. Child., 66, 471-494.
Conservation Society (1978), The Health Effects of Lead on
    Children. Memorandum to the Department of the Environment,
    London.
David, O.J., Clark, J. and Voeller, K., (1972), Lead and hyper-
    activity. Lancet, 2, 900-903.
David, O.J., Hoffman, S., McCann, B., Sverd, J. and Clark, J.,
    (1976), Low lead levels and mental retardation. Lancet, 2,
    1376-1379.
David, O.J., Hoffman, S., Sverd, J. and Clark, J., (1977), Lead
    and hyperactivity. Behavioural response to chelation (a pilot
    study). Amer. J. Psych., 133, 1155-1158.
De la Burde, B. and Choate, M.S., (1972), Does asymptomatic lead
    exposure in children have latent sequelae? J. Ped., 81,
    1088-1091.
De la Burde, B. and Choate, M.S., (1975), Early asymptomatic lead
    exposure and developmental school age. J. Ped., 87, 638-642.
Department of Health and Social Security, (2980) Lead and Health:
    The report of a DHSS Working Party on Lead in the Environment
    (Lawther Report). London: HMSO.
Gregory, R.J., Lehman, R.E., and Mohan, P.J., (1976), Intelli-
    gence test results for children with and without undue lead
    absorption. In: Wegner, G. (ed) Shoshone Lead Health Project.
    Idaho Department of Health and Welfare (Division of Health,
    State House, Boise, Idaho 83270).

Hebel, J.R., Kinch, D. and Armstrong, E., (1976), Mental capability of children exposed to lead pollution. Brit. J. Prev. Soc. Med., 30, 170-174.

Landrigan, P.J., Gehlback, S.H., Rosenblum, B.F., Shoulta, J.M., Candelaria, R.M., Barthel, W.F., Liddle, J.A., Smrek, A.L., Staehling, N.M. and Sander, J.D.F., (1975a), Epidemic lead absorption near an ore smelter: the role of particulate lead. New Eng. J. Med., 292, 123-129.

Landrigan, P.G., Whitworth, R.H., Baloh, R.W., Staehling, M.W., Barthel, W.F. and Rosenblum, B.F., (1975b), Neuropsychological dysfunction in children with chronic low-level lead absorption. Lancet, 1, 708-712.

Lansdown, R.G., Shephard, J., Clayton, B.E., Delves, H.T., Graham, P.J. and Turner, W.C., (1974), Blood lead levels, behaviour and intelligence: a population study. Lancet, 1, 538-541.

Lin-Fu, J.S., (1973), Vulnerability of children to lead exposure and toxicity. New England J. Med., 289, 1229-1233; 1289-1293.

McNeil, J.L. Ptasnik, J.S. and Croft, D.B., (1975), Evaluation of long-term effects of elevated blood lead concentrations in asymptomatic children. Arch. Indust. Hygiene Toxicol., 26, (Suppl.) 97-118.

Medawar, P.B., (1969), Induction and Intuition in Scientific Thought. London: Methuen.

Milar, C.B., Schroeder, S.R., Mushak, P., Dolcourt, J.L. and Grant, L.D., (1980), Contributions of the caregiving environment to increased lead burden of children. Amer. J. Ment. Defic., 84, 339-344.

Moore, M.R., Meredith, P.A. and Goldberg, A., (1977), A retrospective analysis of blood lead in mentally retarded children. Lancet, 1, 717-719.

Needleman, H.L., Gunnoe, C., Leviton, A., Reed, M., Peresie, H., Maher, C. and Barrett, P., (1979), Deficits in psychological and classroom performance of children with elevated dentine lead levels. New Eng. J. Med., 300, 689-695.

Perino, J. and Ernhart, C.B., (1974), The relation of subclinical lead level to cognitive and sensorimotor impairment in black preschoolers. J. Learn. Dis., 7, 26-30.

Perlstein, M.A. and Attala, R., (1966), Neurologic sequelae of plumbism in children. Clin. Ped., 5, 292-298.

Pueschel, S.M., Kopito, L. and Schwachman, H., (1972), Children with an increased lead burden. J. Amer. Med. Assoc., 222, 462-466.

Ratcliffe, J.M., (1977), Developmental and behavioural functions in young children with elevated blood lead levels. Brit. J. Prev. Soc. Med., 31, 258-264.

Rein, M. and White, S.H., (1977), Policy Research: Belief and doubt. Pol. Anal., 3, 239-271.

Repko, J.D. and Corum, C.D., (1976), Critical Review and Evaluation of the Neurological and Behavioural Sequelae of Inorganic Lead Absorption. ITR-74-26. February, 1974. Washington: U.S.D.H.E.W.

Rutter, M., (1980), Raised lead levels and impaired cognitive/

behavioural functioning: A review of the evidence. Develop. Med. Child. Neurol., 22, Supplement No. 42.

Rutter, M., (1983a), Family and school influences: meanings, mechanisms and implications. In Nicol, A.R. (ed) Practical Lessons from Longitudinal Studies. John Wiley (in press).

Rutter, M., (1983b), Statistical and personal interactions: Facets and perspectives. In: Magnusson, D. and Allen, V. (eds) Human Development: An Interactional Perspective. New York: Academic Press.

Rutter, M. (ed) (1983c), Developmental Neuropsychiatry. New York: Guilford Press (in press).

Rutter, M. and Madge, N., (1976), Cycles of Disadvantage: A review of research. London: Heinemann Educational.

Sachs, H.K., Krall, V., McCaughran, D.A., Rozenfeld, I.H., Youngsmith, N.M., Growe, G., Lazar, B., Novar, L., O'Connell, L. and Rayson, B., (1978), IQ following treatment of lead poisoning: a patient-sibling comparison. J. Ped., 93, 428-431.

Silbergeld, E.K. and Goldberg, A.M., (1973), A lead induced behavioural disorder. Life Sci., 13, 1275-1283.

Silbergeld, E.K. and Goldberg, A.M., (1974), Lead induced behavioural dysfunction. An animal model of hyperactivity. Exp. Neurol., 42, 146-157.

Thomas, H.M. and Blackfan, A.D., (1914), Recurrent meningitis, due to lead, in a child of five years. J. Dis. Child., 8, 377-380.

U.S. Committee on Lead in the Human Environment, (1980), Lead in the Human Environment. National Research Council, National Academy of Sciences. Washington, DC: National Academy Press.

U.S. Environmental Protection Agency, (1977), Air Quality Criteria for Lead. EPA-600-8-77-017. Washington, D.C.: US Government Printing Office.

PART 2
Sources of
Lead Exposure

Lead Versus Health
Edited by M. Rutter and R. Russell Jones
© 1983 John Wiley & Sons Ltd.

BRITISH MEGA EXPOSURES TO INDUSTRIAL LEAD

Clair C. Patterson

Division of Geological and Planetary Sciences
California Institute of Technology
Pasadena
California 91125

The attention of most medical investigators and the public has been focused on the probable harm to children resulting from rather small increases of lead exposure, above typical or average levels received by the population as a whole. My colleagues and I have focused on a different aspect of this matter. We have discovered that the magnitude of industrial lead emissions to the environment on a hemispheric scale has been so excessive in relation to the natural occurrences of lead that most people living with industrialised societies contain 500 to 1000 times more lead in their bodies than did their prehistoric ancestors. The extent of this overexposure is so great that it is highly probable that most people are suffering ill effects from it. The identification of the exact nature of these ill effects, however, poses formidable problems since no suitable control populations exist in the modern world.

The principal sources of industrial lead in people are exhausts from leaded gasolines, lead solders in metal food containers, and lead paints. Exhausts from leaded gasolines are the most serious of these because lead from this source enters the body in two ways: through breathing lead polluted air; and through eating foods contaminated by the lead fall-out from lead contaminated air.

Figure 1 compares the relative amounts of lead in three different populations of people, using dots, where each dot represents 3×10^{-4}g Pb/70kg person. In the left hand person there is only one dot. This represents the natural amount of lead occurring in prehistoric people. Because of the ubiquitous distribution of industrial lead over the earth, living representatives of this group of people have not yet been observed.

The central figure with 500 dots represents the average amount of industrial lead found in persons living within industrialised societies today, including the British.

The right hand figure with 2000 dots represents the minimum amount of lead which will cause classical lead poisoning in a significant fraction of people exposed to this degree. This information is based on experimental determinations of prehistoric natural human skeletal Pb/Ca ratios (Elias, 1982; Ericson et al., 1979), measurements of lead in contemporary human skeletons (Ericson et al., 1979), and medical evidence (National Academy of

Science, 1980). Today, most medical investigators are concerned with ill effects in children caused by above average lead exposures within the range between the central and right hand figures. Such investigations have been pursued for a relatively short time; nevertheless, substantial evidence has been obtained showing that haematopoietic and central nervous system dyfunctions are caused in children by modern exposures to industrial lead (Needleman, 1980).

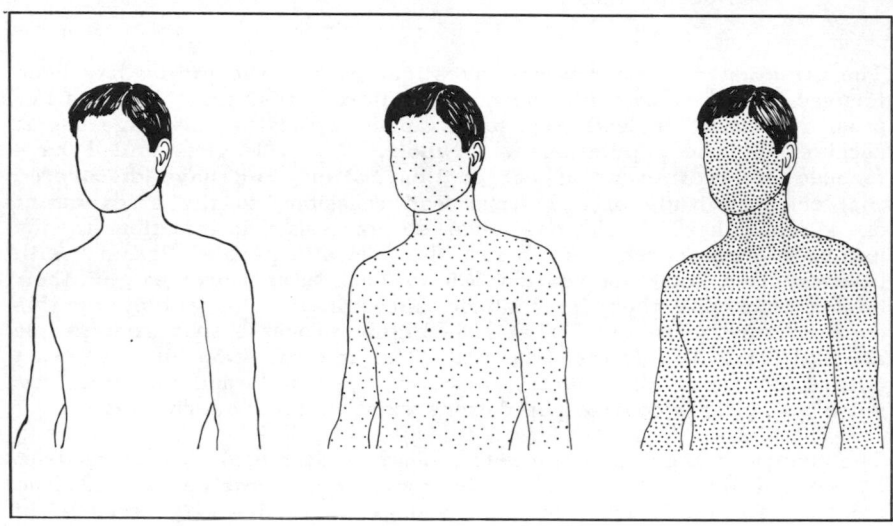

Fig. 1. Comparison of relative amounts of lead in people: natural amount found in prehistoric people on the left (one dot); average amount found in present-day Americans in the middle (500 dots); and minimum amount which will cause classical lead poisoning in a significant fraction of a group of people on the right (2000 dots). Each dot represents a unit of lead equivalent to 3×10^{-4}g Pb/70 kg person, based on a prehistoric natural skeletal value Pb/Ca (atomic) = 6×10^{-8} at age 45 (Ericson et al., 1979).

It is obvious that such ill effects are to be expected because in these dose response investigations involving only four-fold differences in lead exposures, control groups of children are not at natural base-line levels of lead exposures, but are themselves overexposed some 500-fold above base-line levels. At present these investigators have no children available to them as representatives

of a control group depicted by the left hand person depicted in
Fig. 1. In order to obtain such a group, scientists will be
required to construct laboratory sanctuaries nearly free from
industrial lead where experimental animals can be grown and where
studies can be undertaken into natural biochemical reactions within
their cells to observe the difference between these reactions and
the perturbed biochemical reactions now occuring within cells of
extremely lead polluted animals. This is and inordinately difficult
task. It is relatively easy to perform the necessary biochemical
studies on cells and cell extracts taken from such organisms. It is
quite a different matter to grow such organisms in a lead-free
sanctuary and to know unequivocally that this has been done. Not
only must the lead contents of successive generations of organisms
be enormously reduced and nourished by nearly lead-free nutrients,
but analytical control of lead contamination and lead contents of
nutrients and organisms must be far more rigorous than anything
yet attempted. In our laboratory at the California Institute of
Technology, so far only dead tissues and chemicals have been
analysed and purified. No other scientific laboratory in the world
has yet been able to correctly measure lead in a fish muscle (a
possible nutrient), while only a mere handful of scientific
laboratories out of many thousands in the world can correctly
measure lead in their purified laboratory water.

The reason why the contrast in body lead burdens between the left
hand and the central outlined persons in Fig. 1. was not discovered
until recently is that industrial lead has contaminated everything
(including scientific laboratories) worldwide, so that most of the
lead which analysts measure is industrial. They are unaware that
this is the case, however, because the ubiquity of industrial lead
has made it, in effect, "invisible" because it constitutes a constant
background feature. My colleagues and I were drawn to this
discovery more or less by accident. About twenty years ago we
were studying lead isotopes in open ocean sediments as part of an
attempt to work out the evolutionary history of the earth's mantle.
We discovered that far less lead had been leaving the ocean in
pelagic sediments during prehistoric times than was reported by
other investigators to be presently entering the oceans via the
rivers. This might have been a complexity of nature, but if not,
then it meant that industrial lead was contaminating the earth's main
hydrolic cycle on a vast scale. The tonnages involved directed
suspicion to lead coming from gasoline exhausts, because this
source could account for the observation and we published those
suspicions (Tatsumoto and Patterson, 1963). It turned out from
our maticulous measurements made years later that the reports of
lead in rivers were erroneously high, but that enormous excesses of
lead were instead entering the oceans by directed precipitation from
the atmosphere.

The editor of a medical journal asked me for an editorial comment on
our arguments. My paper in response (Patterson 1965) put the
case as follows. To begin with it is apparent that if everything is
contaminated with lead now, one can only infer what the levels of

natural lead must have been in uncontaminated things; that
inference must be by analogy; Barium constitutes an appropriate
analogue of lead in terms of its occurrence in plants and animals
and of its uptake by animals, which is fractional, small, and
independent of amounts already present in the organism. In
addition, Barium is a biological analogue of calcium, although the
fractional uptake of calcium is much greater than for barium.
Therefore if we know the factor by which the Ba/Ca ratio is
reduced in transferring calcium from rock (the ultimate source of
these metals) through plants and animals to ultimate consumers like
humans, we can apply this same reduction factor to the Pb/Ca ratio
in rocks to estimate an approximate value for the prehistoric natural
Pb/Ca ratio in people. Values for lead, barium, and calcium in
rocks, as well as some tentative data for barium and calcium in
plants, human diets, and humans were known. These allowed a
theoretical estimate of the natural lead level in humans to be
calculated. It was 1/100th of the average in present-day
Americans.

When the paper was published in 1965 it raised a furore and helped
fuel a drive to reduce lead in gasoline and paint, but investigators
in the field of environmental occurrences of lead did not show the
slightest interest in scientifically significant pattern of calcium,
barium, and lead in food chains carefully outlined in this paper.
Subsequently, together with a group of co-workers, I set out to
investigate both the extent of industrial lead pollution in the world
and also the natural lead level in humans.

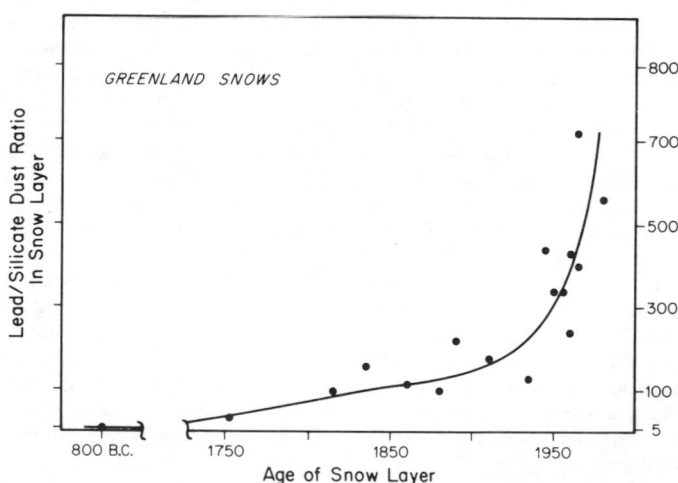

Fig. 2. Increase of Pb/Silicate dust ratio (actual values
multiplied by 10^5 and then plotted in figure) in Greenland
snow during the past 3000 years.

We constructed an array of internally consistent measurements which delineated the world-wide extent of lead pollution as follows. Lead/dust ratios were shown to have increased about 300-fold in north polar snows during the past 3000 years. This change, illustrated in Figure 2, was shown on a mass inventory basis to result from increasing emissions of industrial lead to the atmosphere from smelteries and leaded gasoline exhausts, and from reentrainment of lead deposits on soils and foliage. This provided a natural baseline of lead in the atmosphere and in precipitation and a record of changes caused by industrial lead pollution. We and colleagues from other institutions measured natural lead emissions from volcanoes and sea spray and showed that fluxes from these sources were about 1/100th of the industrial lead emissions to the atmosphere (Ng and Patterson, 1981).

TABLE 1. Observed relation between soluble Pb fluxes and ocean concentration profiles

	South Pacific Easterlies (15°S 150°W)	North Pacific Easterlies (15°N 160°W)	North Pacific Westerlies (33°N 140°W)	North Atlantic Westerlies (34°N 66°W)
present eolian input fluxes (ng/cm^2 yr)	3	7	50	170
ocean concentration (pg/g)				
Depth: 0-100 m	3.5	10	15	34
100-800 m	2.5	8	11	32
800-2500 m	1.2	1.5	3.5	14
2500-5000 m	0.9	0.9	1.1	5
ancient sediment output fluxes (ng/cm^2 yr)	4	4	3	30

Then, as shown in Table 1, present-day rates of atmospheric inputs of lead to the oceans were observed to vary geographically in direct correspondence with variations in rates of upwind emissions of industrial lead from industrial and urban complexes on land. Furthermore, in the North Pacific and North Atlantic, present rates of atmospheric lead inputs to ocean surfaces were found to be 10-fold greater than prehistoric lead outputs from the water column to the sediments in those regions, while in the South Pacific present atmospheric lead inputs were found to be nearly equal to past lead outputs. The atmosphere of the northern hemisphere receives by far the largest share of the world's industrial lead emissions, and since the residence time of industrial lead in air is only a few weeks compared to the several years it takes to mix air between the hemispheres, air in the southern hemisphere contains far less industrial lead. Vertical concentration profiles of lead in the oceans were found to be directly related to present-day atmospheric input fluxes of industrial lead to the surfaces of the water columns in different regions, as shown in Table 1. The residence times of lead in sea water at various depths were worked out and shown to be so brief that lead concentrations should have responded quickly to changes in input fluxes of lead, predicted by the north polar ice record in Figure 2. The data in Table 1 shows that this did happen. The findings provided a scheme for the natural occurrence of lead in the oceans and a record of changes caused by industrial lead pollution (Schaule and Patterson, 1982; Flegal and Patterson, 1982).

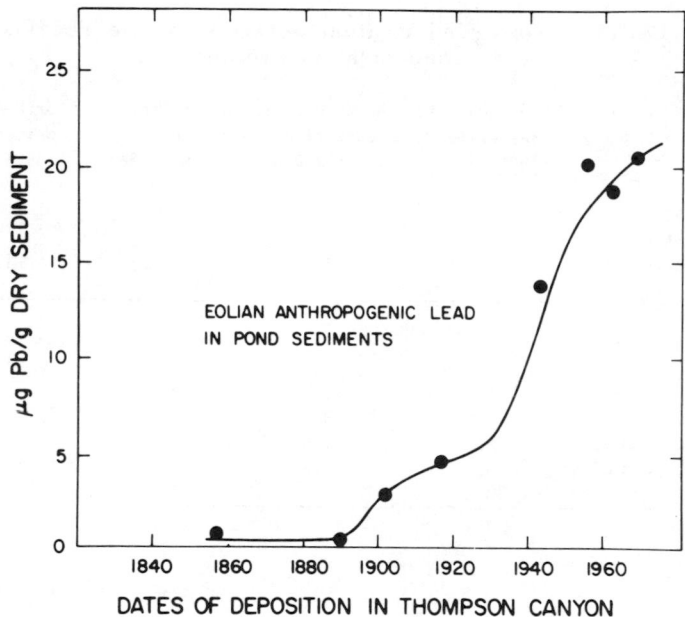

Fig. 3. Increase of industrial lead added from the atmosphere to sediments of a subalpine pond.

These data indicate that ancient river pathways by which lead used to enter the oceans have been overwhelmed in the northern hemisphere by industrial lead inputs via rain and dry deposition directly from the atmosphere. Ordinarily, nutrients and trace metals in seas are supplied from rivers and stored in immense quantities in oceanic depths. Life in surface waters is regulated by the rate at which nutrients are mixed by up-welling into them from the deep, because nutrients are rapidly removed from surface waters by sinking dead creatures and fecal pellets. Trace metal concentrations, therefore, usually are low in surface sea waters where they are consumed and removed by living matter, and highest in deep waters. Lead concentration profiles in northern oceans are not like that at all, being more like concentration profiles of atomic weapons debris, which show surface maxima and deep water minima, and which were introduced recently to the oceans from the atmosphere.

In other studies the inputs of industrial lead via precipitation and dry deposition, output in stream flow, and the extent of industrial lead contamination of soil, plants and animals were determined in a terrestrial ecosystem located in an isolated canyon in a remote, uninhabited region. A record of the increases of industrial lead inputs to this canyon with time, shown in Figure 3, was obtained from pond sediments, which coincided with changes predicted by the north polar ice record in Figure 2 and by the marine flux and water column records in Table 1. It was found that the atmospheric input flux of lead to the canyon had increased about 100-fold in two centuries and now outweighted by about 20-fold the natural input flux from weathering of rock.

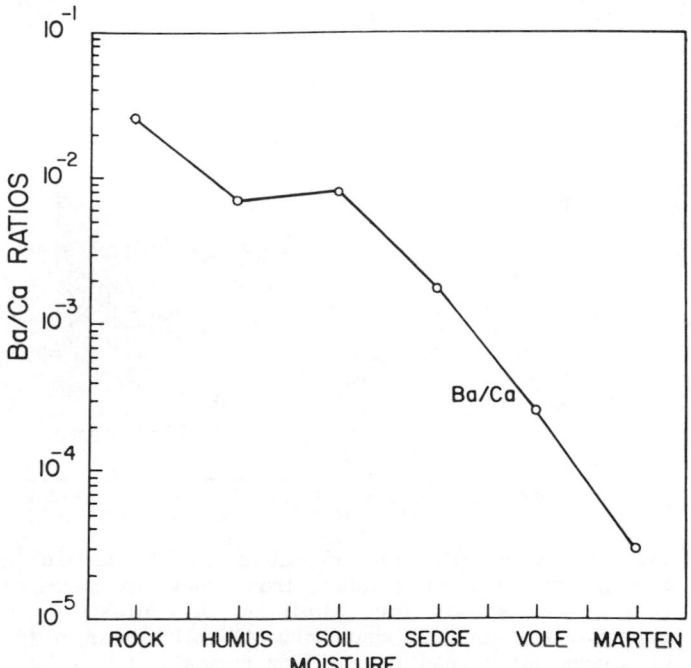

Fig. 4. Biopurification of calcium with respect to barium during transfer of calcium from rock to carnivore in a grazing food chain within a remote subalpine ecosystem (atomic ratios).

The reduction of Ba/Ca in its transfer from source rock through

successive steps of a food chain in the canyon was then
experimentally delineates as shown in Figure 4. The findings
demonstrated for the first time why human and skeletal Ba/Ca ratios
1/800th of those in the soils and established the validity of the
analogue model upon which the theory of reduction of Pb/Ca ratios
through biopurification in food chains was based.

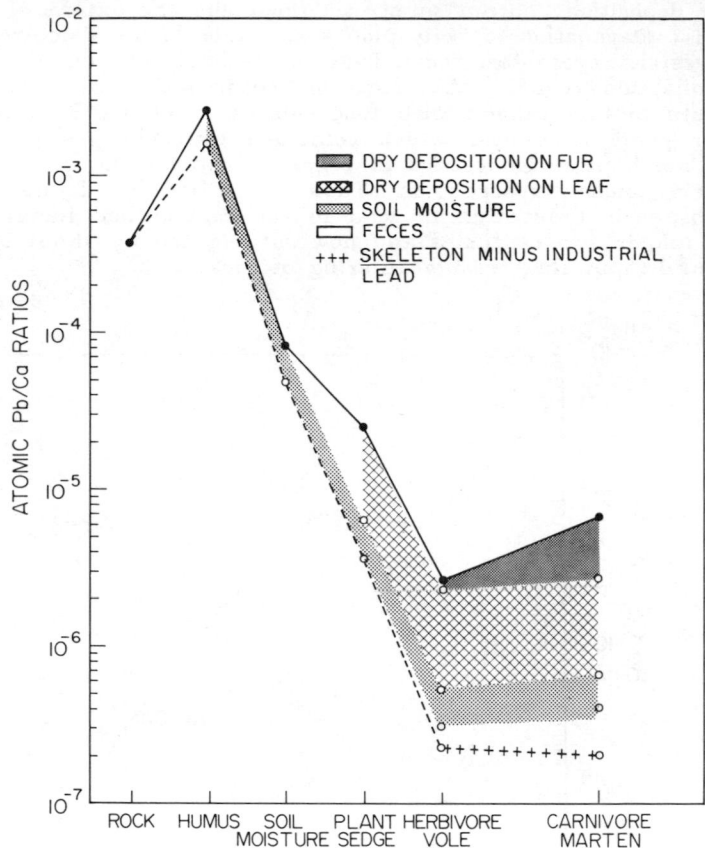

Fig. 5. Biopurification of calcium with respect to lead
during transfer of calcium from rock to carnivore with
corrections shown for additions of industrial lead via
precipitation and dry deposition to soil humus and surfaces
of leaves and animal fur (atomic ratios).

Next, the extent of industrial lead contamination was determined in
each of the components of this food chain, varying from 82% in
plant leaves to 97% in carnivore, to provide after correcting for
industrial contamination, an experimental measure of the natural
step-by-step reduction of Pb/Ca as it transferred from rock to the

ultimate consumer. As shown in Figure 5, this overall reduction was about 1700-fold for the pine marten carnivore, somewhat more than the initial theoretical estimate of 230-fold for humans published in 1965. This provided natural baselines of lead in terrestrial plants and animals and a record of changes caused by industrial pollution (Elias et al., 1982). Similar studies of calcium, barium, and lead in marine food chains and ecosystems showed how lead was transferred from water, through organisms and other substrates, to the ocean floor. The resulting picture indicated the changes caused by industrial lead pollution.

Subsequently, it was shown in other studies that an 1100-fold reduction of the Pb/Ca ratio had indeed been attained in the skeletons of ancient Peruvian Indians who had lived nearly 2000 years ago in an environment free of industrial lead contamination (Ericson et al., 1979), By measuring lead in least-polluted air, in fresh water, and in tuna muscle from remote regions, and by making corrections for contamination by industrial lead in these substances based on mass inventories of industrial lead emissions and estimates of the extent of lead pollution in these remote regions, further inferences were possible. Experimental samples of the foods eaten by the ancient Peruvians were obtained. It was found that, indeed, these foods included the low lead concentrations that were necessary for them to have such low burdens of lead (Settle and Patterson, 1980). These experiments proved that the natural baselines of lead in plants and animals, determined from ecosystem studies, had existed in prehistoric times. Concentrations of lead in old stemwood of trees was measured. These established the magnitude of the reservoir of natural lead in the earth's biosphere, and indicated that the mass of industrial lead annually emitted to the earth's atmosphere today exceeds by 100-fold the mass of natural lead turned over in the earth's biosphere each year during prehistoric times (Settle and Patterson, 1980).

This matrix of experimental data showed that the prehistoric natural level of lead in humans was about 500 times less than that observed in the average American or European today, it outlined essential natural ecosystem relationships between lead in prehistoric people and lead in their environment, and it provided records of changes in these relationships which occurred on a world-wide scale during the past 2000 years as annual amounts of industrial lead dispersed throughout the Northern Hemisphere increased with time.

These measurements comprise all that is available of the core of essential and trustworthy information upon which is based the present scientific view of the natural occurrences of lead in the earth's atmosphere, hydrosphere, and biosphere. They constitute a small fraction of the total available amount of data relating to occurrences of lead in these spheres of the earth. Parts of this larger body of data are approximately correct in numerically expressing lead concentrations in substances when they involve highly contaminated materials from urban regions, as, for example, accurate analyses of lead in urban air, foliage and dusts, and in blood of lead poisoned people. Industrial lead added to such materials via environmental pathways exceeds by some 10,000-fold natural amounts of lead in them. Accordingly large positive errors caused by the addition of more industrial lead during sample collection, handling, and analysis can be avoided by taking reasonable precautions. Such data are useful for the detection of subclinical or overt lead poisoning and identifying sources of exposure, but they have no scientific value when applied to the measurement of natural levels.

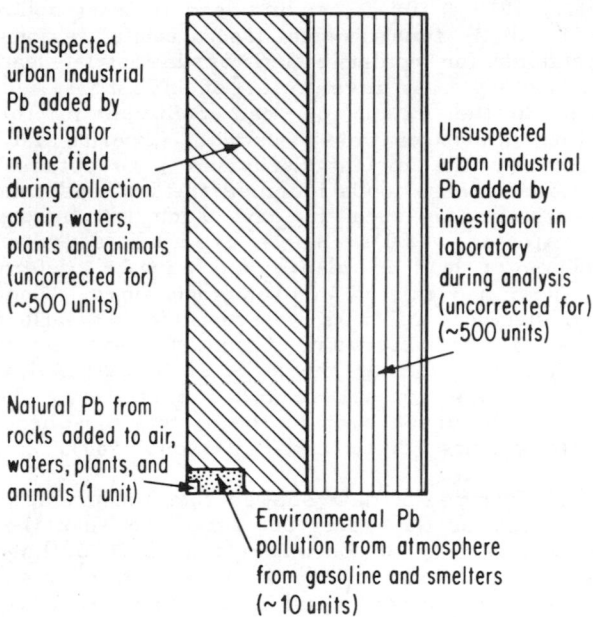

Unsuspected urban industrial Pb added by investigator in the field during collection of air, waters, plants and animals (uncorrected for) (~500 units)

Unsuspected urban industrial Pb added by investigator in laboratory during analysis (uncorrected for) (~500 units)

Natural Pb from rocks added to air, waters, plants, and animals (1 unit)

Environmental Pb pollution from atmosphere from gasoline and smelters (~10 units)

Fig. 6. Typical relative proportions of natural and different kinds of industrial leads actually responsible for results in most erroneous reports of lead concentrations in air, precipitation, waters, plants and animals collected from remote, uninhabited locations. Analysts should have reported only concentrations of the sums of natural and environmental industrial lead pollution in such materials. The proportions of these two different kinds of leads in those materials must be obtained from theoretical reconstructions of natural conditions based on biogeochemical models (such as those which interpret figures 2, 3, 4, 5, and table 1).

The remainder of the larger body of environmental lead concentration data are erronous because the analysed materials were collected from non-urbanised regions where amounts of industrialised lead added via environmental pathways to them were small, although still larger than the natural amounts of lead originally present. This is illustrated in Figure 6, where natural amounts of lead weathered from rocks and then added to water, wood, or animal flesh are represented by the tiny area in the lower left hand corner. The area surrounding it, about ten times larger, represents industrial lead originating from leaded gasoline and smelter fumes which has travelled through the atmosphere for hundreds or thousands of kilometres, and which has added to those materials via rain and dry deposition. Investigators entering these regions bring with them from heavily polluted urban regions such large quantities of industrial lead adhering to their equipment, bodies, life support systems, and transport, that improperly controlled transfer of tiny fractions of this intruded lead to collected samples of materials completely overwhelms the sums of natural and environmentally added industrial lead already in the materials. This is illustrated by the 500-fold larger collection lead contamination area surrounding the original natural lead area in Figure 6. Most investigators fail to properly reduce or subtract this lead they add to samples they have collected. Moreover, generally they have no idea of the proportion between the natural lead and the environmentally added industrial lead originally in the samples. They bring this underfined mixture of three different kinds of leads in samples back to their extremely polluted urban laboratories. Then, swimming in pools of industrial lead, they tend to make blind, incorrect, and insufficient subtractions for "lead blanks" supposedly added to their sample during analyses. Usually they underestimate this laboratory contamination such that the unaccounted excess adds another unrecognised quantity about 500-fold greater than natural lead originally present in the samples.

The result of these combined mistakes is to report excessively large concentrations of lead, as shown in Table 2. Proven inaccuracies are given in Ng and Patterson (1981) and Settle and Patterson (1980). Examples of authors whose work contains blatant errors are Cavalleri and Minoia (1981) and Eisler (1981). An example of false theorising which results from measurement errors is Jaworowski et al., (1981).

For these reasons, considerable time will pass before other scientists will be able to improve their analytical capabilities for lead so that they can make correct measurements similar to those outlined above and therby educate themselves concerning this matter in order to further the development of meaningful and reliable scientific knowledge in this field. Studies of natural biochemical reactions in cells of organisms grown in lead-free sancturies will be exceptionally costly and will require many years of development and testing before scientifically meaningful and significant information can emerge from them, In the meantime, sufficient reliable and scientifically meaningful information is available to show that most Europeans are severely overexposed to industrial lead. It is reasonable and proper that immediate steps be taken to eliminate the major source of this industrial lead, that is, exhausts from leaded gasoline.

TABLE 2. Comparisons between actual and commonly
reported lead concentrations

(nanogram = 10^{-9}g; picogram = 10^{-12}g; femtogram = 10^{-15}g)

Material	actual concentration determined at Cal Tech	reported concentration in the literature
ultra pure laboratory water	100-500 femtograms Pb/g	100-1000 picograms Pb/g
old glacial ice	1 picograms Pb/g	50-5000 picograms Pb/g
deep sea water	1-6 picograms Pb/g	500-10000 picograms Pb/g
remote fresh water	5-50 picograms Pb/g	500-10000 picograms Pb/g
human blood plasma	0.1 nanograms Pb/g	30-300 nanograms Pb/g
marine fish muscle	0.3-0.4 nanograms Pb/g	300-800 nanograms Pb/g
remote tree trunks	1-3 nanograms Pb/g	1000-10000 nanograms Pb/g

As mentioned at the onset, exhausts from leaded gasoline constitute the most important and serious source of the body lead burden in British, Americans and Europeans. It is scientifically meaningless and against the public interest to permit equivocations based on unresolved details in this matter to forestal a useful appreciation of the overall correctness of this view. Lead isotope tracer studies have clearly identified leaded gasoline as the source of most of the lead in the atmosphere in California. There is no substantive difference in environmental factors between Europe and California which would alter this identification. Furthermore, lead isotope studies in California have shown that atmospheric lead inhaled by typical adults accounts for about one third of the lead in the systemic blood (Rabinowitz et al, 1977). Atmospheric lead also contaminates foods by collecting on fruits and vegetables in the form of dry deposition deposits and by contaminating air-dried milled and powdered food products. Although the legacy of poisonous lead deposits from leaded gasoline exhausts will remain in urban regions for many decades, a 5 tp 10-fold reduction of air-lead concentrations would follow within months of the complete cessation of burning lead alkyls in the atmosphere.

DISCUSSION

Goodacre: Has there ever been lead-free air?

Patterson: My paper described the findings from very
                 careful measurements of lead in the prehistoric
                 environment.   There has always been lead in
                 the air from natural sources but the levels in
                 the biosphere were extremely low.   The crucial
                 point is that the current levels of lead in your
                 body and in those of other people in this room
                 are some 500 to 1000 times above those in
                 prehistoric times.   This ratio represents the
                 relative   contributions   from   natural   and
                 industrialised sources to human lead intake.

Carson: How was it possible to take the step of adding
                 lead to petrol without first proving that it was
                 safe?

Patterson: That is an important issue.   Unfortunately,
                 social institutions and the precepts upon which
                 they were founded encourage a viewpoint that
                 permits lead to be used before proof that it is
                 harmless.

Rutter: With respect to your Table 1, I am puzzled by
                 the fact the surface ocean concentrations do not
                 show the same pattern as that exhibited by the
                 eolian input fluxes.   You commented on the
                 huge difference between the South Pacific
                 fluxes (3 ng/cm^{2}yr) and the North Atlantic
                 fluxes (170 ng/cm^{2}yr) - a ratio of 1:57.   Yet
                 the ratio in the shallower depths of 0-100
                 metres was much smaller (less than 1:10) and,
                 furthermore, there was no systematic change in
                 ration according to ocean depth.

Patterson: That is a very perceptive point.   However,
                 although that particular finding appears
                 surprising, it is necessary to pay more
                 attention to the overall pattern.   When we deal
                 with just one latitudinal atmospheric circulation
                 cell, in which all the air is moving in the same
                 direction, we get a good correlation.   But, we
                 do not get a linear correlation between different
                 atmospheric circulation cells, nevertheless, the
                 correlation is positive.

Gallagher: In view of your very serious claims regarding
                 the frequency of large errors in the
                 measurement of lead concentrations today, to
                 what extent would you trust the data that

demonstrates relationships between indices of body lead and health?

Patterson:
Let me focus on the blood lead findings reported by Annest and Billick (chapters 3 and 4). Their results are not subject to the kind of error to which I referred with respect to the comparison of low natural levels and high levels in urban areas. Their data base is reliable just because they apply to people subjected to high lead pollution; with reasonable precautions you can obtain reliable measurements at those high concentrations of lead. However, this is not always the case. If you ask for a routine blood lead analysis in a hospital, there may be a 50% error in measurement, an error of similar magnitude to that made by many past investigators.

Rutter:
As I am sure you would agree that replication constitutes the essence of science.........

Patterson:
No, I would not.

Rutter:
Even if you do not, many scientists would consider replication crucial. Our confidence in science depends on the ability of different researchers to obtain the same findings if comparable methods are used. You seem to imply that your laboratory measurements are different from those of all others. Is that really so, or have other investigators been able to produce comparable results? Perhaps, you could indicate the criteria to be employed in deciding which result to accept and which to reject?

Patterson:
Our data derive from isotope dilution mass spectrometry, used under ultra-clean laboratory conditions – a technique that I developed. This is a very powerful and accurate analytical method for trace amounts of lead. However, it is extremely cumbersome, very costly, and very time consuming: as a consequence it can generate only relatively small amounts of data. After World War II, as a graduate student at the University of Chicago, I was assigned the task of developing this method to measure uranium-lead ages in microscopic minerals. Lead contamination constraints imposed by that work were unavoidable. Geologic ages of gram quantities of uranium-lead minerals had been determined by macroscopic chemical methods,

and we had micro-quantities of minerals in rocks that were geologically associated with those macro-ore minerals. Therefore we had to obtain the same ages for the uranium-lead clocks in the microscopic minerals. Contamination of these microscopic systems became immediately apparent by violation of physical laws if we got the wrong geological age. This was a constraint that provided a unique training; it taught me always to exercise great care to control lead contamination while studying the occurences of lead. But the reason why the method is so powerful is that it is the most accurate method for determining very, very tiny quantities of lead. Lead contamination control is a supremely important thing, and you must be able to measure very tiny amounts of lead if you are going to control your contamination correctly and reliably. These two factors are not involved in most of the thousands of laboratories that ordinarily measure lead. Consequently, there are only a very few laboratories in the world where such analyses can be done accurately. There is one at the University of Paris, another at Caltech, and one in Denver, Colorado. These few other laboratories that are capable of carrying out reliable studies of lead at ultra low concentrations are studying lead in lunar rocks or very exotic cosmological debris. There are two other laboratories that soon will be able to provide accurate measurements of lead in sea water. Another labortary will soon be able to provide accurate measurements of lead fluxes to the ocean. But laboratories that provide most of the official statistics on lead occurrences cannot provide accurate and reliable data concerning the occurrences of lead in other than urban substances. Even the United States Bureau of Standards cannot yet analyse lead in fish muscle correctly. These are very difficult things - I do not know how it impress upon you the enormous dedications and sophistication that is required to do these things correctly.

REFERENCES

Cavalleri, A., Minoia, C. 1981. Plasma lead values: are they accurate? Clin. Chem. 27, 765.
Eisler, R. 1981. Trace metal concentrations in marine organisms, Pergamon Press, New York.

Elias, R.W., Hiras, Y., Patterson, C.C., 1982. The circumvention of the natural biopurification of calcium along nutrient pathways by atmospheric inputs of industrial lead. Accepted for publication in Geochimica et Cosmochimica Acta.

Ericson, J.E., Shirahata, H., Patterson, C.C., 1979. Skeletal concentrations of lead in ancient Peruvians. N. Engl. J. Med. 300:946-951.

Flegal, R., Patterson, C.C., 1982. Vertical concentration profiles of lead in the Western Pacific at N15° and S20°, Manuscript submitted to Earth and Planetary Science Letters.

Jaworowski, Z., Bysiek, M., Kownacka, L., 1981 Flow of metals into the global atmosphere. Geochimica et Cosmochimica Acta, 45:2185-2199.

National Academy of Science 1980. Lead in the human environment, a report prepared by the Committee on Lead in the Human Environment, Environmental Studies Board, Commission on Natural Resources, National Research Council, National Academy of Sciences, Washington DC.

Needleman, H.L., 1980. Low level lead exposure. The clinical implications of current research. Raven Press, New York.

Ng, A., Patterson, C.C., 1981. Natural concentrations of lead in ancient Artic and Antartic ice. Geochimica et Cosmochimica Acta, 45:2109-2121.

Patterson, C.C., 1965. Contaminated and natural lead environments of man. Arch. Environ. Health, II, 344-360.

Rabinowitz, M.B., Wetherill, J.W., Kopple, J.D., 1977. Magnitude of lead intake from respiration by normal man. J. Lab. Clin. Med. 90:238-248.

Schaule, B.K., Patterson, C.C., 1982. Perturbations of the natural lead depth profile in the Sargasso Sea by industrial lead. Trace metals in Sea Water, NATO Advanced Research Institute, Plenum Press, New York.

Settle, D.M., Patterson, C.C., 1980. Lead in Albacore: guide to lead pollution in Americans. Science 207:1167-1176.

Tatsumoto, M., Patterson, C.C., 1963. Concentrations of common lead in some Atlantic and Mediterranean waters and snow. Nature 199:350-352.

Lead Versus Health
Edited by M. Rutter and R. Russell Jones
© 1983 John Wiley & Sons Ltd.

TRENDS IN THE BLOOD LEAD LEVELS OF THE US POPULATION

THE SECOND NATIONAL HEALTH AND NUTRITION EXAMINATION SURVEY (NHANES II) 1976 - 1980

Joseph L Annest, PhD

Geneticist and Statistician
Division of Health Examination Statistics
National Center for Health Statistics
Hyattsville
Maryland

INTRODUCTION

The impact of the changing environment on health constitutes a growing public health concern in the United States. To address this concern, a component of the Second National Health and Nutrition Examination Survey or NHANES II, conducted between 1976 and 1980, was developed to measure the degree of exposure of the US population to certain toxic substances, including lead. In the NHANES II survey, the determination of lead levels in whole blood was used as an index of human exposure to lead. The rationale for measuring exposure to this environmental hazard was to provide information about the distribution of blood lead levels in the general US population, to establish base-line estimates for future studies to monitor changes in such exposure over time, to provide normative data for use in health policy and regulatory decisions and to correlate levels of exposure to this toxic substance with other health and nutritional parameters on examinees in NHANES II. (McDowell et al, 1981).

This study documents the distribution of blood lead levels of persons aged 6 months - 74 years with respect to age, race, sex, annual family income and degree of urbanisation of place of residence. It also presents findings relating to chronological trends in the NHANES II lead data. The findings represent the first national estimates of blood lead levels obtained form a representative sample of the civilian non-institutionalised population of the United States. A more detailed analysis is provided in the National Center for Health Statistics publication. (Annest et al. 1982).

SURVEY, METHODS AND PROCEDURES

A cross-sectional survey was conducted from February 1976 through February 1980 with a probability sample of 27,801 persons aged 6

months - 74 years from 64 areas of the United States.   There was a
deliberate oversampling of certain subgroups in the population that
were of special interest for nutritional assessment and these
included preschool children, persons ages 60 - 74, and persons
living in low income areas.   (McDowell et al. 1981).

Of the total sample of 27,801 persons, 16,563 (chosen on the basis
of a complete sample of children ages 6 months - 6 years and a
half-sample of persons ages 7 - 74 years) were asked to provide
blood specimens for assessment of lead levels.   However, some
parents refused to have their young children examined and/or give
blood.   Among adults, especially the elderly, some were reluctant
or unable to come to the mobile examination units for examination.
Also to a lesser degree, a number of blood specimens were lost
during shipment and processing.   As a result, reliable blood lead
levels were determined for blood specimens from 10,049 examinees.
Blood was obtained from one hundred and thirteen of these
individuals by pricking the fingertip, and on the remaining 9,936
examinees by venipuncture.

Investigation of the distribution of sample persons in the lead
subsample with missing blood lead data showed that they are
distributed randomly with respect to the demographic variables of
interest in this study.   (Annest et al. 1982).

The laboratory determinations were performed by the Clinical
Chemistry Division, Center for Environmental Health, Centers for
Disease Control (CDC), Atlanta, Georgia, and financed by the
Bureau of Foods, Food and Drug Administration, Cincinatti, Ohio.
Lead concentrations of NHANES II whole blood specimens and
quality control specimens were determined by atomic absorption
spectrophotometry using a modified Delves cup micro-method.
(Gunter et al. 1981; Mahaffrey et al. 1979; Barthel et al. 1973).
Specimens were analysed in duplicate with the two assessments done
independently in the same analytic run.   The average of the two
measures was used for this statistical analysis.

The national estimates that follow are based on data obtained on
9,933 NHANES II examinees with blood lead levels ranging from 2.0
to almost 70.0 µg/dl.   All of these individuals had lead determinations from blood specimens collected by venipuncture.   The
potential for contamination during capillary blood collection by
fingerstick is a well recognised problem in the measurement of blood
lead levels (Crisler et al. 1973).   Likewise, preliminary analysis of
the NHANES II data suggested that inclusion of the finger-sticks in
this analysis would have introduced bias into the estimates of mean
venous blood lead levels in children.   Overall, for children ages 6
months - 5 years, the unweighted mean blood lead levels for those
receiving finger-sticks was observed to be approximately 6.0 µg/dl
higher than for those receiving venipunctures.   This observed mean
difference was consistent for black and white children.   Three
examinees who received venipunctures had blood lead levels greater
than 70.0 µg/dl.   These are extreme cases of lead exposure and are

Figure 1

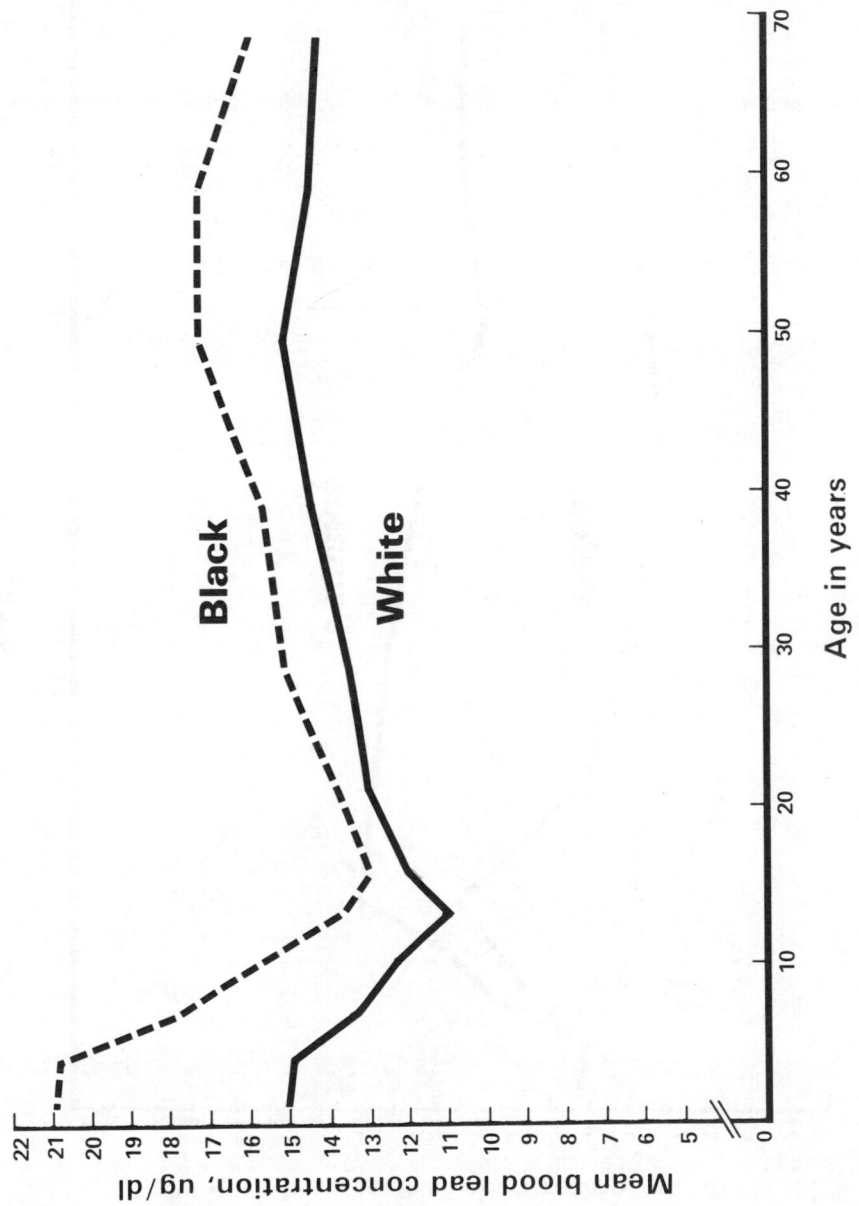

Figure 2

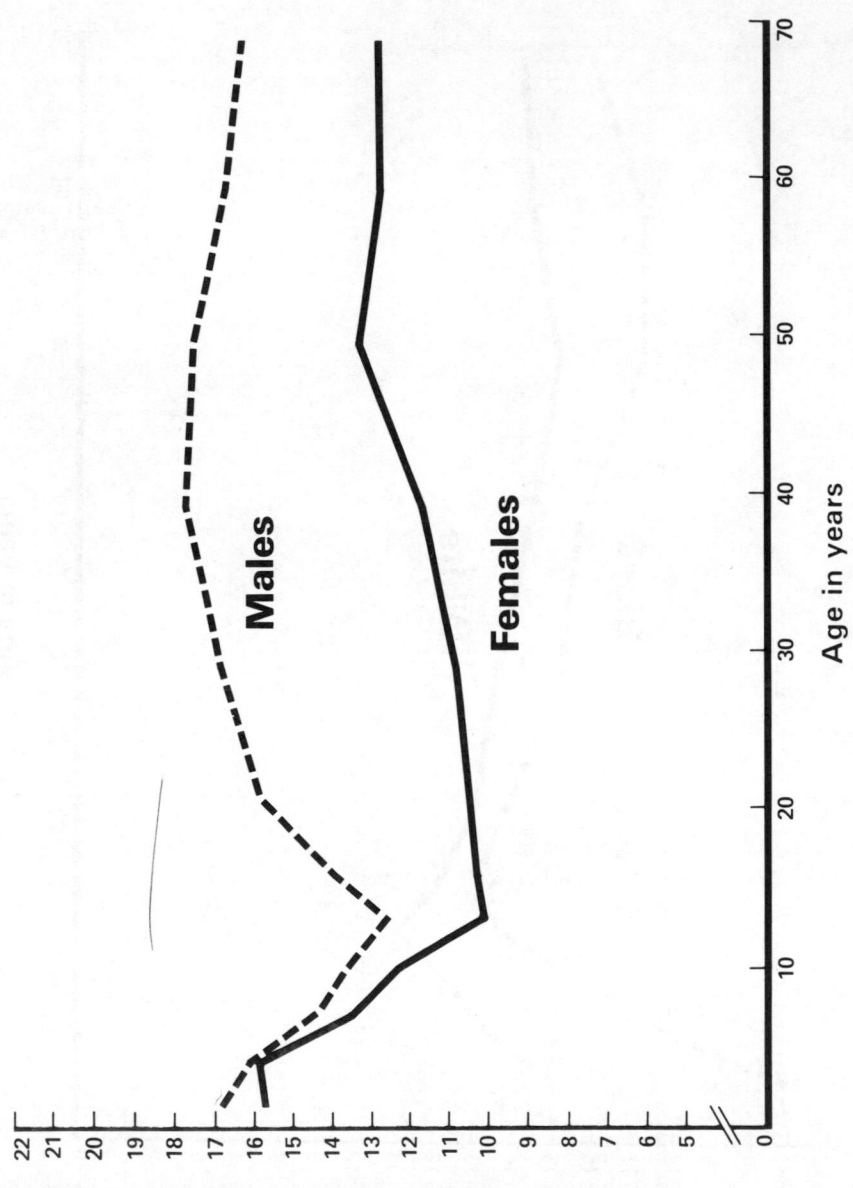

considered a separate part of the distribution of blood lead levels in the general population. Accordingly, the finger-sticks and the three extreme cases were excluded from further stages of the analysis.

For the statistical analyses of blood lead levels with respect to race, sex, income and degree of urbanization of place of residence, the population was divided into three age groups: namely, young child- ren ages 6 months - 5 years, children and youths ages 6 - 17 years and adults ages 18 - 74 years. Computation of the standard errors of weighted means, proportions and regression coefficients were performed using specially prepared statistical computer programs that take into consideration the complex survey design. (National Center for Health Statistics 1979). Using these programs, the analyst can apply the proper statistical methods necessary to provide unbiased estimates of standard errors and reliable tests of significance for comparing means and proportions using regression and generalised least-squares categorical data analysis. Further details on statistical methods are presented in the advance data report (Annest et al. 1982).

RESULTS

Mean Blood Lead Levels by Age, Race and Sex   Mean blood lead levels by age and race and by age and sex are shown in figures 1 and 2. Lead levels are recorded in micrograms of lead per deciliter of whole blood. For tests of significance, the 0.05 level of probability was used unless otherwise specified.

For children under 6 years, there was no statistically significant association between age and mean blood lead level. For children and youths ages 6 - 17 years, there was a statistically significant relationship between age and mean blood lead concentration. In general, mean blood lead values declined with increasing age until late adolescence (about ages 15 - 17 years). Among adults ages 18 - 74 years, too, there was a significant trend in blood lead level with age: that is, mean blood lead levels are positively associated with age until middle age, followed by a moderate decline in the older age groups.

Race and mean blood lead level concentrations were significantly associated within each of the three age groups used for analysis. Thus average blood lead levels were consistently higher for black than white persons across all ages (see figure 1). Overall, for children ages 6 months - 5 years, blood lead levels of black children were, on the average, 6 micrograms per deciliter higher than those of white children.

Blood lead concentrations were not significantly different for boys and girls under six years of age. Among children and youths ages 6 - 17 years, the difference in mean blood lead levels between males and females progressively increased with age. For adults, 18 - 74 years of age, mean blood lead concentrations were consistently

and significantly higher for men than women across all age
groupings.

Mean Blood Lead Levels for Children by Income and Degree of
Urbanization   The associations of family income and of the degree
of urbanization with blood lead levels were generally consistent
across all three broad age groups in the population, with lower
mean blood lead levels among the more affluent than among the
poor, and among those in rural than in urban areas.   These
associations were most pronounced, however, in children ages 6
months - 5 years.   The relationship of blood lead to these two
demographic variables will therefore be presented in relation to the
findings amongst pre-school children.

The mean blood lead levels of children in low moderate and high
family income categories are shown in Figure 3.   In 1978, the
income level of $6,000 was near the poverty threshold for a family
of four as determined by the US Bureau of Census (1980).   The
three income categories were also selected to ensure subsamples of
adequate size for computing national estimates.   In each income
group, mean blood lead levels for black children were significantly
greater than those for white children.   There was also a significant
decrease in mean blood lead levels with increase in income.

Similarly with respect to degree of urbanization, mean blood lead
levels were significantly different between white and black children
within the large urban (with one million persons or more), and
smaller urban (with fewer than one million persons) areas (see
figure 4).   The mean difference between these racial groups was
also observed in rural areas but was not statistically significant due
to the small sample number of rural black children.   Also, mean
blood lead levels were higher in urban than in the rural areas for
white and black children, with statistically significant differences
only for white children.   The relatively higher mean blood lead
levels for black compared to white children in all three urban-rural
groups suggests that the observed racial effects are not simply a
function of the degree of urbanization.   No clearcut explanation for
this racial difference can be given from the results of this study;
how- ever the findings in the NHANES lead data are consistent with
results from other studies (Billick et al. 1979, Cohen et al. 1973,
Simpson et al. 1972).

Further investigation of blood lead levels in the large urban areas
revealed that mean blood lead levels of black children living in the
central cities were 3.9 and 4.8 µg/dl higher than black children
living in non-central city and rural areas, respectively (see figure
5).   These differences were not statistically significant, probably
because of the small number of black children in the sample who
were living in non-central city and rural areas.

However, within the central cities, the mean blood lead level of
black children was significantly higher than that of whites.   Other
studies indicate that exposure to lead in inner city children may be

Figure 3

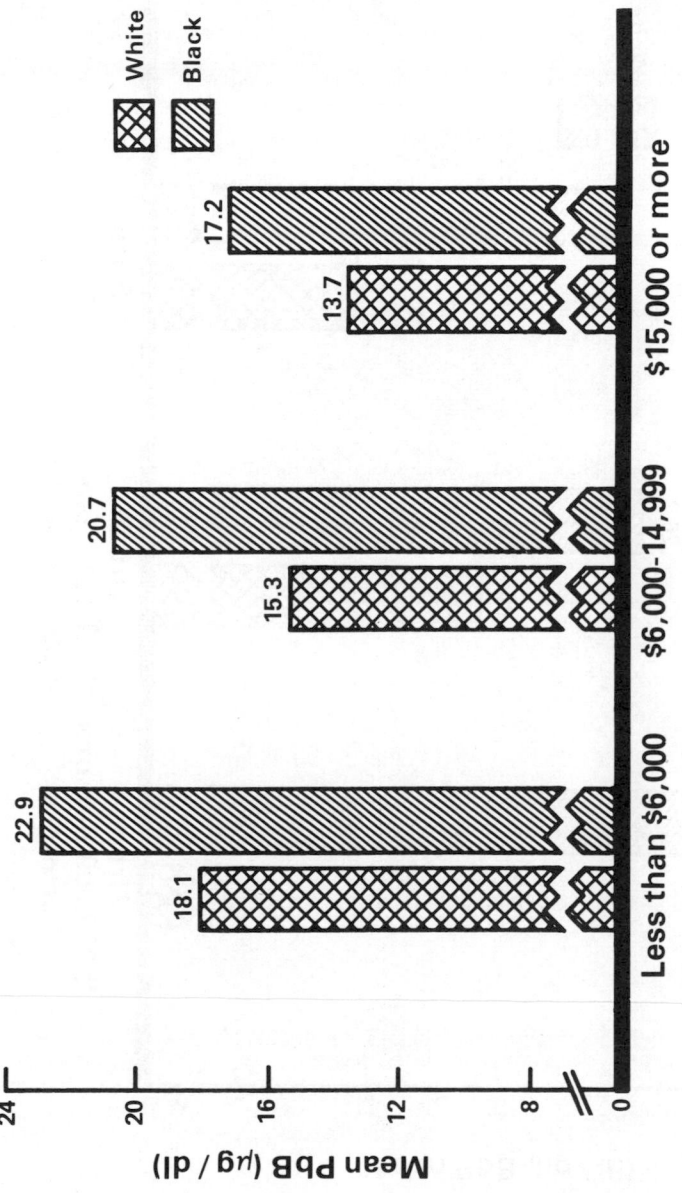

SOURCE: National Health and Nutrition Examination Survey, National Center for Health Statistics

Figure 4

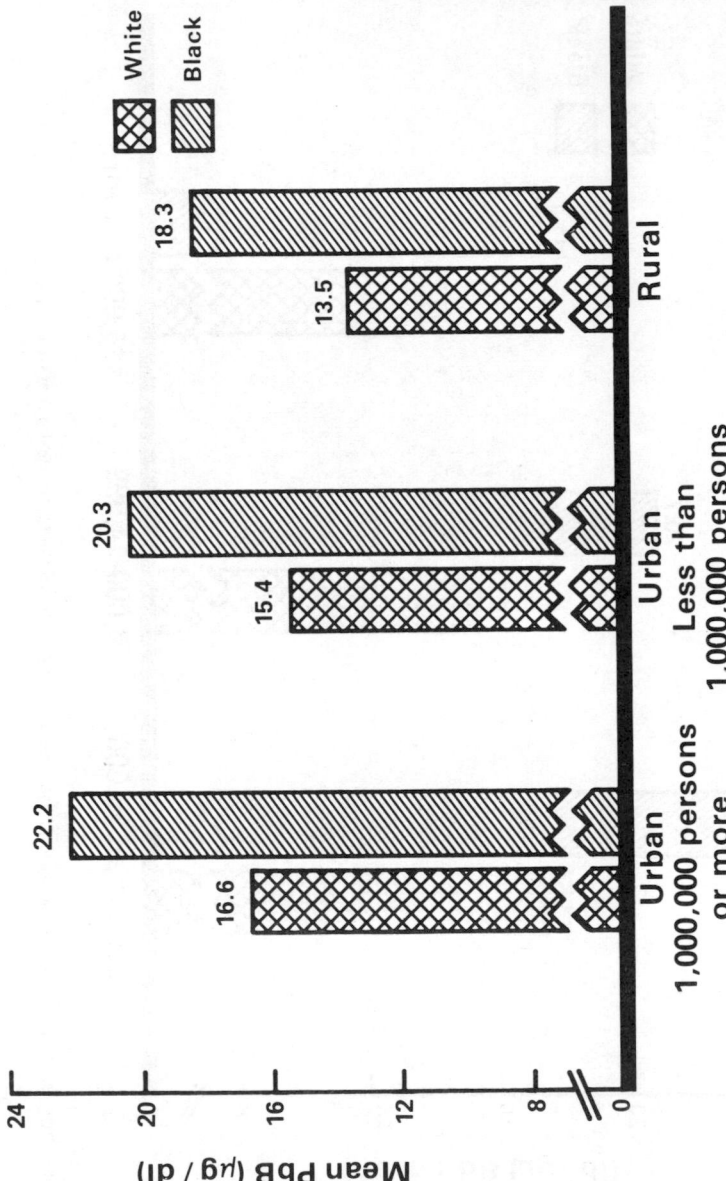

SOURCE: National Health and Nutrition Examination Survey, National Center for Health Statistics

associated to some degree, with socioeconomic factors (Lin Fu 1975). In this study, 43 percent of black compared with 22 percent of white children living in the central areas were from households with annual family incomes of under $6,000.

Levels of undue exposure to lead for children by income and degree of urbanization   The consistent black-white difference in children ages 6 months - 5 years and the presence of higher blood lead levels among those in the low income group and large urban areas is also reflected in the percent of children with blood lead levels of 30μg/dl or more.   According to the Centers for Disease Control guidelines established in 1978, 30μg/dl is the cut-off used in CDC community-based lead poisoning prevention program for referring children for medical attention and follow-up.   (Centers for Disease Control 1978).

Overall, an estimated 4.0 percent or approximately 675,000 US child- ren ages 6 months - 5 years showed evidence of excessive or undue, absorption of lead.   Among these children, 12.2 percent of blacks compared to 2.0 percent of whites had blood lead levels of 30 μg/dl or more (figure 6).   This black-white difference was significant for boys and girls.   The percent of elevated blood lead levels was slightly higher in boys than in girls, but this difference was not statistically significant.

There was a significant decrease in the proportion of children with elevated blood lead levels with increase in income (figure 7).   This relationship was strong for both black and white children.   Based on CDC guidelines (30.0 μg/dl or more), almost one out of five (18.5 percent) black children from low income families, the group with the highest proportion of elevated blood lead levels, showed evidence of undue lead absorption.   For white and black children, the percent of elevated blood lead levels was lowest in the high income group.

The percent of children with undue blood lead levels by degree of urbanization is shown in figure 8.   In the central cities, the percent of children with elevated blood lead levels was significantly higher for blacks than whites, with approximately a four-fold difference between these racial groups.   This racial difference was significant even in the smaller urban and rural areas (combined) with 10.0 percent of black children compared to less than 2.0 percent for white children having elevated lead levels.   (The 3.3 percent estimate for non-central city black children is unreliable because of the small number of sample persons (less than 50) in that cell).

Chronological trend in the NHANES II Blood Level Data   The remainder of this paper concerns the 37 percent reduction in the overall mean blood lead levels from February 1976 through February 1980 as reported in the CDC publication, Morbidity and Mortality Weekly Report March 19, 1982.   (Centers for Disease Control 1982).

Figure 5

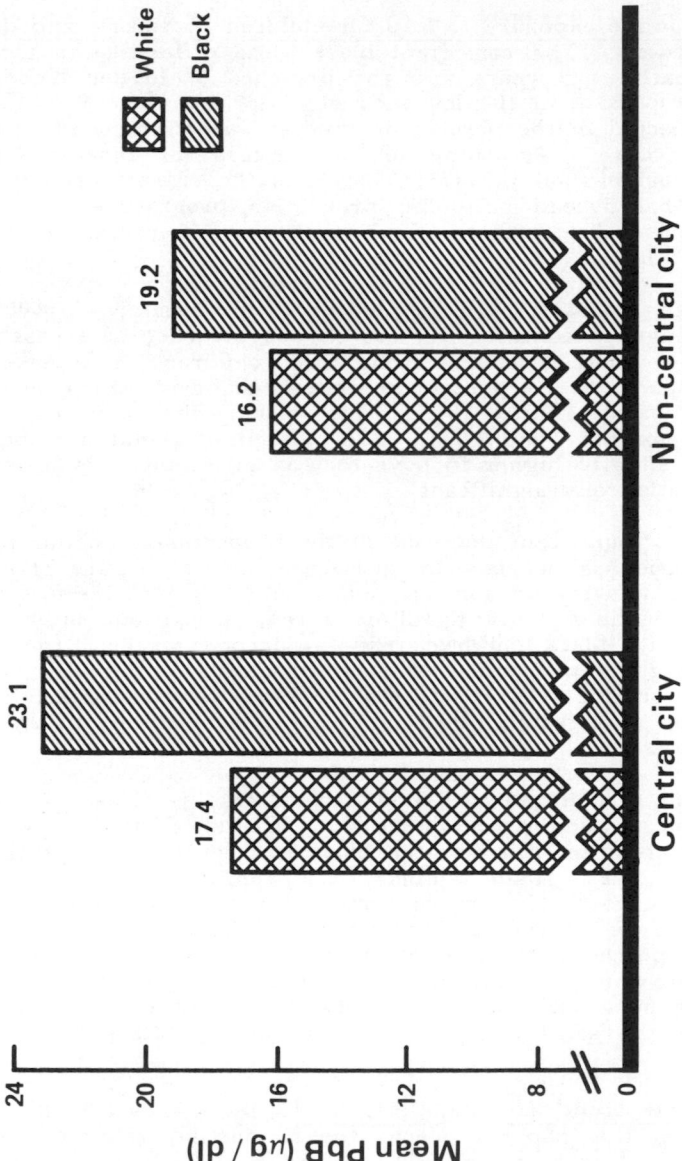

SOURCE: National Health and Nutrition Examination Survey, National Center for Health Statistics

Figure 6

	Race	
	White	*Black*
Both sexes	2.0	12.2
Males	2.1	13.4
Females	1.8	10.9

SOURCE: National Health and Nutrition Examination Survey, National Center for Health Statistics.

The statistical analyses of the chronological trend over the 4 years of the survey were conducted in two phases. Phase one was an analysis of the trend in blood lead data for blood specimens drawn from the quality control blood pools, and Phase two was an analysis of the trend in the observed blood lead data from the NHANES II specimens. These analyses were a collaborative effort between the Center for Environmental Health of CDC and the Division of Health Examination Statistics of NCHS. My main collaborator at CDC was Dr James Pirkle.

The quality control analysis was conducted first to rule out the possibility that the observer chronological trend in the NHANES II lead data was due to measurement error in the laboratory. This was accomplished through an analysis of blood lead determinations from "blind" quality control specimens. The "blind" quality control specimens were drawn from two pools of bovine blood with known quantities of lead, one of which had a lower amount of lead than the other (Gunter et al. 1981). These pools were set up at the beginning of NHANES II and used throughout the course of the survey. The "blind" quality control specimens were placed in vials, labelled and processed in duplicate so as to be indistinguishable from regular NHANES II specimens.

Blood lead data for the two sets of "blind" quality control specimens were standardized (Z=(Pb - mean Pb)/Std. Dev.) separately for the high and the low pools; then the resulting data having a mean of zero and standard deviation of one were pooled for analysis of the "time" trend. The "time" variable was defined to denote the chronological order of processing of the quality control and corresponding NHANES II specimens. Using a simple linear regression of these standardized lead values on the "time" variable, a test of the hypothesis of no chronological trend in these standardized blood lead values was conducted. This hypothesis could not be rejected even at the 0.25 level of probability. There was no indication of any chronological trend, upward or downward, in the these quality control blood lead data.

Next, a statistical analysis of the observed NHANES II lead data was conducted that took into consideration the complex survey design and sampling within population subgroups defined by demographic and socioeconomic factors previously reported (on the NHANES II data and in the literature) to be associated with blood levels in the general population. The weighted mean blood lead values of persons ages 6 months - 74 years by a chronological "time" variable from the beginning to the end of the survey (February 20, 1976 - February 27, 1980) is shown in figure 9. The "time" variable was based on the date of examination (which was also the date the blood specimens were collected) of the NHANES II examinees. This ordered the blood lead data according to 28-day periods. Using this definition, the chronological "time" variable ranged from 1 to 53. Figure 9 shows a linear relationship between the weighted mean blood lead levels and the "time" variable with a change in slope occurring, approximately, in the fall of 1978 (the

Figure 7

Annual family income	Race	
	White	*Black*
Under $6,000	5.9	18.5
$6,000-14,999	2.2	12.1
$15,000 or more	0.7	2.8

SOURCE: National Health and Nutrition Examination Survey, National Center for Health Statistics.

Figure 8

Degree of urbanization	Race	
	White	*Black*
Urban, 1,000,000 persons or more		
Central city	4.5	18.6
Non-central city	3.8	3.3
	4.0	15.2
Urban, less than 1,000,000 persons	1.6	10.2
Rural	1.2	10.3

SOURCE: National Health and Nutrition Examination Survey, National Center for Health Statistics.

35th "time" period). Mean blood lead values were observed to be
higher during the summer months than during the winter months,
except for the summer of 1979 when values fell. Coincidently, the
summer of 1979 was when the petroleum crisis brought on a gasoline
shortage in the United States.

Using the specially designed regression program that took into
consideration the complex survey design that is, clustering and
over-sampling in selected groups (Holt 1977), tests of the hypothesis of no chronological trend in the mean blood lead levels over
the four year course of NHANES II were conducted. To account
for the change in slope that was observed, a piecewise (or segmental) linear regression model was used. (Neter and Wasserman
1974) Regression analyses of blood lead levels on the "time"
variable were conducted for all persons ages 6 months - 74 years
and for white and black persons, separately. Regression analyses
were also conducted for selected subgroups within the general
population. (Note: this could not be done for black persons due to
small sample sizes among the subgroups). These subgroups were
defined by age, sex, degree of urbanization of place of residence,
annual family income, region and season. Overall, and for all but
one subgroup - white persons living in large urbanized areas (one
million or more population) - the hypothesis of no chronological
trend was rejected at the 0.001 level of probability. For white
persons living in large urbanized areas, this hypothesis could not
be rejected at the 0.05 level of probability.

Using the regression equations obtained from these analyses, the
predicted reduction in mean blood lead levels from February, 1976
through February, 1980 was computed overall and within each
subgroup. The predicted percent change in blood lead levels was
consistently equal to or greater than 30 percent for subgroups by
race, sex and age, (figure 10) and for subgroups by degree of
urbanization, annual family income, region and season, except for
white persons in large urbanized areas where the percent reduction
was estimated to be 19.1 percent (figure 11). The lack of trend in
the laboratory data and the degree of consistency in the downward
trend in blood lead levels over the 4-year period for these
subgroups led us to conclude, with considerably confidence, that
the reduction in NHANES II mean blood lead levels was not due to
laboratory-measurement error, or chance.

DISCUSSION

Several factors may have contributed to the downward trend in
blood lead levels in the general US population including 1)
community awareness programs on lead toxicity, 2) federally-funded
lead screening programs, 3) occupational safety programs regarding
exposure to toxic substances, 4) efforts to alleviate lead from the
diet, and 5) a phasedown in the use of lead as an octane-booster in
gasoline.

An example of a community awareness program is the extensive

Joseph L. Annest

Figure 9

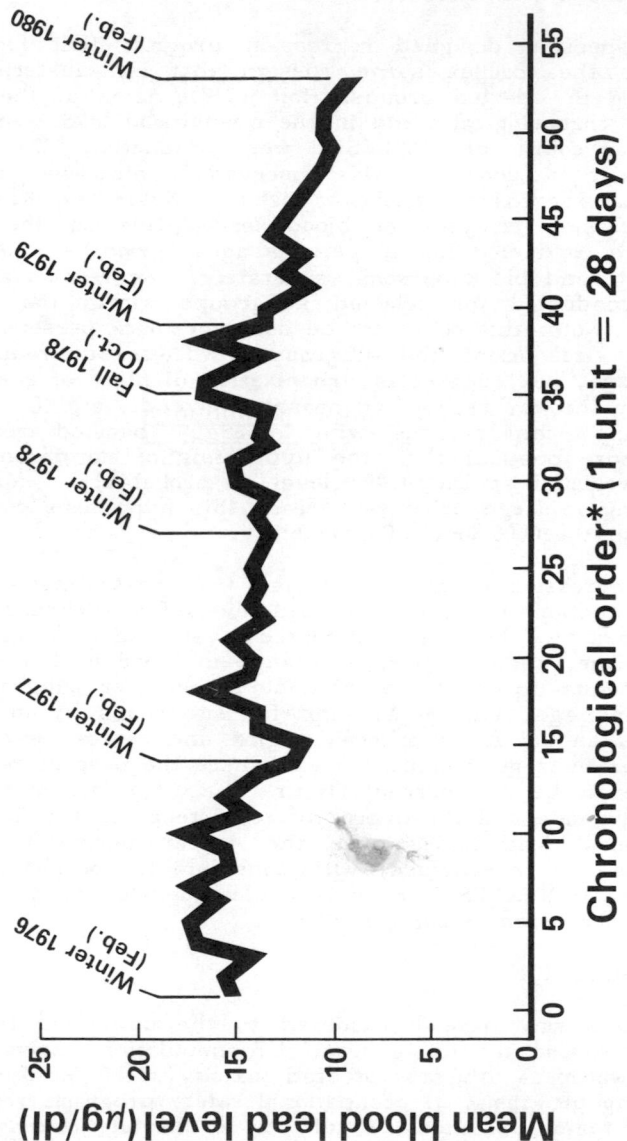

*Based on dates of examination of HANES II examines with blood lead determinations
SOURCE: National Health and Nutrition Examination Survey, National Center for Health Statistics

Figure 10

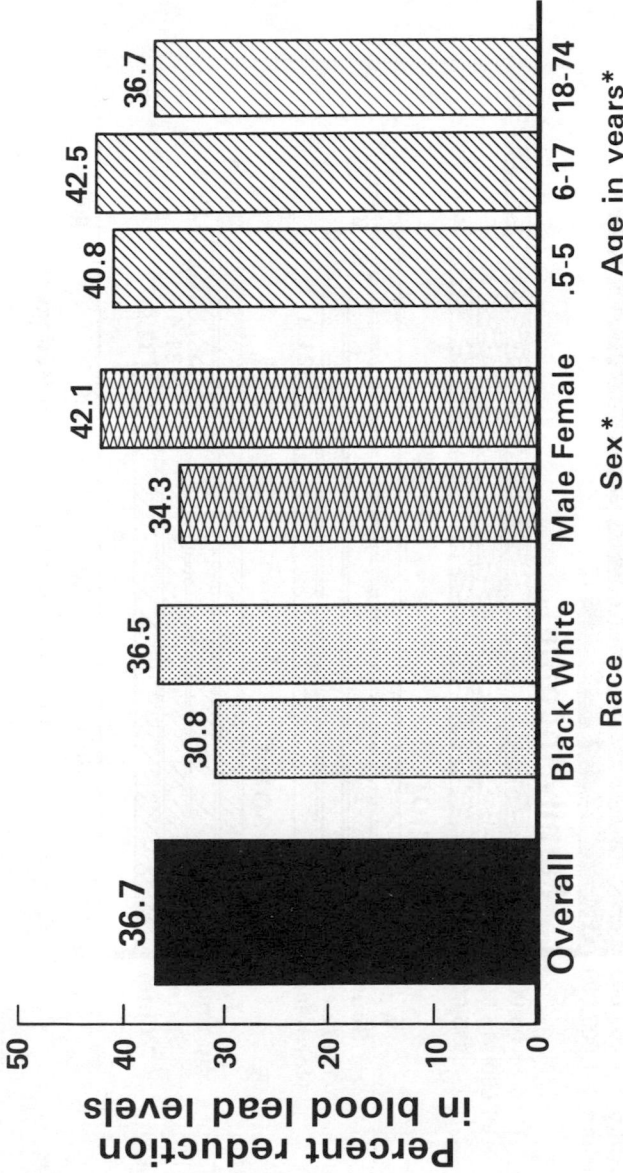

*For white persons only
SOURCE: National Health and Nutrition Examination Survey, National Center for Health Statistics

Figure 11

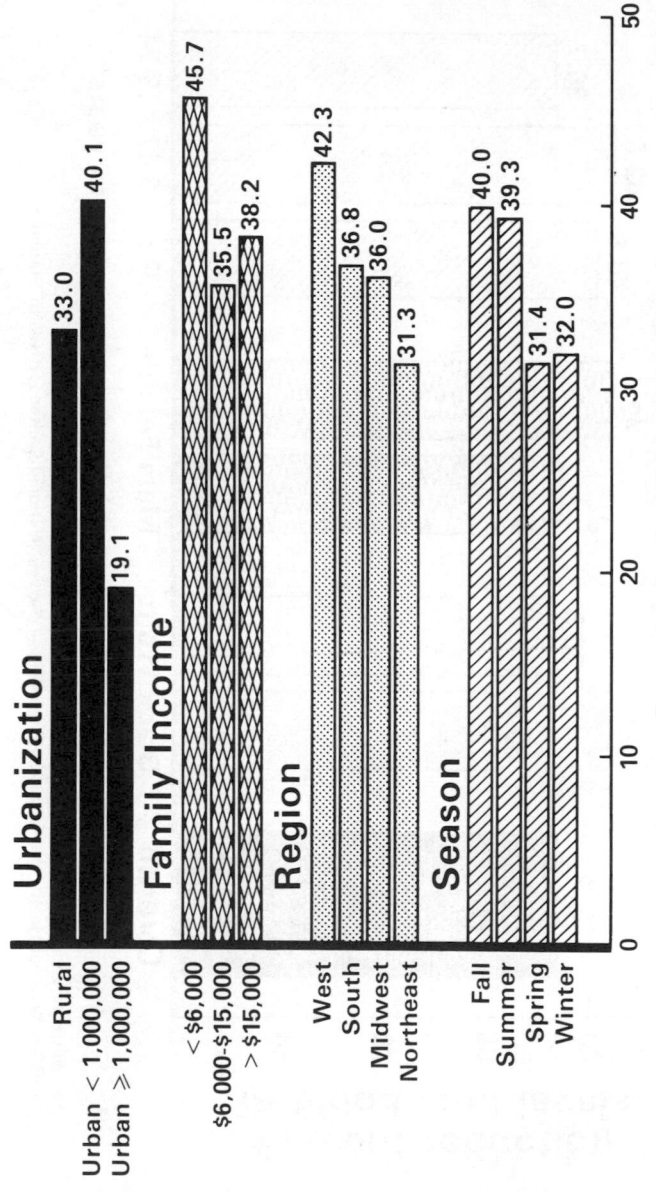

[1]For whites only
SOURCE: National Health and Nutrition Examination Survey, National Center for Health Statistics

efforts by an advocacy group called the "Committee for Lead
Elimination Action in the District of Columbia" abbreviated L.E.A.D.
It is likely that these public awareness efforts have had a
significant role in explaining a decrease in the proportion of
children with elevated blood lead levels observed in the district.
Lead screening programs located throughout the district are
currently finding approximately 5 times fewer children ages 6
months - 5 years with elevated blood lead levels than was found in
1976. In 1976, 16,090 children living in Washington DC were
screened, of whom 10 percent had blood lead levels of 30 micrograms per deciliter or more. In 1981 until present, 18,948 children
were screened, with 1.6 percent having elevated blood lead levels.
(Ehrnman, K., personal communication). From fiscal year (FY)
1973 through FY 1980 federally-assisted projects funded through
CDC screened 3,350,000 children and uncovered 221,000 (6.6
percent) with confirmed undue lead absorption. For FY 1981,
535,000 children were screened of whom 22,000 (4.1 percent) had
undue lead absorption. (Centers for Disease Control 1981).

Findings from surveys of non-infant canned foods carried out by
the US Food and Drug Administration (FDA) indicate that the mean
lead levels in a sample of 13 popular canned adult foods, commonly
eaten by young children, dropped from 0.38ppm in 1974 to 0.21ppm
in 1980. (Jelinek 1982) Data developed by FDA and others
indicate that about 1/3 of lead in the American diet comes from
canned foods. The decrease of lead in canned foods is attributed
to a shift by the food-processing industries from the use of
lead-soldered three piece cans to either welded three-piece cans or
two-piece steel cans.

Similarities in chronological trends in the NHANES II blood lead data
and the amount of lead used in the production of leaded gasoline
have been presented by Dr Vernon Houk, Director of the Center
for Environmental Health of the Centers for Disease Control, at
public hearings concerning regulation on lead phasedown in gasoline
held by the US Environmental Protection Agency on April 15-16,
1982 (US Environmental Protection Agency 1982). NHANES blood
lead data for person ages 6 months - 74 years, presented in figure
12, show that the decrease in the weighted mean blood lead levels
computed by 6 - month intervals almost parallel the amount of lead
used in the production of gasoline in the United States from
February 1976 through February 1980. Figure 13 shows that the
product-moment correlation between these mean NHANES II blood
lead values and lead used in gasoline production was 0.95.
Although these data do not prove a cause and effect relationship,
the correlation does require explanation and is consistent with
findings from a study of blood lead levels in New York school
children for the period 1970 to 1976 (Billick et al. 1979).

Exposure to environmental lead occurs via lead in air, food, dust,
dirt, soil, water supply, and lead-based paint. Over 90% of
atmospheric lead is derived from vehicle emissions, but the extent
to which lead in air contributes to lead in food and lead in dust is

Joseph L. Annest

Figure 12

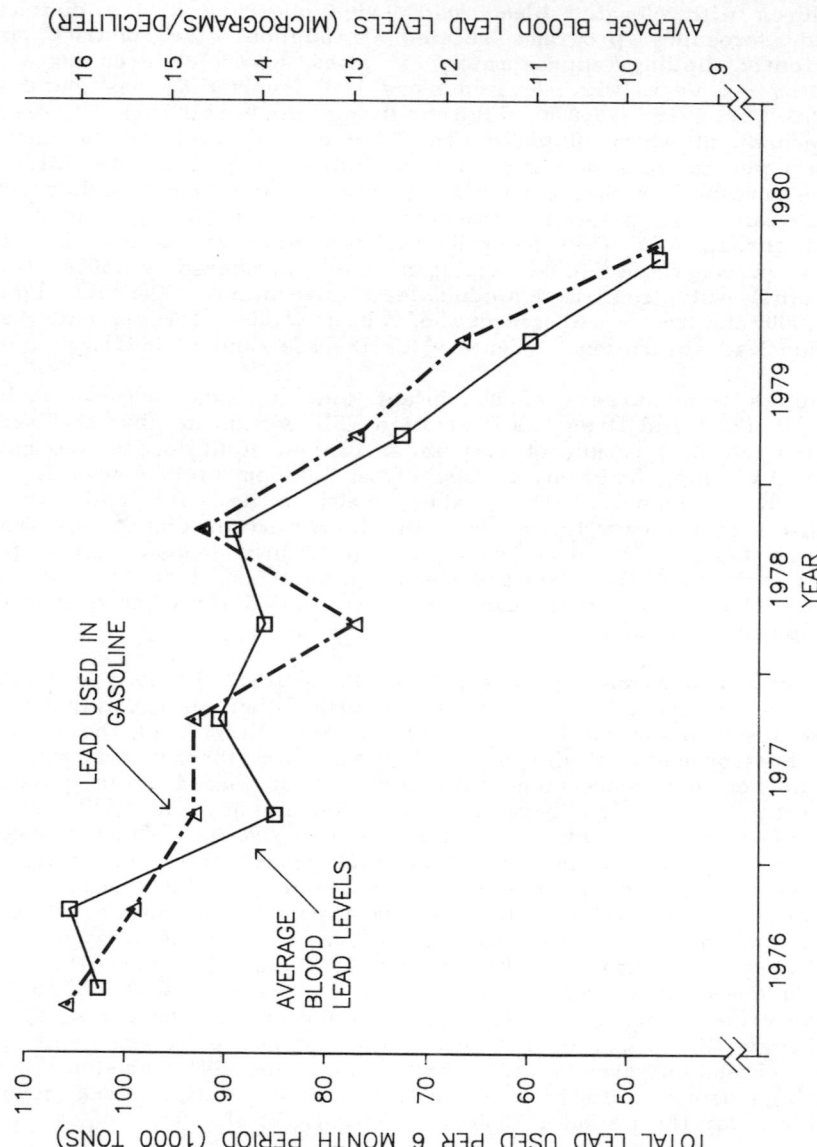

Figure 13

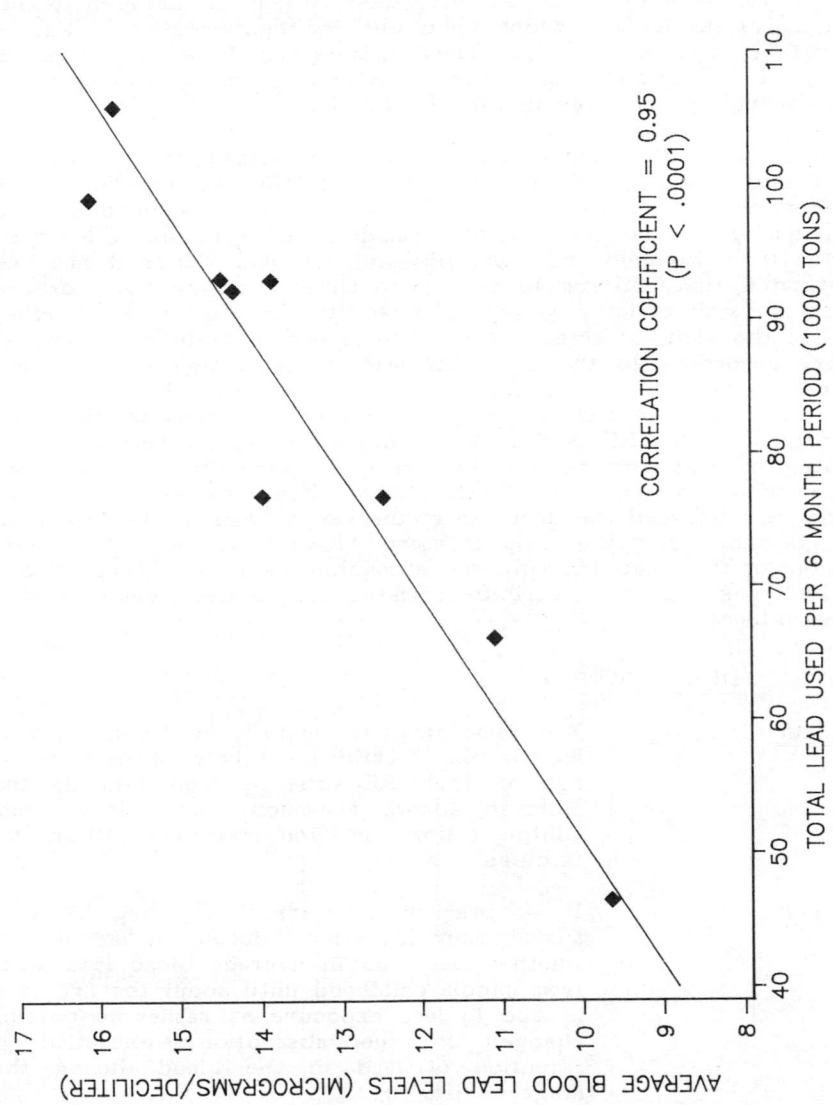

still controversial. (US Environmental Protection Agency 1977).
Most lead gains access to the human system by ingestion or
inhalation, and the relative contribution of each will vary depending
upon individual circumstances. Very young children have a higher
rate of gasto-intestinal absorption of lead than do adults and they
are more likely to ingest lead rich dust, which has adhered to their
hands or to objects which they put in their mouths. (National
Academy of Science 1980). These factors may have had an important role in explaining the changes in average blood lead levels for
pre-school age children in the NHANES II.

The rate of absorption of airborne lead in relation to age is not so
well understood. (US Environmental Protection Agency 1977). The
percentage of inhaled lead retained will vary depending upon
particle size, and the amount inhaled by each person will depend
upon their metabolic rate and physical activity. Thus it has been
estimated that children inhale two to three times as much airborne
lead per unit of body weight as do adults (Lin Fu 1975). Furthermore, the value of alpha, which is the blood lead/air lead ratio, will
vary according to the base line lead concentration so that alpha
tends to fall as air lead and blood lead increase. (Hammond et al.
1979). All these factors need to be taken into consideration when
interpreting the NHANES II data. Consequently the relative contribution of lead from gasoline to human exposure cannot be precisely
quantified from the NHANES II study. Nevertheless, the striking
similarity between the decrease in the use of lead in the production
of gasoline, and the drop in mean NHANES II blood lead levels
suggests that lead entering the atmosphere from the combustion of
leaded gasoline can contribute significantly to the level of lead in
human blood.

DISCUSSION

Walker:

You demonstrated a significant decline in blood
lead levels in children of both sexes until the
age of 16. Subsequently you told us that
children absorb at much higher levels than
adults. How do you reconcile these two
findings?

Annest:

It is pre-school children who are likely to
absorb more lead than adults. It is not clear
whether the drop in average blood lead levels
from middle childhood until about the age of 16
is due to less exposure or rather to possible
changes in the absorption, excretion or
retention of lead in the blood during that
stage of life.

Bryce-Smith:

To what extent do you feel the the differences
between the blood lead levels of black and
white populations reflect, on the one hand,
differences in exposure because all black
people live in city centre areas; and, on the

| | other hand, differences in the metabolic handling of lead which is perhaps genetically determined? |

Annest: That is not yet known. However, the National
                 Center for Health Statistics is about to begin a
                 Hispanic HANES survey that is family oriented
                 and designed to answer some of those
                 questions. In addition to other survey
                 components, blood lead data will be obtained
                 for an average of 3 to 4 persons living in the
                 same house. A family aggregation study on
                 these data could be informative regarding the
                 role of genes and household environment in
                 explaining variations in blood lead levels in the
                 population.

Russell Jones: The figure for the contribution of petrol lead
                 to body lead burdens on which the British
                 Government is currently operating is 10%. On
                 that basis, the predicted reduction in your
                 study should have been no more than 5.5%
                 since there was a 55% reduction in the amount
                 of leaded gasoline used over a four year
                 period. The observed reduction was 37%.
                 Could you comment on your figures in relation
                 to the Government's position?

Annest: I am not really in a position to comment on
                 policy making decisions using these data.

Rutter: I appreciate your caution with respect to
                 public policies but can I press you a little with
                 respect to some of the scientific findings. As
                 I see it, your study raises two rather separate
                 issues. The first is the question of whether
                 the drop in population levels of lead was true
                 or artefactual (perhaps as a result of shifting
                 laboratory standards). The findings appear
                 clear-cut in showing that laboratory standards
                 had not altered and hence that the drop was
                 true. The second question is whether the
                 drop was caused by the phasing out of lead
                 from petrol. If it was, then one might expect
                 a greater drop in urban centres than in rural
                 areas. In fact, to the extent that there was a
                 trend, it went in the opposite direction. How
                 does that affect the inference that the
                 reduction of lead in petrol was responsible for
                 the fall in blood leads?

Annest: Although I agree that that does appear
                 puzzling at first sight, there are possible

explanations. In the first place, in so far as the lead in petrol enters the body through the contamination of food (rather than through the breathing of polluted air), any reduction should be reflected equally in urban and rural populations. Secondly, with respect to the slightly smaller fall in large cities, it is possible that the changeover to new cars using unleaded fuel may have taken place more slowly there. Finally, there continues to be considerable traffic congestion in urban areas, and since the relationship between air lead and blood lead is not linear, you might expect less of a drop in cities.

Question:

Were the same individuals measured year after year, or were there separate groups of individuals each year?

Annest:

Each year group does not constitute a representative sample of the United States but the entire set of data from 1976 until the end does provide a representative sample of the United States. In NHANES II, persons were sampled cross-sectionally from 64 different locations, based on a probability sample design over the course of four years. Collectively, when weighted using the census information on population estimates, the sample is then representative of the United States. Thus, the data for each year represent different individuals.

Goodacre:

It worries me that, according to Patterson, the measurement of blood lead can involve as much as 50% error.

Annest:

The way that statisticians deal with measurement error is that they compute the coefficient of variation based on quality control data. In this study, the coefficient of variation ranged from 7-15%.

Delves:

With respect to Patterson's claims, the error rate is not as high as 50%. Quality control data show that the results are accurate. The use of such data is being adopted in Britain as well as the United States in order to provide demonstrably good quality control.

Annest:

Certainly, since 1970, the techniques for measuring blood lead levels have improved considerably. I reviewed the quality control

programme that was used with the NHANES
data and I am convinced that the laboratory
technicians did just about as well as they
possibly could have done.

REFERENCES

Annest J L, Mahaffey K R, Cox D H, Roberts J (1982). Blood lead
    levels for persons 6 month - 74 years of age: United States,
    1976-80. Advance Data From Vital Health Stat, No. 79. DHHS
    Pub. No. (PHS) 82-1250. Public Health Service, Hyattsville,
    Md.
Barthel W F, Smrek A L, Angel G P , Liddle J A, Landrigan P J,
    Gehlbach S H, Chisolm J J, Modified Delves cup atomic
    absorption determination of lead in blood. J Assoc. Off. Anal.
    Chem. 56:1253-56.
Billick I H, Curran A S, Shier D R (1979) Analysis of pediatric
    blood lead levels in New York City for 1970-1976. Environ.
    Hlth. Perspect. 31:183-192.
Centers for Disease Control (1978) Preventing lead poisoning in
    young children. J. Pediatr. 93: 709-720.
Centers for Disease Control (1981) Surveillance of childhood lead
    poisoning - United States. MMWR 31(9): 118-119, Public Health
    Service, Atlanta. US Government Printing Office.
Centers for Disease Control (1982) Blood lead levels in US
    population. MMWR 31(10):132-134 DHHS Pub. No. (CDC)
    82-8017, Public Health Service, Atlanta. US Government
    Printing Office.
Cohen C J, Bowers G N, Lepow M L (1973). Epidemiology of lead
    poisoning, a comparison between urban and rural children.
    JAMA 226:1430-1433.
Crisler J P, Lao N T, Tang L C, Serrano B A, Shields A (1973).
    A micro-sampling method for the determination of blood lead.
    Microchem J. 18:77-84.
Gunter E W, Turner W E, Neese J W, Bayse D D (1981).
    Laboratory procedures used by the Clinical Chemistry Division,
    Centers for Disease Control, for the second National Health and
    Nutrition Examination Survey (NHANES II). Public Health
    Service, Atlanta, Ga.
Hammond P B, O'Flaherty E J, Gartside P S (1979). The impact of
    air lead on blood lead in men. A critique of the recent
    literature. Paper presented at the International Conference on
    Management and Control of Heavy Metals in the Environment,
    London.
Holt MM (1979) SURREGR, standard errors of regression coefficients
    from sample survey data. Unpublished. Research Triangle
    Institute, North Carolina.
Jelinek C F (1982). Levels of lead in the United States food
    supply. J. Assoc. Off. Anal. Chem. 65:942-946.
Lin-Fu J S (1975). Undue lead absorption and lead poisoning in
    children - an overview. In: Proceedings, Int. Conf. on Heavy
    Metals in the Environment, pp 29-52. Toronto, Canada, Oct.

27-31.

McDowell A, Engel A, Massey J T, Maurer K (1981). Plan and operation of the second National Health and Nutrition Examination Survey, 1976-1980. Vital Health Stat. Series 1, No. 15, DHHS Pub. No. (PHS) 81-1317. Public Health Service, Washington. US Government Printing Office.

Mahaffey K R, Annest J L, Barbano H E, Murphy R S (1979). Preliminary analysis of blood lead concentrations for children and adults : NHANES II 1976-1980. Trace Substances in Environmental Health - XIII. pp 37-51, Ed. Hemphill D D, Univ. of Missouri, Columbia.

National Academy of Science (1980). Lead in the Human Environment. National Academy of Sciences pp. 34-43 Washington D.C.

National Center for Health Statistics (1979) Statistics needed for determining the effects of the environment on health, report of the technical consultant panel to the United States National Committee on Vital and Health Statistics. Vital Health Stat. Series 4. No. 20. DHEW Pub. No. (PHS) 79-1457. Public Health Service. Washington. US Government Printing Office.

Neter J, Wasserman W (1974) In: Applied linear Statistical Models. Ed. Irwin R D. pp 313-315. Homewood, III. 60430.

Simpson J M, Clark J L, Challop R S, McCabe E B (1972). Elevated blood lead levels in children, a 27-city neighbourhood survey. Health Service Report 88:419-422.

US Bureau of Census (1980) Consumer Income. Characteristics of the population below the poverty level: 1978. Current Population Reports. Series P-60, No 124. Washington. US Government Printing Office.

US Evaluation Protection Agency (1977). Air quality criteria for lead. EPA Pub. No. 600/8-77-017, Office of Research and Development. Washington US Government Printing Office.

US Evaluation Protection Agency (1982). Regulation of Fuel and Fuel Additives. Federal Register. Vol. 47 No. 35:7812-7814.

SOURCES OF LEAD IN THE ENVIRONMENT

Irwin H. Billick

Program Manager
Lead Poisoning Research
Environmental Research Group
Department of Housing and Urban Development
Washington DC
USA.

Although the toxic nature of lead had been known for thousands of years, it is only recently that is has been recognised as a ubquitous environmental pollutant. Historically efforts to control lead poisoning have been centred mainly on well defined high level sources such as lead glazed food utensils or occupational exposure. Furthermore, these efforts focused on the detection and elimination of lead poisoning in which the victim exhibited the chronic and observable symptoms of the disease.

Only in about the last twenty years has concern about lead exposure been extended to include detection and control of both symptomatic lead poisoning and asymptomatic, but unacceptably high, lead levels in the general population, particularly children. In the United States, during the mid-1960's and early 1970's public health professionals, local officials and the public, became increasingly aware of increases in the number of cases of lead poisoning and of high lead levels in urban children. At that time, this was attributed almost exclusively to ingestion of lead-based paint (Lin-Fu, 1970). Some cities (such as Chicago in 1965, and New York in 1970) began large scale screening programmes to identify children at risk and to remove lead-paint from the dwelling units of children with high lead levels. Following the passage of the Lead-based Paint Poisoning Prevention Act, in 1971, a grant in aid program from the Federal Government established similar lead poisoning screening and control programmes in over 60 other local communities.

Other Federal Agencies also increased their activities related to lead pollution from sources that fell under their jurisdiction; by the mid-1970's a number of new regulations governing lead exposure of the population in general had been implemented. These included not only regulation of allowable lead levels in paint, but also the direct regulation of permissable levels of lead in food, water and air. Furthermore, the amount of lead discharged into the environment from the combustion of petrol was controlled directly by regulations that limited the average level of lead per gallon of petrol, as well as, indirectly by the requirement of lead-free petrol for automobiles manufactured after 1975, which used catalytic converters to control other air pollutants.

For the most part these efforts were all independent and
uncoordinated, but the overall net effect has been a decrease in the
average lead level in the environment which, in turn, is reflected
in the lead levels in the population where measurements are
available.   From both a public policy and a public health point of
view, it would be desirable to know which of these sources of lead
are the most critical and which control programmes (or combinations
of control programmes) are the most effective.   Unfortunately, the
determination of the relative importance of each of the different
sources is not a simple exercise (Billick, 1981).

Only recently, has it been appreciated that the problem of lead in
the environment is a complex and inter-twined system.

Figure 1 is a diagram of lines, arrows, boxes, circles and numbers,
which described the uses, products, transport media and pathways
of human exposure to lead (National Academy of Sciences, 1979).
It certainly illustrates the complexity of the system but whether it
clarifies or confuses the understanding of what is happening is
questionable.

A major source of information about the problem of sources of lead
exposure to children is provided by the vast data bases that have
been created as a result of the local screening programmes.   While
these were not rigorously designed epidemiological studies, the data
from these programmes contain a great deal of information about the
lead levels in the populations considered to be at the highest risk.
Analysis of the changes in lead levels with time, along with the
demographic characteristics of the population and changes in levels
of lead in the environment have yielded valuable insight and
understanding into the nature and extent of the problem.

TABLE 1. DATA BASE CHARACTERISTICS - GENERAL

	New York	Chicago	Louisville
Time Period	1970 - 1979	1967 - 1980 (QTR 2)	1974 (QTR 4) - 1976 1978 - 1979
Sampling Technique	Venous	Venous	Fingerstick
Analytic Technique	Atomic Absorption	Atomic Absorption	Anodic Stripping
Laboratory	In House	In House	Commercial/In House
Race Classification	unknown White Black Hispanic Other	White Black	White Black other
Raw Data	Decade Grouped	Ungrouped	Ungrouped

Fig. 1.   Sources and pathways for environmental lead.
(From National Academy of Science, 1980).

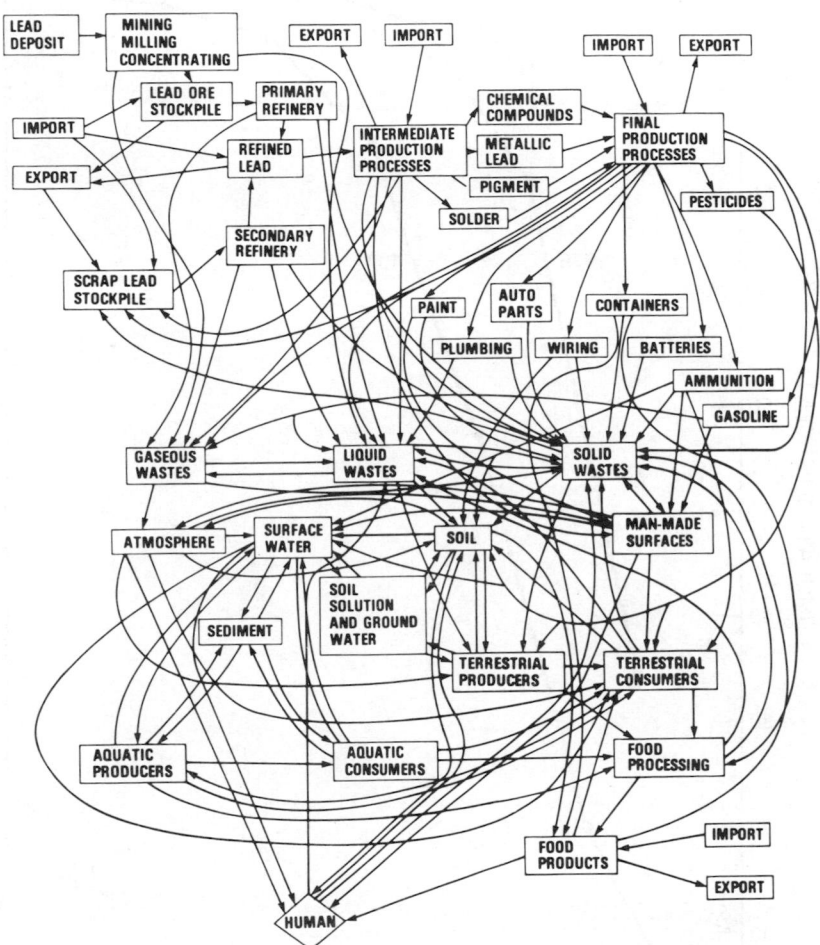

Irwin H. Billick

Fig. 2.   Data from Billick et al, 1979.

CUMULATIVE DISTRIBUTION OF BLOOD LEAD LEVELS FOR BLACKS,
25 - 36 MONTHS, JULY - SEPTEMBER SAMPLING DATE

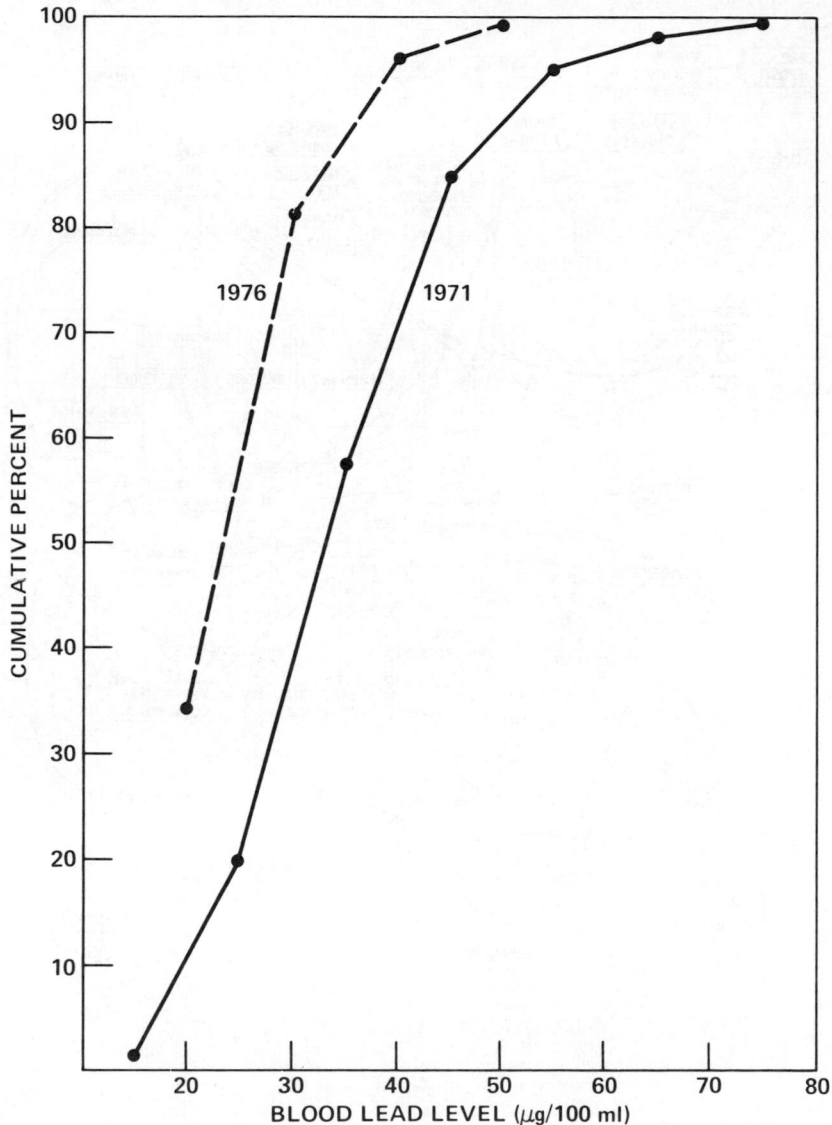

Fig. 3.   Data from Billick et al, 1979.

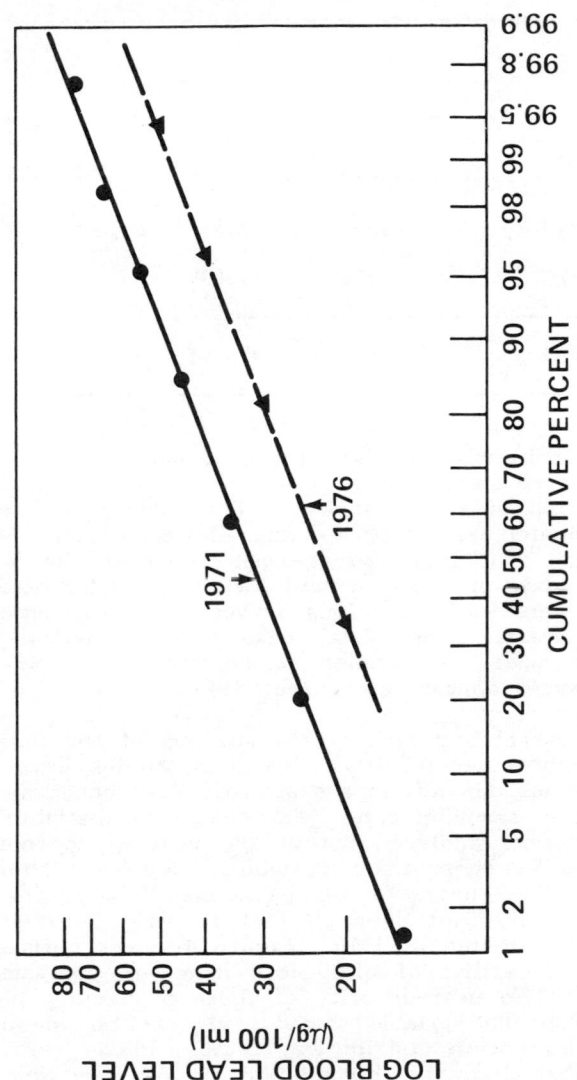

TABLE 2.   DATA BASE CHARACTERISTICS - NUMBER
OF OBSERVATIONS

Race	New York Screening Status Unknown	New York Screening Status Known	Chicago	Louisville
Unknown	69,658	43,891		11
White	5,922	9,446	6,459	3,864
Black	51,210	83,680	20,353	8,929
Hispanic	41,364	57,112		
Other	4,398	5,036		109
TOTAL	172,552	199,165	26,812	12,913

This chapter summarises the analysis of the lead screening data
from three cities in the United States: Chicago, Illinois, New York,
and Louisville, Kentucky. The primary independent variable
investigated was blood lead in children, usually below the age of 84
months. All three programmes reported the amount of lead in
blood, date of collection and somewhat similar demographic data but
there were some variations between the programmes. Tables 1 and
2 summarize the data base characteristics from the three
programmes; a detailed discussion of their similarities and
differences appears elsewhere (Billick, 1982).

The general approach to the analysis of the data was to consider
each city independently. Previous studies have shown that blood
lead levels depend, in a systematic way, on ethnic group, age, and
quarterly sampling date. Therefore, the distributions of blood lead
levels were analysed within the more homogenous subpopulations
defined by these three variables. Figure 2 shows the cumulative
distribution curves for children, age 23-36 months, who were tested
during July-September of 1971 in New York city and a similar
subgroup tested in 1976. Figure 3 shows normal probability plots
of the logarithm of blood lead level for the same two subpopulations. The near-linearity of these probability plots indicates that
the response variable (blood lead) can be adequately represented
by a log-normal distribution (Billick, 1982). Analogous figures for
the other distinct subpopulation groups from New York, as well as
the two other cities, showed similar findings. These plots also
illustrate a pronounced shift of the distribution curves to lower lead
levels with time. It is apparent from the curves presented in
Figures 2 and 3 that the shifts reflect the entire behaviour of the
lead levels in subgroup, rather than a change in the relative

Fig. 4.   Time dependence of blood lead in black children
          aged 24-35 months.

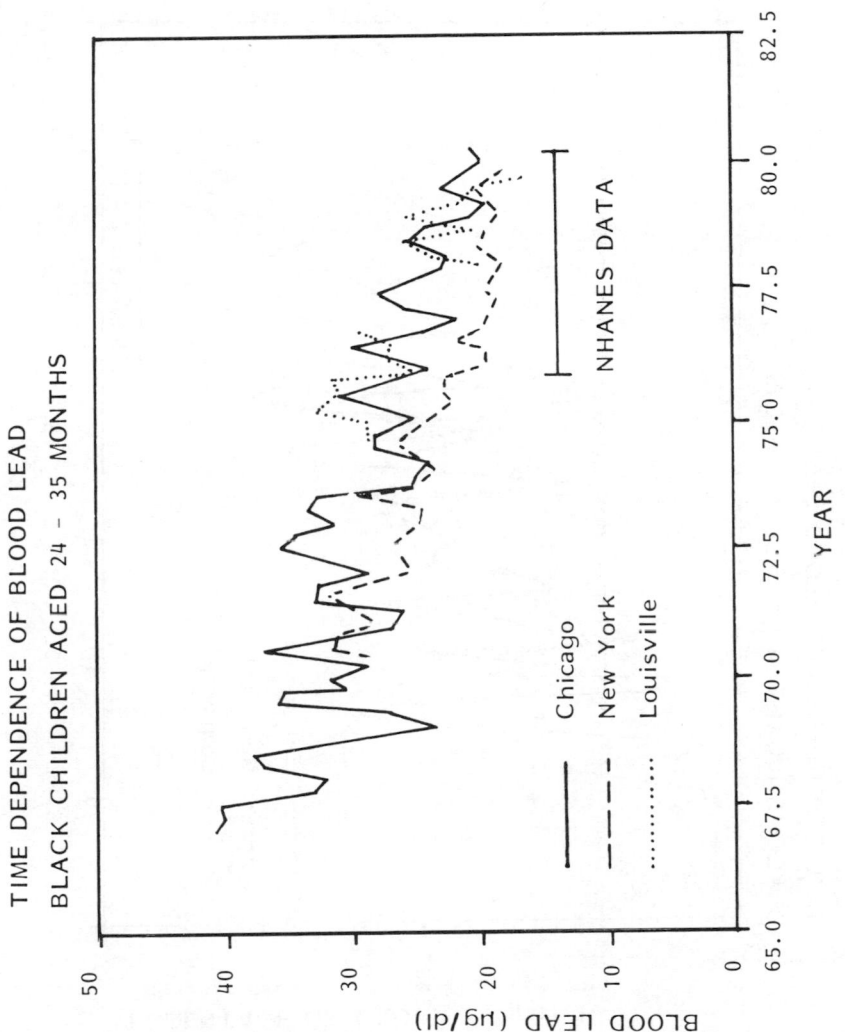

Fig. 5. Time dependence of blood lead in black children
         aged 24-35 months.

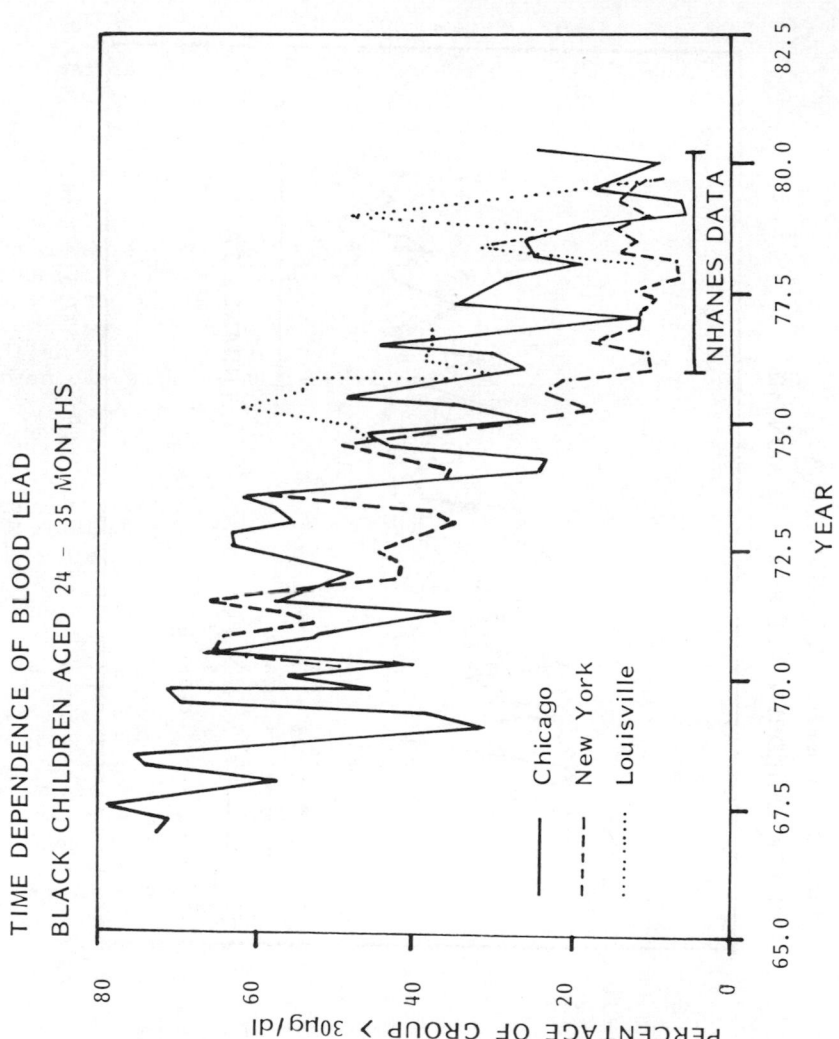

frequencies of higher or lower lead within the subgroup. Similar shifts with time have recently been reported in the cumulative distribution of umbilical cord blood lead concentrations (Rabinowitz and Needleman, 1982).

The time dependence of the blood lead levels, from all three cities, showed a similar pattern. This is illustrated in Figure 4 and 5 where data from three cities are presented for a single comparable age-race population. The 24-35 month, black subpopulations was selected for illustration since this subgroup appears to be the most sensitive. Figure 4 documents the changes in geometric mean blood lead with time for this group and demonstrates that the changes recorded in all three cities are equivalent. Figure 5 documents the effects of these changes on the percentage of black children ages 24-35 months with blood lead levels greater than 30 µg/dl. The 30 µg/dl level was chosen since it is currently considered to be the maximum safe limit by the US Environmental Protection Agency and the Department of Health and Human Services (US Environmental Protection Agency, 1978). Between 1970 and 1980 the proportion of black children with blood lead levels above 30 µg/dl fell from above 50% to below 20% in all three cities. Even if one disregards the possible adverse effects of lead levels below 30 µg/dl, the benefits to health of such reductions require no emphasis.

An independent measure of blood lead levels in the US population was obtained from the results of the Second National Health and Nutrition Examination Survey (NHANES II) carried out between 1976 and 1980 (chapter 3). This survey provided a comparison for checking the range and representatives of the blood lead levels obtained through the childhood lead screening programs used in our studies (Annest et al, 1982). The NHANES II study reported that, for centre city black children between the ages of 6 months – 5 years, the 1976-1980 mean blood lead level was 23.1 µg/100 ml, while for a similar group of white children the mean blood lead was 17.4 µg/100 ml. The urban average values for percent of observed blood lead over 30 µg/100ml were 18.6 and 4.5 respectively. The urban populations survey, the method of blood lead sampling and the analysis were all comparable to those used in the New York and Chicago screening programs. The agreement between the studies is rather good, considering possible differences that may exist either between the programs or between the methods of data analysis. A more recent study of umbilical cord blood lead (Rabinowitz and Needleman, 1982) also reported a similar temporal decrease and summer-winter cyclic behaviour to that which we have observed in screening data.

The observed variation in the screening programmes, blood lead levels have been related to the demographic, programmatic or environmental factors. Some of the variation may be attributed to differences in age or race of the population. For example, Figure 6 shows both the variations of geometric mean blood lead levels with age and ethnic group for New York city in 1971 (Billick et al, 1979). Generally speaking, all three cities showed that blacks had higher blood lead levels than whites; the age trends for New York and Chicago were comparable and the overall pattern was similar regardless of reporting period.

Fig. 6.   Variation   of   blood   lead   with   age   and   ethnic group.   Data from Billick et al, 1979.

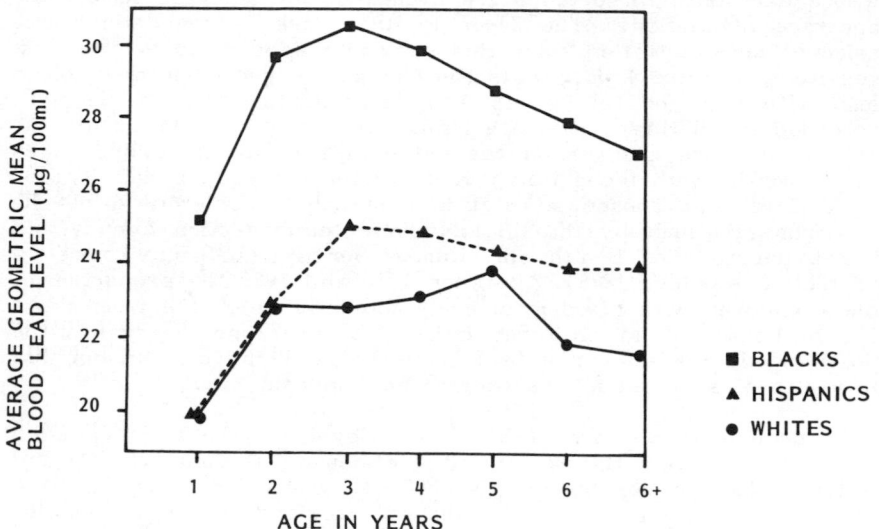

Indications of the reasons for the very dramatic decrease in blood leads with time, however, are of greatest interest.   Unfortunately, with a system as complex as environmental lead, together with the added handicap of retrospective analysis, one can only look for statistically   valid   correlations   between   historical   trends   in environmental   lead levels and blood lead levels.   Even when such correlations are found it is not possible to assume definitive cause and effect relationships on the basis of statistical analysis alone. We are left with the problem that there are many unknown or unquantifiable factors that may influence lead levels beyond those included in our analyses.

In trying to relate temporal blood lead changes to environmental lead, we first attempted to link changes in blood lead level to changes in exposure to lead based paint.   For the most part this was unsuccessful due to lack of data on changes in lead paint exposure in any of the three cities.   To the best of our knowledge, however,   there   were   no   large   scale   programmes   to   remove lead-based   paint   as   a   preventative   measure,   for   the   general population.   Normally, lead-based paint hazards are removed after the child is identified as having unacceptable high lead levels.

Several studies have been carried out both to assess the extent of paint containing lead in the dwelling units of the population at risk and to determine if a correlation existed between the lead level in paint and the blood lead of the children living in the dwelling unit. The results of one such study, which investigated the distribution of lead paint in dwelling units in Pittsburgh, Pa, is shown in Figures 7 and 8 (Shier and Hall, 1977).   Figure 7 shows that lead in a paint, at some measurable level, was present in the vast majority of homes.   However, as is shown in Figure 8, little or no statistical correlation existed between the children's blood lead and the fraction of the surfaces in the dwelling unit with paint lead levels greater than 2 mg/cm^2 (Urban, 1976).   Exposure to lead in paint might contribute to episodic occurrences of high lead exposures but in the absence of continuing efforts to remove lead paint, it cannot explain either the uniform decrease in distribution of blood lead level with time or their cyclic variation.

Pica for paint has often been afforded a major role in lead intake among children, but normal oral exploration and hand-to-mouth activity with the resultant ingestion of lead containing soil and dust has also been cited as a significant source of lead intake (Lin-Fu, 1973; US Environmental Protection Agency, 1977).   The highest incidence of pica overlaps that age bracket (18-30 months old) where other studies, as well as our own, find the highest prevalence of elevated blood lead levels (Lin-Fu, 1973).   While normal or abnormal ingestion may explain these higher blood lead levels in the 18-30 month group, it does not explain the seasonal variation in blood lead levels, which is virtually the same in very young children (1-12 months) as it is in older children (over 72 months).   The latter two age groups are not usually considered to be those in which pica is a common occurrence.   Nor does pica by itself account for the decrease in lead levels over time, which is similar in all age groups.

Seasonal variation in the number of children with elevated blood lead levels has been previously observed (Hunter, 1977).   Our analysis shows that this fluctuation is a characteristic of the entire screened population, represented by uniform shifts in the population distribution curves.   Explanations for this seasonal variation have, for the most part, been speculative.   It may be that sunlight increases the absorption of lead from the intestine (Chisolm, 1971).   On the other hand, seasonal variations in blood lead values may also result from seasonal variations in lead exposure.   The similarity in seasonal patterns and the temporal trends for the different age groups in different cities suggests that the reasons for the variation (e.g. exposure, metabolism) should be ones that are shared by all geographical areas.

Irwin H. Billick

Fig. 7   Data from Shier and Hall, 1977.

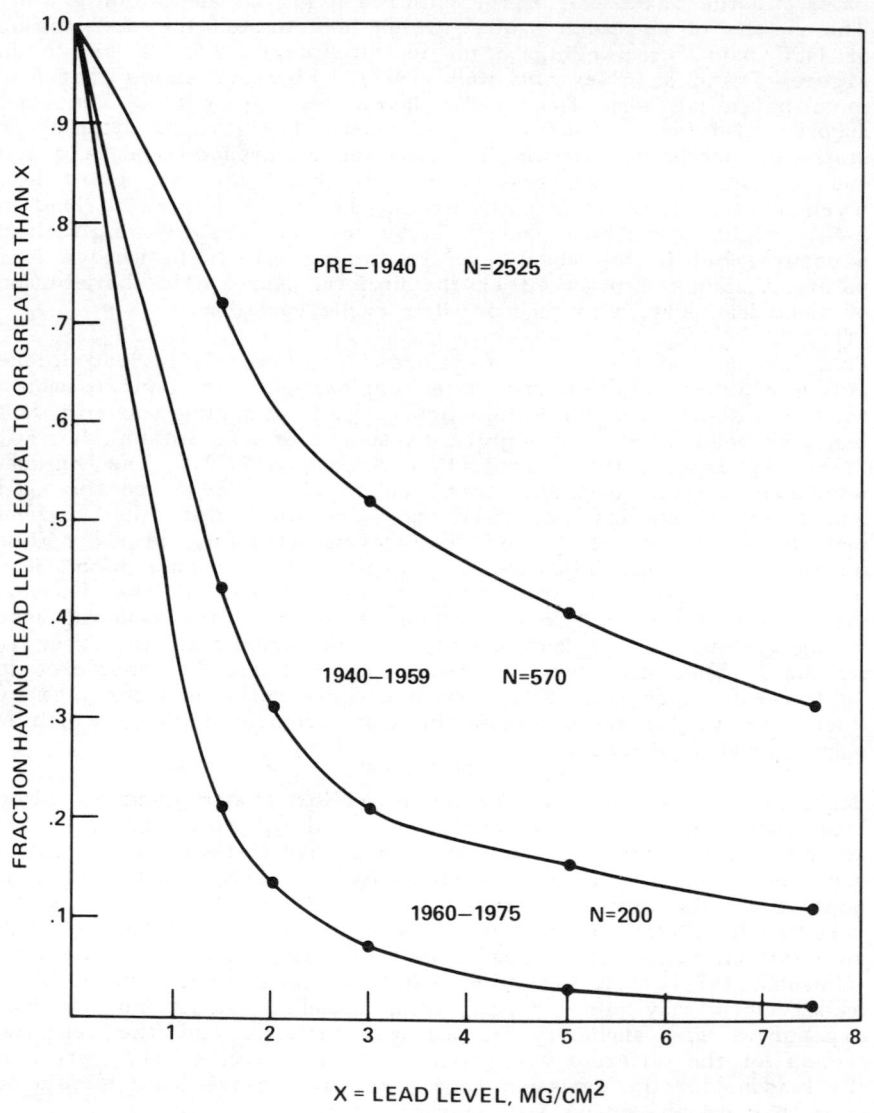

CUMULATIVE DISTRIBUTION OF HIGHEST LEAD
LEVELS ON DWELLING UNIT WALLS

Fig. 8. Date from urban, 1976.

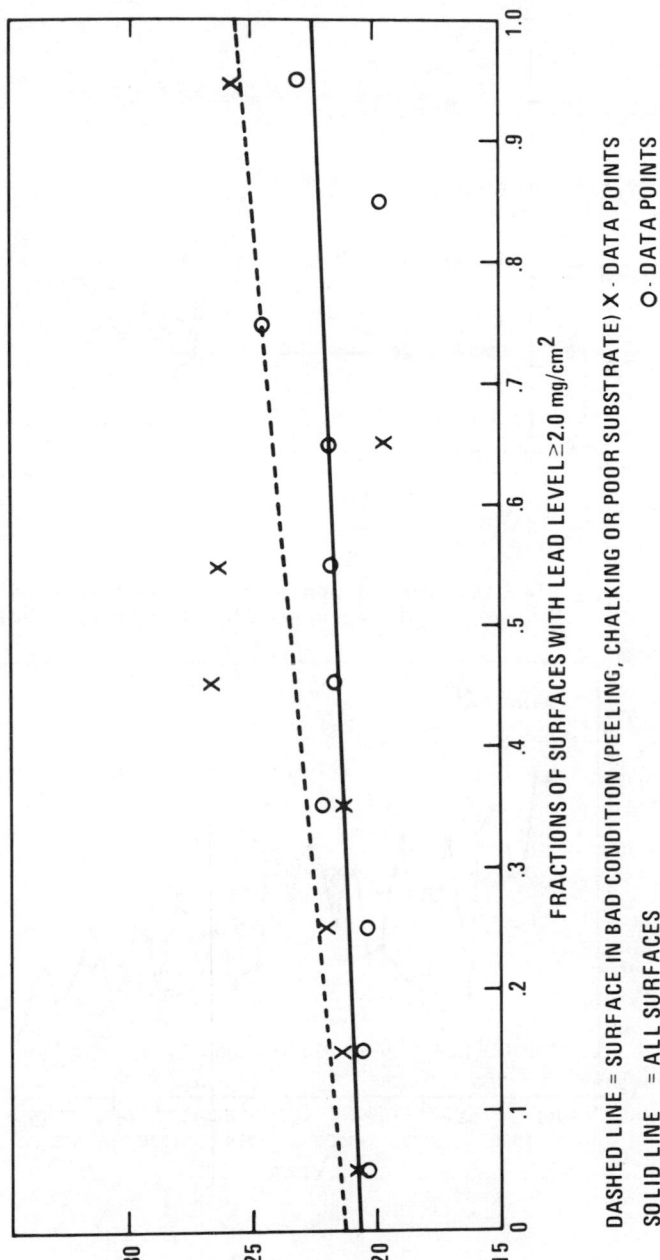

PLOT OF CHILDREN'S BLOOD LEAD LEVELS AGAINST FRACTION
OF SURFACES IN DWELLING UNIT WITH LEAD LEVELS AT LEAST 2.0 mg/cm^2

FRACTIONS OF SURFACES WITH LEAD LEVEL ≥2.0 mg/cm^2

CHILDREN'S BLOOD LEAD LEVELS -μg/100 ml

DASHED LINE = SURFACE IN BAD CONDITION (PEELING, CHALKING OR POOR SUBSTRATE) X - DATA POINTS

SOLID LINE = ALL SURFACES   O - DATA POINTS

Fig. 9.   Time dependence of blood lead and gasoline lead,
          black children aged 24 - 35 months, New York.

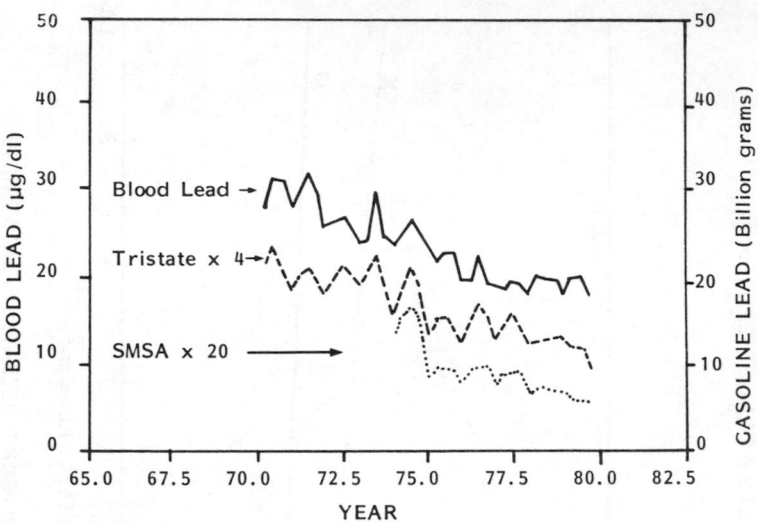

Fig. 10. Time dependence of blood lead and air lead, black
         children aged 24 - 35 months, Chicago.

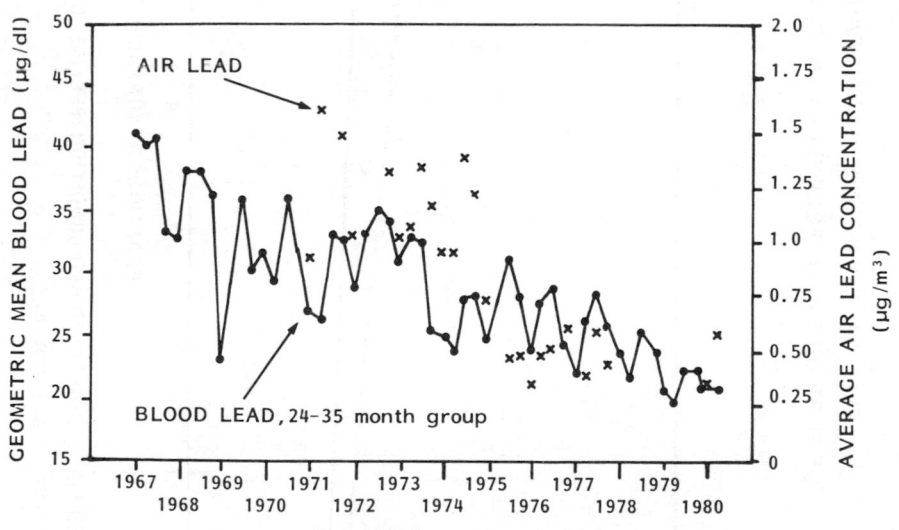

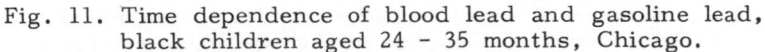

Fig. 11. Time dependence of blood lead and gasoline lead,
black children aged 24 - 35 months, Chicago.

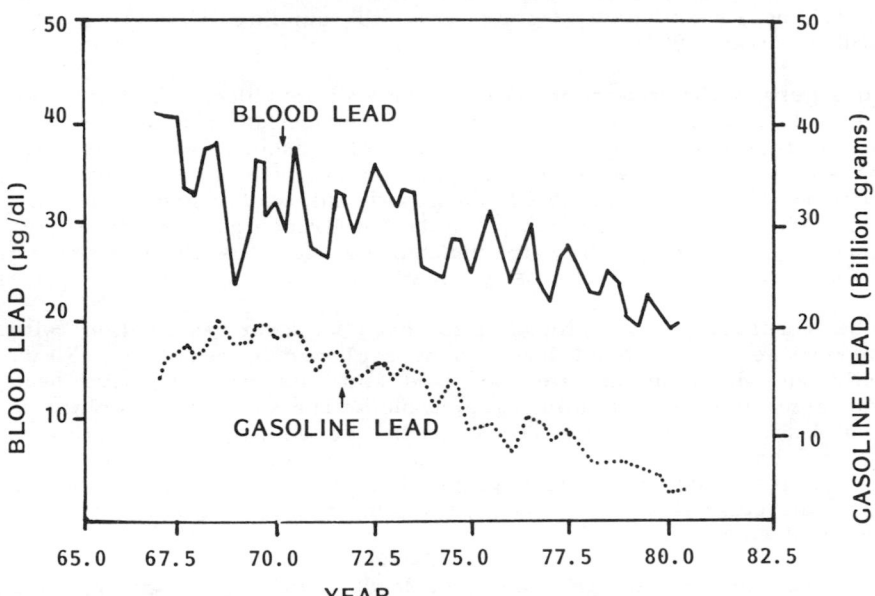

The main source of lead released into the environment comes from
the combustion of lead containing petrol additives. Approximately
24 per cent of petrol lead is retained in the car, and the remainder
is emitted to the atmosphere where it is deposited or removed by
the wind. Of the total lead originally consumed, approximately 50
per cent is deposited while 26 per cent remains in the ambient air.
(Huntzicker et al, 1975). In consequence, over 90 per cent of air
lead derives from the use of organo-lead petrol additives (Jenkins,
1976). Despite decreases in the amount of lead used in petrol,
automotive exhausts still represent the most important dynamic
source of lead in the environment. Research into its effects on
humans have been rendered unnecessarily complex by attempts to
quantify the contribution of individual pathways to human lead
intake, rather than examining the relationships between primary
sources of exposure such as petrol lead, and biological response
such as blood lead. Studies that relate blood lead levels and
proximity to road-ways represent a more satisfactory appraoch to
the problem (US Environmental Protection Agency, 1976) but the
most direct method is to correlate changes in petrol-lead
consumption with changes in blood lead.

In our original study of the changes in blood lead levels in New
York city between 1970 and 1976, we found that a correlation

existed between air lead variations and lead in children (Billick et al, 1979). However, this relationship was less impressive than that between the geometric mean blood lead and the amount of lead in petrol consumed in a 3-state area surrounding New York city (Billick et al, 1980).

In Figure 9 the geometric mean blood lead for black children aged 24 to 35 months is plotted against the petrol-lead consumption data as a function of time. Two sets of gasoline lead data are presented, the tristate consumption data used in the previous analysis (Billick et al, 1980) along with the lead consumption data reported at the level of the standard metropolitan statistical area (SMSA). The qualitative relationship between the blood lead and either set of petrol-lead data is apparent.

The observation that blood lead had a closer association with petrol-lead than with air-lead can be explained in two ways. First, only one air sampling site was used and this may not have been representative of the city as a whole. The second possibility is that lead in air may give access to the human system by pathways other than direct inhalation. For example, lead in air may contribute substantially to lead in dust and lead in food, whereas air lead concentrations provide only an indirect measure of these two pathways.

Analysis of the petrol-lead/blood-lead data from Chicago and Louisville produced broadly similar results to our New York studies (although the associations were less close). Fig. 10. demonstrates the relationship between air lead and blood lead in Chicago blacks aged 24 to 35 months. However, this is less impressive than the relationship between petrol lead and blood lead for the same sub-population (Fig. 11). In Chicago data from 20 air-lead sampling stations were available, but not all have been operating at the same times or over the entire period where blood-lead data exists. The air-lead data shown in Fig. 10 represents the average of five stations so even here data is incomplete before 1970 and between 1978 and 1979. Despite these reservations, the data confirm that blood-lead correlates more closely with petrol-lead than with air-lead and indicates a substantial input from petrol-lead via pathways other than direct inhalation.

Regression analysis on both the mean blood lead and the percent observations over 30 $\mu g/100$ ml produce highly statistically significant correlations (Billick, 1982). Using the values for the regression coefficients with age, race, season, and petrol lead as independent variables it is possible to predict the expected change in blood levels with changes in lead in petrol levels. Such predictive equations are useful to regulatory agencies such as the US Environmental Protection Agency in arriving at regulatory decisions related to the permissable levels of lead.

While we have discussed the general problem of the relationship between changes in blood lead levels, as measured by community screening programs, and environmental or other factors, it should not be assumed that the list is exhaustive. For example, socio-economic factors (Stark et al, 1982) or even the existence of a screening program itself (Oberman et al, 1977) may change the blood lead levels of the population. However, analyses of these data bases have provided valuable insights into the possible factors that contribute to children's lead levels, and such studies should continue to increase our understanding of the lead problem which, in turn, will provide the informed guidance to policy makers for the development and operation of cost-effective programmes and actions to minimise lead levels in the populations at risk.

DISCUSSION

Barry:

It is striking that the reduction in blood lead began as early as 1967 and has continued ever since in spite of the fact that the introduction of lead-free gasoline was not until 1974.

Billick:

Gasoline lead consumption started to decrease about 1970, probably because of a change in the buying habits of the American automobile consumers. High compression engines which use premium gasoline with a high lead content were replaced by low compression engines using regular gasoline with a lower lead content. The second change, as you indicate, was the introduction of lead-free gasoline which was introduced in 1975. Then. later, about 1978, the EPA regulations called for a phase-down in the allowable lead in gasoline. The decrease therefore was not solely determined by the introduction of leadfree gasoline.

Duck:

The data presented by Annest and Billick show an encouraging downward trend in community lead levels. However, as Annest pointed out, this coincided with an effective public campaign to prevent the lead contamination of foods and to get rid of lead paint. How can you be sure that the reduction was largely due to the elimination of lead from petrol?

Billick:

In my paper I emphasized that the reduction of blood lead levels probably stemmed from many different programmes. However, the campaign to reduce lead in paint from houses was not one of the more ambitious programmes in the United States. The number of dwelling units that have had the lead paint removed has not changed dramatically over time and it does not fluctuate seasonally. It is more difficult to assess the effect of an educational campaign. I cannot deny that the existence of the public health programmes, particularly the CDC screening programme, may have influenced the decrease in blood lead levels. However, this is conjecture. All that we have are highly significant statistical correlations between the timing of a fall in blood lead levels and the timing of changes in lead in gasoline. That does not prove a causal relationship (only direct experimentation can do that), but it suggests that a causal inference is reasonable.

Annest: It is useful in that connection to compare our general population data with Billick's data in high risk groups. Both showed the same pattern. Whatever it was that contributed to the downward trend in both studies must be something that affected both high risk and low risk populations. Certainly, lead in gasoline must be a major suspect as one of the key factors involved.

REFERENCES

Annest, H.L., Mahaffey, K.R., Cox, D.H., Roberts, J. (1982), Blood Lead Levels for Persons 6 months - 74 years of Age: United States 1976-1980. Advance data from Vital Health Statistics, No. 79. Pub. No. (PHS) 82-1250. Public Health Service, Hyattsville, Md.

Billick, I.H., (1981), Lead: A Case Study in Interagency Policy-Making. Environ. Health Perspect. 42, 73-79.

Billick, I.H., (1982) Prediction of Pediatric Blood Lead Levels from Gasoline Consumption. Report to the EPA, US Department of Housing and Urban Development, Washington, DC.

Billick, I.H., Curran, A.S., Shier, D.R. (1979), Analysis of Pediatric Blood Lead Levels for New York City 1970-1976. Environ. Health Perspect. 31, 183-190.

Billick, I.H., Curran, A.S., Shier, D.H. (1980) Relation of Pediatric Blood Lead Levels to Lead in Gasoline. Environ. Health Perspect. 34, 213-217.

Chisolm, J.J., (1971), Lead Poisoning. Sci. American 224 (2): 15-23.

Hunter, J.M., (1977), The Summer Disease: An Integrative Model of the Seasonality Aspects of Childhood Lead Poisoning. Soc. Sci. Med. 11: 691-703.

Huntzicker, J.J., Friedlander, S.K., Davidson, C.I. (1975), Material Balance for Automobile-Emitted Lead in Los Angeles Basin, Environ. Sci. Technol. 9: 448.

Jenkins, D.W., (Ed.) (April 1976), Design of Pollutant-Oreinted Integrated Monitoring Systems. A Test Case: Environmental Lead. EPA -600/4-76-018, US Environmental Protection Agency, Las Vegas, Nevada.

Lead-Based Paint Poisoning Prevention Act.   PL 91-695, January
    13, 1971.
Lin-Fu, J.S.   (1970), Lead Poisoning in Children.   PHS Pub.
    2108-1970, US Department of Health, Education and Welfare,
    Washington, DC.
Lin-Fu, J.S., (1973), Vulnerability of Children to Lead Exposure
    and Toxicity. N. Engl. J. Med. 289: 1289 - 1293.
National Academy of Sciences 1980, Lead in the Human Environment,
    NAS, Washington, DC.
Oberman, J.W., Karsten, S., Peacock, B. (1977), The Impact of a
    Community Action Programme Against Childhood Lead Poisoning:
    Three Year's Experience of a Neighborhood Pediatric Clinic,
    Clin. Proceed. Child. Hosp. 33, 27 - 37.
Rabinowitz, M.B., Needleman, H.L., (1982), Temporal Trends in
    Lead Concentrations of Umbilical Cord Blood.   Science 216,
    1429-1431.
Shier, D.R., Hall, W.G., (1977), Analysis of Housing Data
    Collected in a Lead Based Paint Survey in Pittsburgh, PA, Part
    1, NBSIR 77-1250, National Bureau of Standards, Washington,
    DC.
Stark, A.D., Quah, R.F., Meigs, J.W., DeLouise E.R. (1982), The
    Relationship of Envrionmental Lead to Blood-Lead Levels in
    Children. Environ. Res. 27, 372-383.
Urban, D., (1976), Statistical Analysis of Blood Lead Levels of
    Children Surveyed in Pittsburgh, PA, NBSIR 76-1024, National
    Bureau of Standards, Washington DC.
US Environmental Protection Agency (1977), Air Quality Criteria for
    Lead.   EPA-600/8-77-017.   Washington DC: US Government
    Printing Office.
US Environmental Protection Agency (1981) National Ambient Air
    Quality Standard for Lead, 40 CFR Section 50.12.   For
    preamable, see Fed. Reg., Vol. 43, 46246 (1978).

Lead Versus Health
Edited by M. Rutter and R. Russell Jones
© 1983 John Wiley & Sons Ltd.

LEAD EXPOSURE AND WATER PLUMBOSOLVENCY

Dr. Michael R. Moore

Senior Lecturer in Medicine
University of Glasgow
Department of Medicine
Western Infirmary
GLASGOW
G11 6NT

HISTORY

In the middle of the last century, it was realised that Glasgow, as a burgeoning industrial city, would have to procure for its inhabitants a more satisfactory water supply than the wells then currently in use. Various problems had been linked with the water supply including endemic typhus and epidemics of typhoid and cholera (Hamilton, 1981). It was therefore decided to implement a plan that utilised the very pure soft water supplies from Loch Katrine, through holding reservoirs at Mugdock and Craigmaddie, to supply the whole of the city (Burnet, 1869). As was standard practice at that time and as it had been for many centuries throughout the world, lead piping was used to distribute domestic water supplies. The opinion had been voiced that some problems might accrue from the dissolution of lead by such pure waters (Christison, 1844) and the city fathers wisely decided to invite the opinions of pre-eminent engineers of the time, amongst whom were numbered Stevenson and Brunel. Their conclusion at that time was that no ill-effects would accrue.

INITIAL FINDINGS

From the opening of the Water Works in 1859 by Queen Victoria until the early 1960's it was generally accepted that such pure clean water supplies would be unlikely to be associated with adverse health effects. However, there had been many pointers from studies dating from the turn of the century that there might be ill-effects (Oliver, 1914). Our initial findings established firstly that a potential problem did exist in relationship to over exposure from lead-affected water supplies, as evidenced both by increased blood lead concentrations and diminished activity of ALA deyhdratase in people living in high water lead exposure situations (Addis and Moore, 1974; Beattie et al, 1972), and secondly that there were very pronounced relationships between plumbosolvency pH, temperature, calcium concentrations in water supplies (Moore, 1973). Of these effects, pH was the most pronounced and it was significant that at the time our studies commenced the mean pH of the water supply to Glasgow lay around 6.3, a point very much on the ascending portion of the graph relating pH and pumbosolvency (Richards et al. 1980; Richards and Moore, 1982). Following on the studies in Glasgow, we found that similar relationships could be found in other parts of Scotland (Forteath, 1981; Sherlock et al, 1982) and indeed that also this applied in many other parts of the world (Moore, 1977; Berlin et al, 1977). An interesting feature of the relationship was that the distribution of blood lead concentrations was a skewed one, in which a tail of subjects had blood lead concentrations greatly in excess of the then current acceptable limits (Figure 1). Around 5% of our population had blood lead concentrations greater than 40 μg/dl (Moore et al. 1979; Department of the Environment, 1981). Corresponding to this skewed distribution we found similar relationships between various health states and this over-exposure to lead in the water supplies (Goldberg, 1974; Moore, 1977). Principal amongst these was the relationship found between excessive exposure to water lead and mental retardation (Beattie et al, 1975) which we subsequently linked with increased infant blood lead concentrations (Moore et al, 1977). There were, however, clear indicators that these effects were manifest in other systems such as the effects upon the kidney (Campbell et al, 1977), with increased incidence of renal insufficiency and gout (Campbell et al, 1978). The potential relationship between lead and its effects upon the heart was investigated (Moore et al, 1975; Kopp et al, 1980; Khan et al, 1977) and it was suggested that a link between this over-exposure and ischaemic heart disease would be found as well as that found between lead and hypertension (Beevers et al, 1976, 1980).

NEUROLOGICAL EFFECTS

Of all these effects, however, the ones we felt to be of the greatest long term consequence were those that were likely to be found upon the nervous system. The situation described by George Bernard Shaw in Mrs Warren's Profession at the turn of the century, "they expected to get their hands a little paralysed", represented that very obvious tip of the iceberg of effects upon the nervous system. We were more concerned at the time of investigation into those insidious long term effects of lead upon the nervous system which inevitably involve large numbers of subjects in whom the effects might be almost immeasurably small. The problem and the effects would almost certainly be of greatest consequence in the newly born infant (Moore, 1980) because at that stage in development children absorb considerably greater quantities of lead from their diet than they do in adult life (Alexander et al, 1974).

In addition one cannot neglect 'in utero' exposure of the foetus. Exposure in these circumstances is equivalent to the exposure of all other maternal soft tissues because the placenta is a poor barrier to lead (Figure 3). A consequence of this is that at birth cord blood lead concentrations are very similar indeed to those found in the mother.

Fig. 1. Frequency distribution of blood lead concentrations in Glasgow. 5% of subjects had blood lead concentrations in excess of 40 μg/dl (2 μmol).

FREQUENCY DISTRIBUTION of BLOOD LEAD in GLASGOW

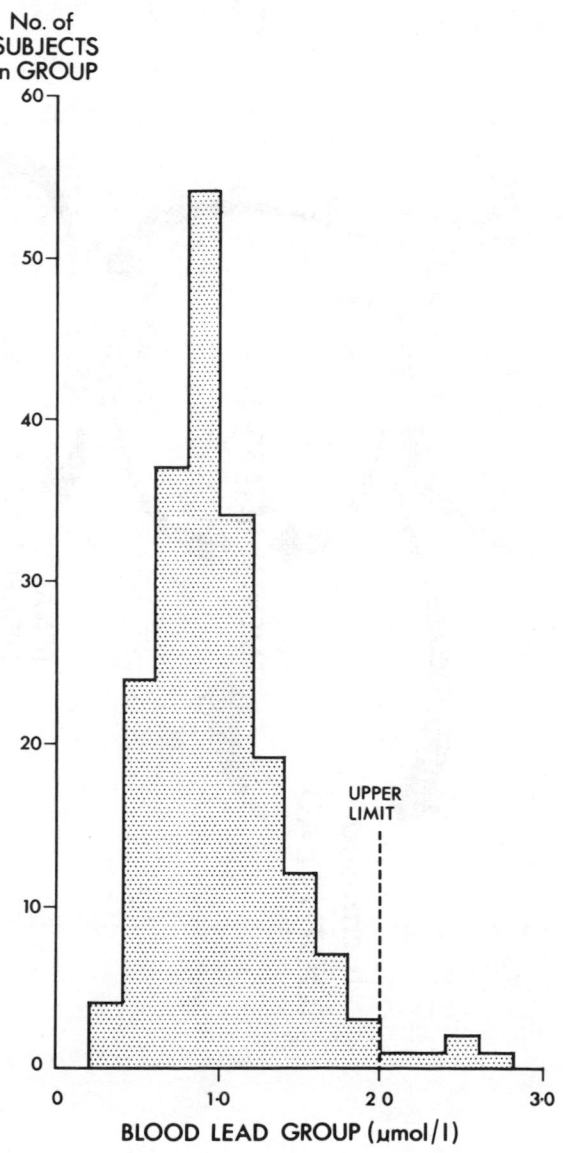

Dr. Michael R. Moore

Fig. 2.   The health effects of water lead exposure.

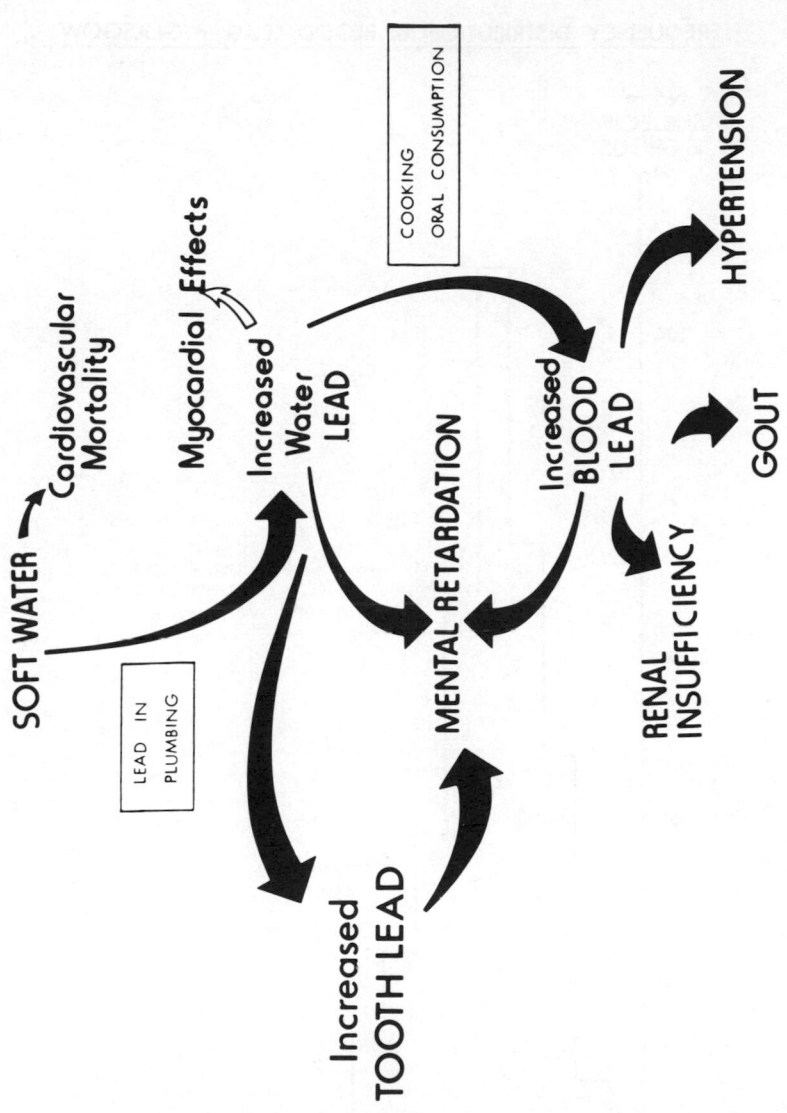

Fig. 3.   The dynamic equilibrium between lead intake and excretion.   Nearly all ingested material is excreted with only around 10-20% of ingested material absorbed.   This is then distributed to the soft tissues with around 9 µg daily in adults being stored in bone.   The principal mode of excretion is through the kidneys.   The greatest concentration of lead will be found in the bone plus all soft tissues including the foetus have similar concentrations within them.

UPTAKE and DISTRIBUTION of LEAD in the BODY

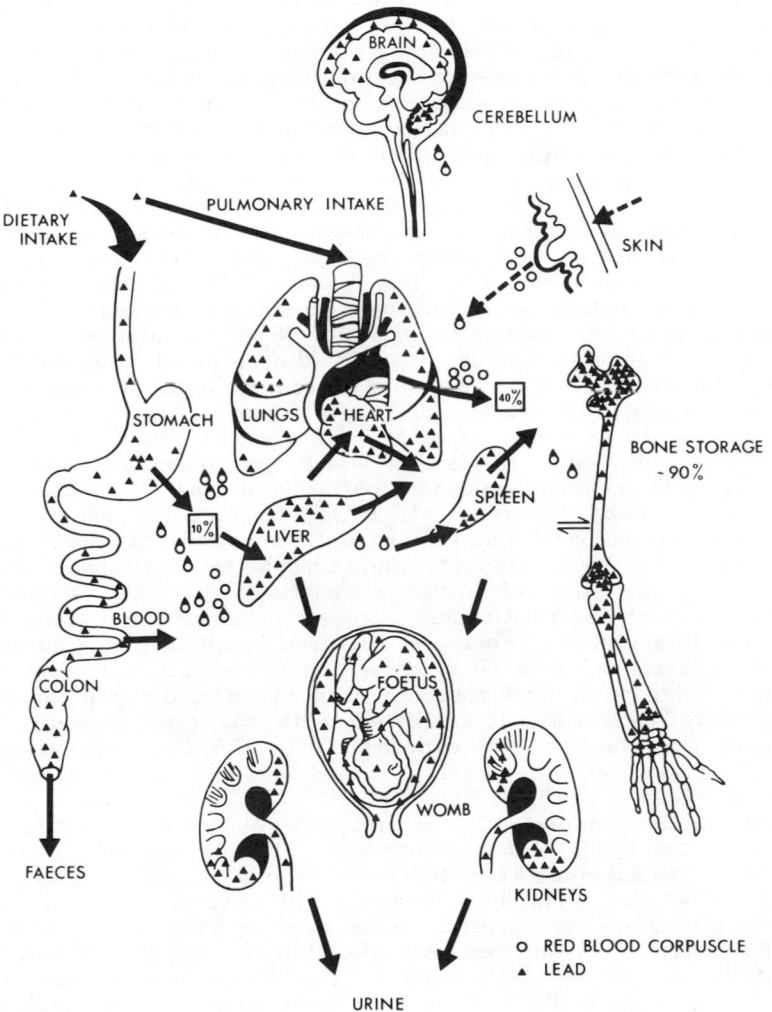

DIETARY STUDIES

Dietary exposure immediately after birth can take one of two forms. If the child is breast fed lead exposure will be relatively small since breast milk contains around 1/10th of the maternal blood lead concentration (Moore et al., 1982). In these circumstances it has been shown through Duplicate Diet Studies that breast fed children, even where the mothers are over exposed to lead, will almost certainly get less lead in their diet than they would if they were fed by the other technique of re-constitution of dried milk feeds (Sherlock et al., 1982; Department of the Environment, 1982). Lead concentrations in all proprietary dried milks are low. Where however, these dried milks are re-constituted with water in which there are variable, but often considerable, concentrations of lead, the child is being exposed to very high concentrations of dietary lead at a time in his life when he is most susceptible to the toxic insult of this metal on his or her developing tissues. Where the concentrations of lead in water are high, as we have found in the West of Scotland, the child is exposed to concentrations of dietary lead which on a weight per kilogram basis are greater than are likely to be experienced at any other time in life and furthermore when at least twice as much of the dietary lead will be absorbed. This type of over-exposure of the children does not stop at weaning. It is not commonly realized that food does in fact accumulate lead from water during cooking. There is a tenfold or greater accumulation of lead by vegetables cooked in water containing high concentrations of lead. The converse situation is true if a vegetable product utilised during food preparation is discarded; in that case the ultimate concentration of lead in the food is lowered. An example of this is when tea or coffee is made with tea leaves or coffee grounds. There is a rapid loss of lead from the liquid into the solids which are discarded leaving a beverage with a lower concentration of lead than the water from which it was made (Moore et al, 1979a; Smart et al, 1981). This type of accumulation is not restricted to vegetable products but is also shown by meat products and cereals in a similar fashion. Conclusive evidence of this association can be found in consideration of the relationship between tooth lead and water lead exposure in children. When we measured tooth lead concentration in 109 children living in Glasgow we found a significant association between molar tooth lead concentrations and the domestic drinking water lead concentrations, consistent with the type of water lead exposure the children had experienced in the first 5-6 years of their life (Moore et al., 1978).

In the earlier studies of the relationship between water lead exposure and blood lead concentrations, it was generally assumed that the association between these two would be linear (Addis and Moore, 1974). On closer examination this proved to be a gross over-simplification. An overall examination in 1977 of our evidence (Moore et al, 1977) together with the findings of others (Berlin et al, 1977) led us to the conclusion that there was a curvilinear relationship - probably a cube root relationship where blood lead

concentrations varied with the cube root of the water lead concentration (Figure 4). This relationship was eventually applied to
the information accumulated by the Duplicate Diet Studies carried
out in Glasgow (Department of the Environment, 1982) and in Ayr
in the West of Scotland (Sherlock et al, 1982). These studies of
dietary lead exposure and blood lead concentrations showed a
relationship similar to that found between water lead concentrations
and blood lead concentrations.

The equations were of the form

A   Infant Blood lead $= 5.5 + 3.3 \sqrt[3]{}$ Kettle water lead (μg/l)
    (μg/dl)

B   Infant Blood lead $= 2.5 + 26 \sqrt[3]{}$ Weeks intake dietary lead
    (μg/dl)   (mg)

One conclusion from these studies was that where water lead
concentrations were around 100 μg/l then 50% of all dietary intake
would be coming from water. The results also showed that where
children were consuming water of this level, then the quantity of
ingested lead taken would be in excess of 500 μg/week, a figure
that the Duplicate Dietary Study Group had settled upon as being
reasonably concordant with the WHO recommendation of no greater
than 3 mg lead/week in an adult diet (World Health Organisation,
1977). At this level of exposure this group of children had a mean
blood lead concentration of 24 μg/dl.

NEUROCHEMISTRY

It is clear that in these circumstances over exposure is taking place
and equally clear that this is likely to involve adverse sequelae on
health. The gross toxic effects are obvious when over exposure is
marked. As shown by the studies described in this volume, the
effects include changes in neuropsychological performance.
However, the precise consequences of different degrees of change
in body lead burden have yet to be defined.

The toxic effects of lead upon the nervous system are biphasic.
Firstly there is an effect upon cell morphology, development and
growth which has been described as a 'hard wiring defect'. This
kind of change is almost certainly irreversible and will result in
permanent neurological change, especially when the exposure has
taken place early in life. Secondly, lead has specific effects upon
various biochemical systems. Where alterations to the normal
function of biosynthetic pathways take place, alterations can occur
in the concentrations of neuroactive metabolites. This type of
change is potentially reversible. Typical of this kind of effect is
the influence that lead has upon haem biosynthesis, where inhibition
of delta-aminolaevulinic acid dehydratase and subsequently inhibition
of coproporphyrinogen oxidase and ferrochelatase, diminishes
concentrations of free haem and causes a negative feedback increase
in the activity of the rate limiting enzyme of the pathway,

Dr. Michael R. Moore

Fig. 4.   The cube root relationship between blood lead
concentration and water lead concentrations.

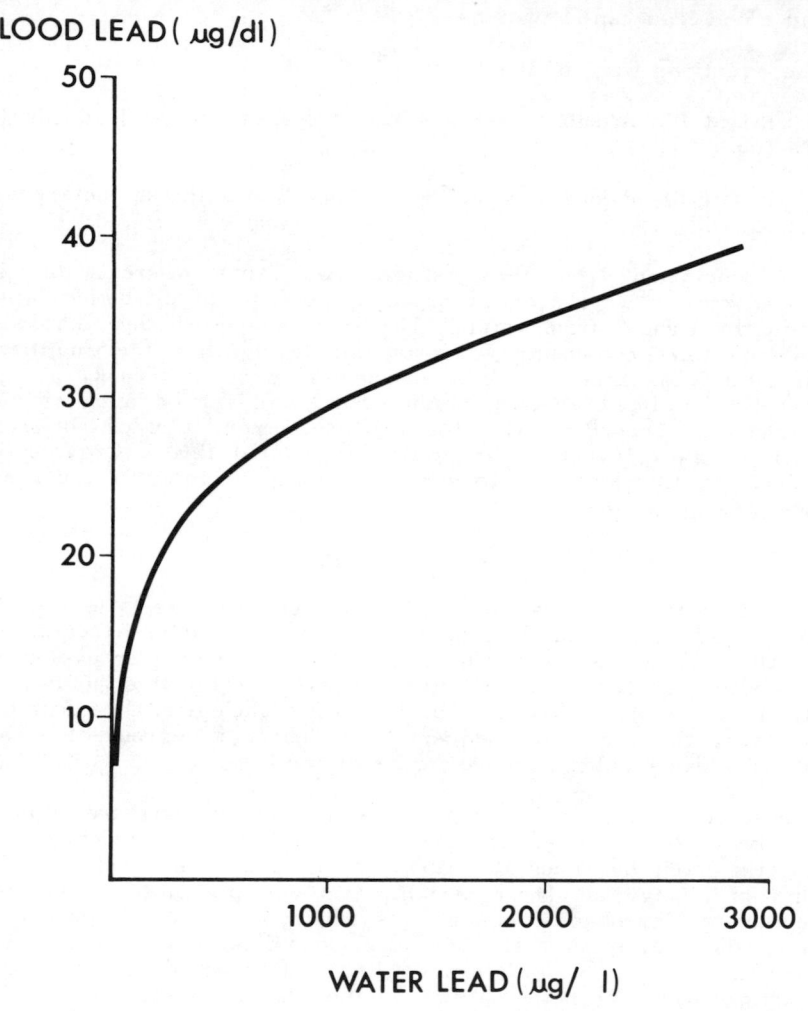

delta-aminolaevulinic acid synthase (Goldberg, 1972; Moore et al, 1980) (Figure 5) with consequent increases in the concentrations of delta-aminolaevulinic acid (Meredith et al, 1978) (Figure 6). This compound has been shown to be neuroactive (Moore and Meredith, 1976; Meredith et al, 1981) and to have specific pharmacological effects on isolated organ systems. We have also found that it will cause behavioural change in small rodents (Cutler et al, 1979) and this leads us to believe it to be one of the compounds central to the neurotoxicity of lead. It should not be forgotten, however, that the nervous system has a high requirement for energy production and the availability of haemoproteins is central to all oxidoreductive energy producing reactions. It is possible therefore that some of the neurological effects of lead are mediated through diminished availability of haem by the same mechanisms that will cause rises in ALA. Whether increased ALA concentrations or decreased haem concentrations or indeed other factors are of greater consequence in the secondary neurotoxicity of lead remains to be proven.

TABLE 1. Effect of acute and chronic lead exposure on the steady state levels of catecholamine synthesising enzymes in the anterior hypothalamus. Acute experiments were carried out at the given dose level daily for 14 days. In chronic studies animals were allowed access adlibitum to water containing 2 mM lead

	NORADRENALINE (nmol/mg protein)	ADRENALINE (nmol/mg protein)	DOPAMINE (nmol/mg protein)	TYROSINE HYDROXYLASE (nmol DOPA/mg protein/h)	PHENYLETHANOLAMINE -N-METHYL TRANSFERASE (pmol N-methyl phenyl ethanolamine/mg protein/h)
Acute Controls	70.0 ± 21.6	4.5 ± 3.7	44.0 ± 16.0	1.28 ± 0.48	1.34 ± 0.50
Acute (5 μmol/kg)	139 ± 29.0**	5.0 ± 4.1	50.7 ± 17.7	0.85 ± 0.31	1.23 ± 0.41
Acute (20 μmol/kg)	171 ± 36.5**	21.4 ± 15.6*	68.0 ± 21.0*	0.80 ± 0.23*	1.38 ± 0.70
Chronic Controls	90.0 ± 14.2	4.3 ± 2.5	49.6 ± 19.7	1.68 ± 0.20	1.11 ± 0.30
Chronic (8 weeks)	134 ± 30.2	4.8 ± 2.5	54.0 ± 30.0	0.98 ± 0.18	1.14 ± 0.19
Chronic (26 weeks)	60.3 ± 13.5*	3.6 ± 1.8	21.6 ± 8.7	0.95 ± 0.31*	1.28 ± 0.31

Results are expressed as mean of six ± S.D.; significance ** $p < 0.005$; * < 0.05.

In addition to the effects upon haem biosynthesis, lead has effects on other neurotransmitters (Hrdina et al, 1980). Most work in this sphere has concentrated upon the effects of lead on adrenergic and cholinergic nervous transmission. Our current research (Meredith et al, 1981) has demonstrated that lead will considerably alter the concentrations of brain amines and the activities of the enzymes synthesising them, especially within hypothalamus (Table 1). This is associated with changes in mouse behaviour (Donald. et al, 1981) (Table 2). Central to this biosynthetic pathway is the activity of

Fig. 5.   The Effect of Lead Upon haem biosynthesis.
Lead inhibits the activity of ALA dehydratase (ALAD)
coprophyrinogen   oxidase,   (Copro   oxidase)   and
ferrochelatase thus diminishing the sysnthesis of haem.
Lead also increases the breakdown of haem by haem
oxygenase   (HAEM   O).   The   resultant   lowered
concentrations of free haem feeds back upon the initial and
rate limiting enzyme of the pathway, delta-aminolaevulinic
acid synthase with consequent large increases in the
concentrations of delta-aminolaevulinic acid, ALA.

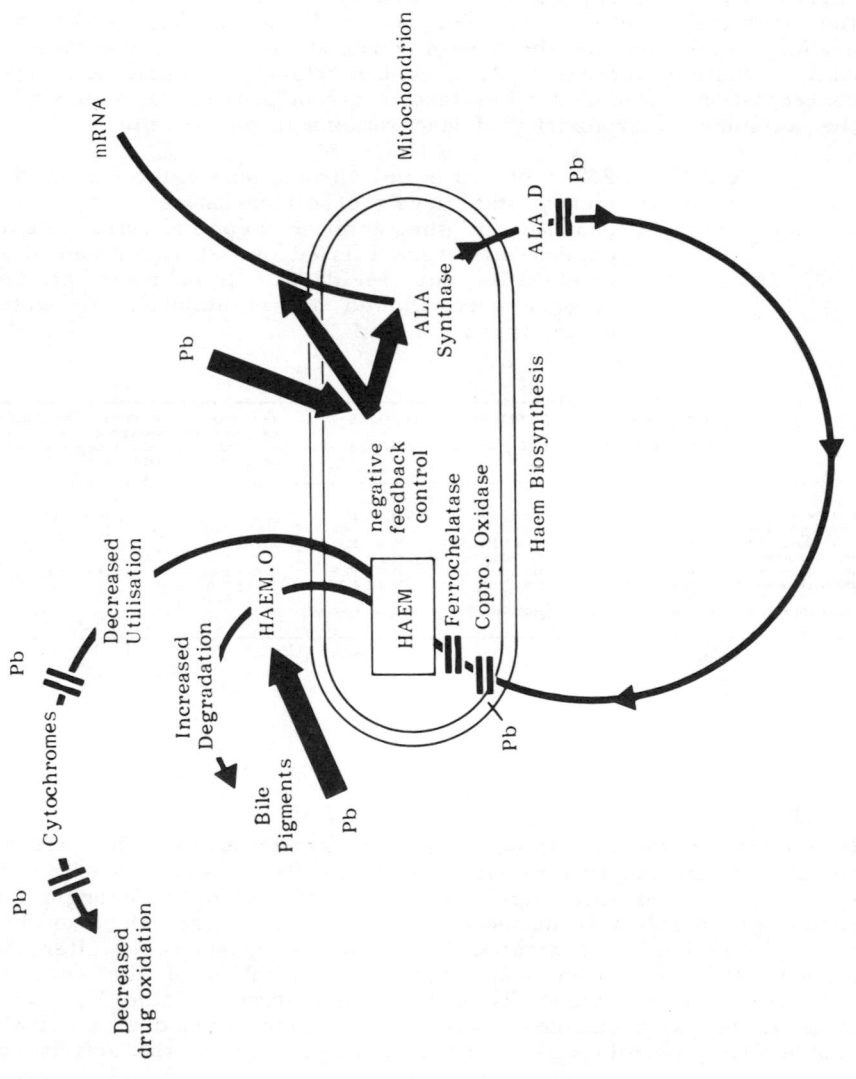

tyrosine hydroxylase and, in concurrent studies, we have shown that one essential cofactor for the activty of this enzyme, tetrahydrobiopterin, is influenced by the presence of lead (Blair et al, 1982). Studies in adults and in children have demonstrated that increasing lead concentrations brought about significant increases in the concentration of plasma biopterins. These were consistent with inhibition of dihydrobiopterin reductase and indeed consistent with the changes in activity of tyrosine hydroxylase seen in animal studies.

TABLE 2. Effects of post natal administration on behaviour of adult mice encountering an unfamiliar mouse of the same and opposite sex. Lead exposed were given access adlibitum to water containing 2 mM lead

Sex	Male		Female	
Treatment	Lead Exposure	Control	Lead Exposure	Control
Same Sex				
Frequency (5 min)/duration secs				
All non-social				
Activity	94.7*/253*	77.6/224	89.8*/236	73.7/237
Explore	41.4	34.7	41.5*	33.6
Scan	37.5	33.1	34.5*	26.3
Other non-social elements	15.8	9.8	13.8	13.8
Immobility	0.7/3.0	1.7/11	0.5/3	1.1/6
Social and Sexual				
Investigation	32.7/44**	37.8/64	39.1/60	33.3/56
Flight	0.3/0.3	0.1/0.1	0/0	0.1/0.1
Aggression	0/0	0.2/0.5	0/0	0/0
Opposite Sex				
Frequency (10 min) duration secs				
All Non-social				
Activity	156.0/426	135.7/413	174.8/407	140.9/422
Dig	20.1*	11.9	24.6	20.2
Other non-social elements	135.9	123.8	150.2	120.7
Immobility	2.0/9	3.4/19	3.3/19	6.5/40
All Social and				
Sexual investigation	96.2/164	87.1/162	81.7*/160*	61.3/110
Attend	27.9*	22.8	26.3	25.7
Investigate	25.4	24.1	23.2*	14.9
Follow up push-under	10.8	9.8	8.1*	1.8
Mount and attempted mount	2.1	2.7	0.1	0
Other social and sexual investigation	30.0	27.7	24.0	18.9
Flight	0.5/0.9	0.8/1.2	3.3/8.3	7.3/21
Aggression	0.3/0.4	2.4/3.0	4.8/54	5.4/5.5

(significance : Mann - Whitney 'U' - ** p < 0.01; * p < 0.05)

A PROSPECTIVE STUDY ON CHILDREN

In view of the interest in the studies that have shown changes in IQ and diminished attention span in school age children, it is appropriate to comment upon our current prospective study of the neurological effects of lead in children. Our research group (comprising clinicians, biochemists, psychologists and paediatricians) has been examining children identified as part of the Duplicate Diet Study in Glasgow. It was essential in setting up this work to be certain that the study was well controlled since the principal criticisms of previous work revolved around the problems of control and of assessment. Our hope is that this longtitudinal prospective study will provide clear and unequivocal evidence on the relationship between lead exposure levels and psychological impairment, as well as a clearer defination of possible specifications in the psychological and behavioural effects.

Our study aimed to follow a group of children from birth through to school age with regular testing at defined ages. We have therefore sought information that will highlight psychological functioning of the child at different ages and that will adequately describe relevant environmental factors. We initially identified three groups of women around the 12-15th week of pregnancy with high lead exposure (blood lead greater than 30 µg%), medium lead exposure (15-25 µg%) and low lead exposure (less than 10 µg%). The families were matched with respect to social class and housing stock in order to avoid the effects of the known relationship between lead exposure and socio-economic background. The children that these mothers bore, have now been studied up to the 2nd year of life. Continuing assessment is planned on a longtitudinal basis and will be extended to include early scholastic performance. Lead exposure is being assessed annually on the basis of measurement of blood lead, erythrocyte ALA dehydratase, blood protoporphyrin and serum biopterin levels. Additionally, deciduous tooth lead concentrations will be measured around the 5-6th year of life. All children are being checked for developmental milestones and growth in order that an allowance can be made for non-lead related change in development. Psychological assessment is based on detailed individual testing with a wide range of measures based on standardised techniques and questionnaires. Especial care has been taken in matching and control of relevant variables such as social class, parental education and housing stock. This is necessitated by the knowledge that children exposed to lead tend to come from backgrounds rich in factors disadvantageous to child development. To date no analysis has been made of the results from these studies (Moore and Bushnell, 1982).

Previous studies of Glasgow children had shown us that there were significant regressions of blood lead from both mothers and children on the cube root of their water lead exposure and that there were annual fluctuations in maternal blood lead concentrations with the highest values being found in the autumn. Most importantly, however, we noted that there was a significant negative correlation of blood lead with gestational age which would be consistent with increased placental lead concentrations observed previously in still-birth (Moore et al, 1982; Wibberley et al, 1977; Bryce-Smith et al., 1977) (Table 3).

TABLE 3. The multiple regression analysis of maternal and foetal blood lead on water lead concentrations, gestational age and parity

MATERNO-FOETAL LEAD STUDY

MULTIPLE REGRESSION ANALYSIS

(1)   Log maternal blood lead

	Regression Coefficient	Significance Level (P<)
$\sqrt[3]{\text{First flush Water Lead}}$	0.573	0.001
Gestational age	-0.056	0.01
Total parity	0.267	0.01

(2)   Log foetal blood lead

	Regression Coefficient	Significance Level (P<)
$\sqrt[3]{\text{First flush Water Lead}}$	0.658	0.001
Gestational age	-0.047	0.05

CURRENT INVESTIGATIONS

At this point the story turns once again to the water works at Mugdock. Following the investigations that demonstrated excessive exposure in children and in adults, it was decided that water treatment would be undertaken to diminish plumbosolvency by increasing pH. Initial pilot studies in the east of Glasgow indicated that this could be achieved successfully through the addition of lime to the water supplies at a rate of around 3 parts per million (Richards et al, 1980). A fully automatic closed loop lime dosing plant was built at Mugdock and went into operation in April 1978. These additions of lime brought the pH up to levels of around 7.8. It was realised, however, that this did not give a sufficiently large increase in the pH to achieve minimum plumbosolvency at the distal

Dr. Michael R. Moore

Fig. 6. The relationship between blood concentrations of lead and blood concentrations of delta-aminolaevulinic acid (ALA). In this figure, control subjects are shown by a solid circle and lead workers by an open square.

REGRESSION OF BLOOD ALA ON BLOOD LEAD

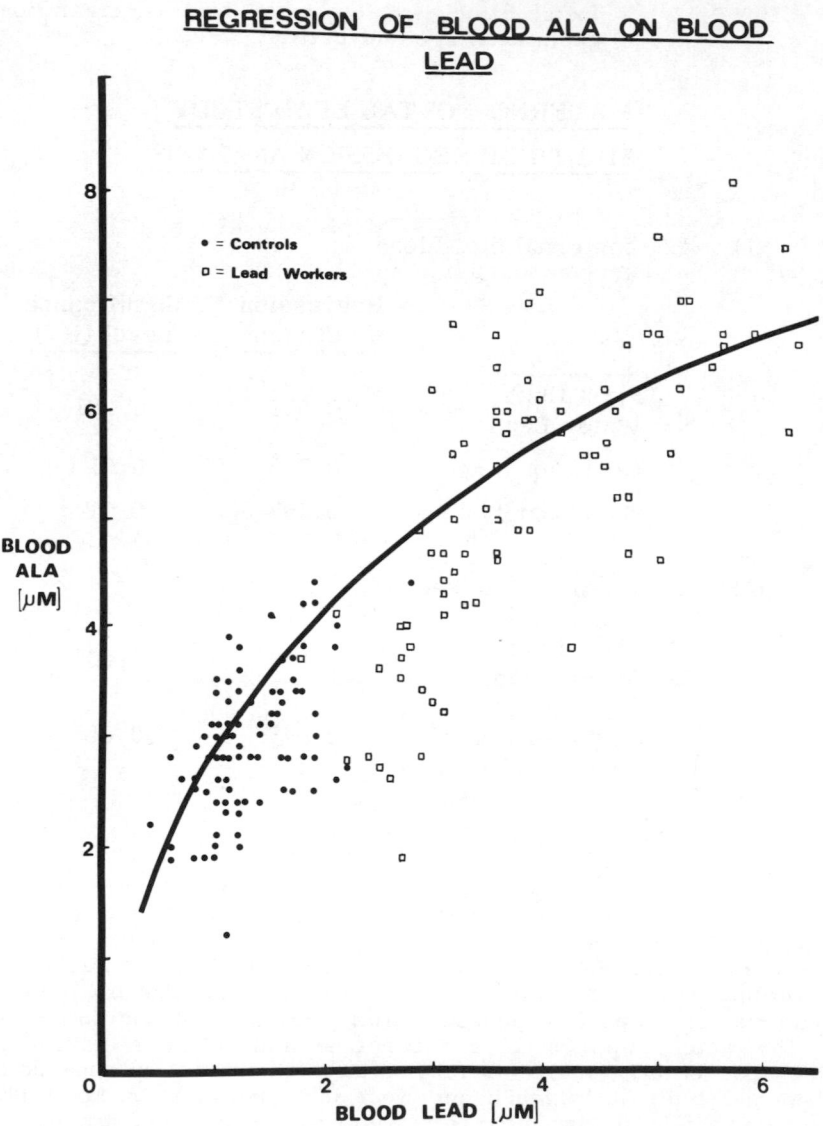

portions of the distribution system and consequently, in 1980, the rate of lime addition was increased to around 5 parts per million giving a pH rise of around 9.0 and a further decrease in plumbosolvency. Before these remedial actions were taken on the water supply, less than 50% of random water samples taken in the city contained less than 100 μg lead/l (Richards and Moore, 1982) which was consistent with previous findings (Department of the Environment, 1977). Levels were frequently greater than 100 μg/l and it was not uncommon to find concentrations of greater than 1000 μg/l.

In the town of Ayr the problem was even worse and in 1980 sampling of the water supply to all mothers in the Seafield area of the town with children under the age of 5, showed that the water pH lay between 4.5 - 5.5. 72% of the samples exceeded 100 μg/l and the mean water lead concentration was 466 μg/l with maximum values of 3070 μg/l. (Table 4).

Following lime dosage, at least 95% of random samples of the Loch Katrine supplies have given figures less than 100 μg/l. A similar figure was obtained in Ayr when treatment was instituted at the Knockjarder treatment works, taking the pH to a level of 9. Laboratory scale investigations indicated that the addition of orthophosphates to the water could further stabilise pH and further reduce plumbosolvency. Following pilot plant experiments in the South of Glasgow, it was found that orthophosphate dosage produced a further 75% reduction quantity of lead present in the water (Richards and Moore, 1982).

CHANGE IN BLOOD LEAD FOLLOWING WATER TREATMENT

To determine the effects that this could have on the population, we examined maternal blood leads in the postnatal wards of one Glasgow hospital. Prior to lime dosage in the autumn and winter of 1976/77, 236 mothers were found to have a geometric mean blood lead of 14.6 μg/dl, with 6% of these mothers having a blood lead concentration of greater than 35 μg/dl. In the autumn and winter of 1980/81, when the water supply pH was raised to 9, a further population of 475 mothers in the same wards of this hospital were found to have a geometric mean blood lead of 8.1 μg/dl and none of them had a blood lead concentration greater than 35 μg/dl (Moore et al, 1981). Similar findings were made in a general adult population (McIntosh et al, 1982) (Table 5). This dramatic reduction in blood lead concentrations in Glasgow supports the evidence from Duplicate Diet Studies that individuals exposed to low concentrations of lead in water will exhibit low blood lead concentrations. (Figure 7).

The studies described here have concentrated upon the effects of one particular vector of over exposure which is of obvious importance in the West of Scotland. One can confidently state, however, that other exposure vectors will exert influences upon the organism which are no less malign. It is, therefore, individious to concentrate exclusively upon one source of over exposure to the detriment of action to be taken in respect of others.

Fig. 7.   The   change   in   blood   lead   concentrations   in
mothers in Glasgow between 1976 and 1980 following water
treatment.

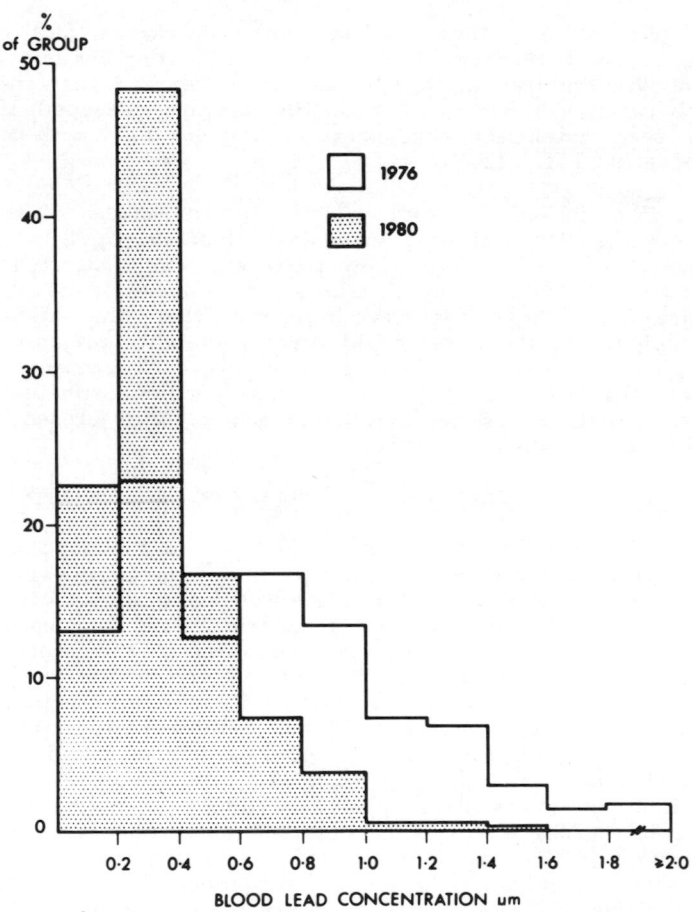

DISTRIBUTION of BLOOD LEAD CONCENTRATIONS in MOTHERS in GLASGOW

TABLE 4. Blood lead and water lead concentrations for adult women living in Ayr

Blood lead (µg/100 ml)	Water lead (µg/l)							Total
	≤10	11–99	100–299	300–499	500–999	1000–1499	≥1500	
≤ 10	8	5						13
11–15	4	7	3	2			1	17
16–20	1	3	12	3	3			22
21–25		4	9	7	5			25
26–30			2	4	4	2		12
31–35			2	1	2	2	3	10
36–40				1	1	1	1	4
≥ 40				1	4	3	3	11
Total	13	19	28	19	19	8	8	114

TABLE 5.   Blood lead concentration in Glasgow during
1979 and 1981

Year	Sex	No.	Geometric Mean ± Geometric Deviation (µg%)		
1979	M	97	19.9	±	30.80
	F	99	15.3	±	33.5
1981	M	82	16.1	±	30.0
	F	118	14.7	±	33.3

There is a multiplicity of sources of over exposure to lead. The
Duplicate Diet Studies in Glasgow and Ayr would suggest, as has
always been thought in the past, that dietary lead exposure is that
source contributing most to the body burden of lead. In the
equation linking adult dietary lead intake over one week and blood
lead concentration. [Adult blood lead (µg/dl) = -1.4 + 19.0
$3\sqrt{}$weekly intake of lead (mg)] the intercept is not significantly
different from zero (Figure 8). As a consequence pulmonary
exposure must be of less importance in this population. That is not
to say that contamination of dietary sources by airborne lead is of
little consequence. It is certain from the studies carried out in
Italy and in the USA described in other chapters that such
contamination of dietary sources contributes very significantly to
the total exposure to lead in the environment. The exact
proportion that this comprises in any specific situation is variable
and contingent upon a number of sociological, climatic and geological
factors. It would therefore be naive to attribute any precise
number to this relationship. It is better by far to merely state
that it is appreciable and to act upon that information to abate all
sources of exposure.

LIMITS OF EXPOSURE

In the development of concordant recommended limits of exposure,
the equations developed from the Duplicate Diet Studies can be of
considerable assistance. Previous regulatory levels for
concentrations of lead in blood, water, air and diet have been
arrived at by rule of thumb methods. There is no equivalence
between any of these measures. If one applies the regulatory limit
of 50 µg/l for lead in drinking water to the Duplicate Diet Study
equations, the calculated blood lead concentrations of 17 µg/dl are
nowhere near the advocated upper limit of blood lead concentration
of 35 µg/dl; nor indeed is there any equivalence with the World

Fig. 8.   The cube root relationship between dietary lead intake over 1 week and blood lead concentrations.

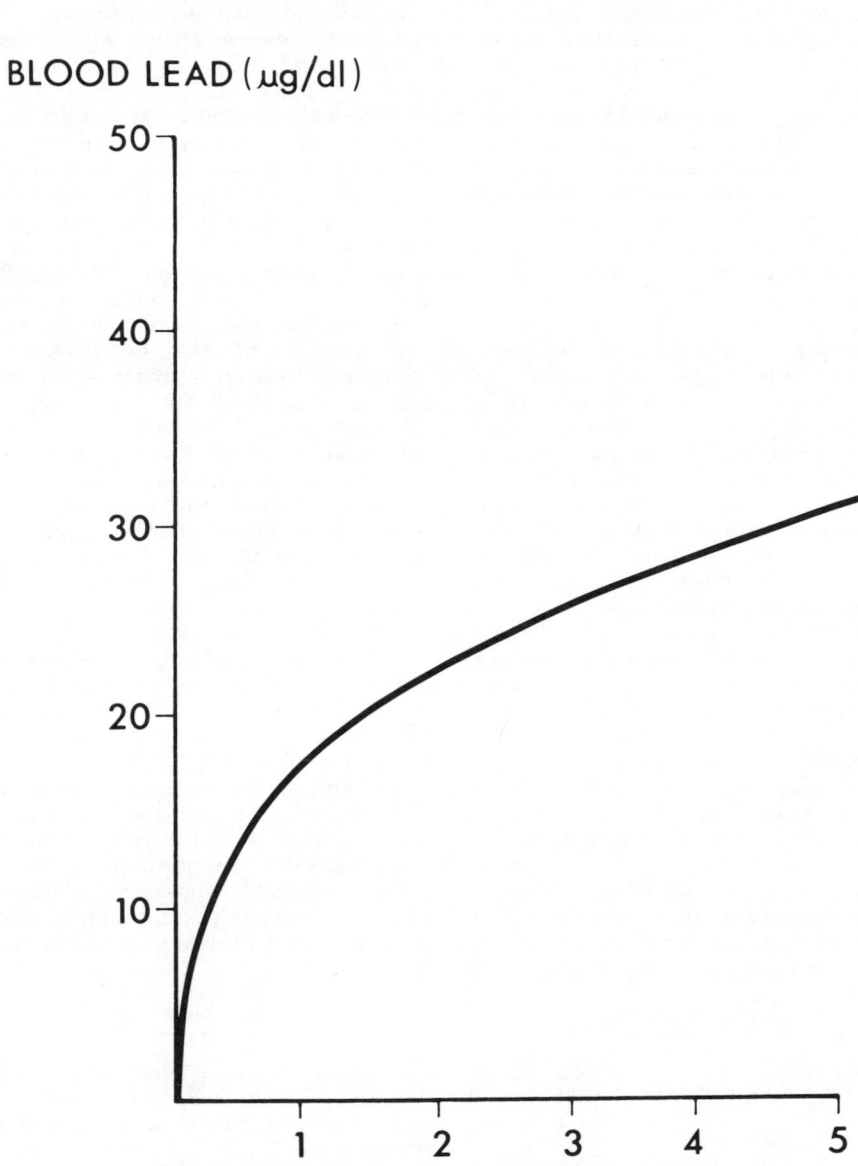

Health Organisation standard of 3 mg/week as the upper limit of dietary lead intake. These equations can be used to develop concordant regulatory values. For this water lead concentration of 50 µg lead/l, equivalent mean blood lead concentrations would be around 17 µg/dl and this would correspond with weekly dietary intakes of lead in adults of less than 1 mg and in children less than 200 µg. Many would consider these values too high. It would be reasonable to suppose that a much more satisfactory way of defining regulatory levels of exposure would be to base them upon biological change corresponding with some value of blood lead concentration. The Environmental Protection Agency in the USA has calculated that if the geometric mean of a population blood lead is set at 15 µg/dl, then 99.5% of children will have blood leads less than 30 µg/dl (Environmental Protection Agency, 1980). Fifteen µg/dl is an interesting figure since it also represents the point at which biological change can be seen in the activity of ALA dehydratase and indeed is the start point for erythrocyte protoporphyrin increase. If this figure is applied to the Duplicate Diet Study equations it would imply that water lead concentrations should be no greater than 10 µg/l and that the mean dietary lead intake per week should not exceed 650 µg for leads for adults and 100 µg for infants. Similar figures could be developed from the relationships between blood lead and air lead discussed in other chapters. It is surely much more satisfactory to base regulatory limits upon proven biological change than to base them upon non-equivalent arbitrary numbers.

The obvious question to be asked in these circumstances is whether the economic toll of setting limits of this sort is too great. We have shown in a very highly exposed area that very effective measures can be taken in abatement of over exposure to lead. The changes in water lead exposure that have been achieved in Glasgow were by no means cheap but certainly were not excessivley expensive either, and much less expensive than doing nothing. The economic burden on society of an unhealthy community is almost immeasurably high and much greater than the cost of proceeding expeditiously with abatement of all forms of over exposure to lead. Politics in these circumstances can stand on the side lines waiting avuncularly for science to seek nobly for truth whilst medicine ethically pressed by experience must act on the available evidence.

DISCUSSION

Question: You have made clear the various strategies that can be employed with lead water pipes. How do you view the possibility of alternative plumbing systems to replace those with soldered joints?

Moore: There is no doubt that if one has badly soldered joints there is a quantity of fluxed solder which passes into the lumen of the water pipe; this raises water lead concentrations proportionate to the number of soldered joints in the run of piping. There are some instances of this being so in certain large public institutions in our city where the values of lead in the water supply were at least as bad as those seen in a lead-plumbed household. So if a copper joint is misused, then certainly one gets an excess of solder in the pipe and therefore lead in the water. This should not occur with properly used joints.

Russell Jones: You mentioned that Professor Christison became worried about plumbosolvency in 1844. At the beginning of this century there was widespread agreement in the British medical profession that areas with a soft water supply had a very high rate of stillbirths and miscarriage, and this was attributed to the use of lead pipes. Now, given that there was so much widespread agreement about this hazard, why has it taken 140 years for anything to be done?

Moore: The problems associated with lead in water are not easily perceived by the general population. There is what can only be described as "roaring apathy". This is a clear case of action being taken by authority in spite of the lack of interest of the general population. People obviously care about the incidence of stillbirths and the like but that type of information is only available to the medical profession. People only tend to worry about things that they can see, like filthy air. You see petrol fumes, and you worry about it. But you see crystal clear water which everyone keeps telling you is the best water in the world; you are not going to damn that water as being bad for you. In fact, in our own area we have an incredible degree of apathy about what should be done to water supplies. Hence the lack of action until the present.

Waldon: You mentioned lead water storage tanks in domestic properties and you also pointed out that replacement grants are not currently available in England. I wonder if you could give some advice for people in domestic housing in England.

Moore: The lead storage tank represents a large static reservoir of water which is usually open to the atmosphere and will therefore dissolve carbon dioxide and become acidic, which in turn enhances the potential plumbosolvency of the water. It therefore creates a sort of background value of lead in the plumbing system which contributes very strongly to exposure, not only by direct uptake from the tank itself but also by its acidity which promotes plumbosolvency on the way to the tap. It is, however, not always the practice to use such tanks. This practice very often relates to specific areas or to specific local authority building ordanances. As far as I know, no specific grant aid is available in England for replacing lead plumbing.

Bailey: I am worried by your findings because in Dublin there is extensive use of lead water pipes. Also, the lead content of Irish petrol is 0.65 grams per litre, which is higher than the EEC directive on this issue.

Moore: The lead content of running water is lower than the first flush samples, but the drop is not massive and definitely not enough in bad exposure situations. I must also emphasise that there is a synthesis of exposures from a number of different sources. I do not think that because, in our cube root equations, there was no apparent residue in the equation linked with pulmonary exposure, that there was no exposure from air lead. It is likely that there was exposure from air but that this occurred primarily through the gastrointestinal route: that is, through the dietary vector, rather than through the pulmonary vector. Of course, obviously the pulmonary vector is of consequence when you go into large industrial conurbations. This is reflected in the difference in the residues between a town, "Ayr" on the west coast, where there is a lower traffic-density and cleaner air, and the situation in Glasgow, which is a largely industrial city with a lot of airborne pollution.

Jackson: You commented on the long time taken to bring about action with respect to lead-polluted water. The British Government has been aware of the general problem and has tried to quantify it and to determine the relevant patterns. This has involved government spending on research and monitoring, including a project of your own. With respect to quantification, it is important that the general survey of 1975/6 showed that lead tanks were not a problem in England, although they were in Scotland. So far as grant availability for plumbing alterations is concerned, it is not true that grants are not available south of the border. Under the "Home Improvements" system, if a local authority considered that pipe replacement was justified as part of a broade scheme then a grant would be available within the system. Furthermore, there are statutory changes on the stocks that will make it possible to get grant aid for pipe replacement plumbing alterations separately from other aspects of the "Home Improvement Grant Scheme", but still within the same system. Lastly, the Government has announced a very large increase in the amount of money in the "Home Improvement Grant" system - between £50 million and £100 million. Local authorities can use that money at their discretion for the replacement of lead pipes. The decision on whether they should do so will be local but the Government is changing the rules to allow that decision.

Moore:
I had no intention of denigrating the essential role played by local government, Scottish government and central government in the development of our own studies. In fact they would not have gone ahead if there had not been such a high degree of collaboration with all these authorities who showed great concern for the problem. Nevertheless, the grant situation within Scotland is really quite different from the set-up in England. In Scotland money has been specifically ear-marked by the Scottish Office for the purposes of handling plumbosolvency. There was £6 million this year for this purpose, together with a further £1 million for education. I do not think that any specific sums as yet have been set aside in England, although I accept that "Home Improvement Grants" represent one way of handling the problem.

Ranson:
Can you give us some indication of the water lead level in Loch Katrine reservoir itself?

Moore:
Unfortunately, we do not have access to Dr. Patterson's superb facilities, so that we have

had great difficulty measuring the lead level in Loch Katrine, which is extremely low. Water authorities have a statutory requirement to supply water that does not contain lead. The initial source of lead in the water supply in these circumstances is almost invariably negligible. Most of the input is linked with the distribution system.

Holmes:

Dr. Moore stated that water could become plumbosolvent in tanks because of dissolved carbon dioxide, etc. Now lots of people do drink water out of tanks, so this could be quite a national problem. Is that so?

Moore:

It is hard to say. Tanks open to the atmosphere are usually linked with hot water supplies. Unfortunately, people still use hot water for drinking; this is very inadvisable since hot water will dissolve very much greater quantities of lead (and other undesirable substances) from any lead or copper system with soldered joints.

Patterson:

At very low pH's your curves seem to indicate almost unbelievable solubilities of lead - of the order of grams per litre. I have some difficulty accepting those figures. My second point concerns your curve which shows an exponential relationship between blood and dietary lead. This model seems rather simplistic. The skeletal return of lead can be appreciable and has a long relaxation time in the blood; your curves need to be modified to take this into account.

Moore:

The equations are really a mathematical attempt to produce the best fit to the available data. That is not to say that they are absolute. The duplicate diet studies show that although there is a moderate amount of disagreement as to whether the lines should be straight or curvilinear, the best fit is achieved with some form of curve such as our cube root equation.

Barry:

We have heard a lot about lead fallout in the last few days and the low lead content of Loch Katrine does rather suggest that this is not a significant factor in your area.

Moore:

Loch Katrine is north of the city and therefore would not receive much fallout from the city as the prevailing winds are mostly from the southwest and west.

Edwards: I was interested to note the 10:1 differential between lead in blood and lead in breast milk. Does a similar purification scheme operate in the cow?

Moore: Yes. Any lacating animal will show a similar effect, though the figures may not be exactly the same. 95% of blood lead is carried by red blood cells and transfer of lead to breast milk takes place through the bio-available component in plasma. Hence, there is a filtering effect and one would anticipate some diminution in exposure among breast fed infants. Our duplicate diet sheet studies indeed demonstrated that breast fed infants have a lower level of exposure, even in households where mothers were over-exposed, when compared with children fed with dried milk feeds made up with tap water.

REFERENCES

Addis, G., Moore M.R., 1974. Lead levels in the water of surburban Glasgow. Nature, 252, 120-121.

Alexander, F.W., Clayton, B.E., Delves, H.T., 1974. Mineral and trace-metal balances in children receiving normal and synthetic diets. QJ Med, 43, 89-111.

Beattie, A.D., Moore, M.R., Devenay, W.T., Miller, A.R., Goldberg, A., 1972. Environmental lead pollution in an urban soft-water area. BR. Med. J. i, 491-493.

Beattie, A.D., Moore, M.R., Goldberg, A., Finlayson, M.J.W., Mackie, E.M., Graham, J.F., Main, J.C., McLaren, D.A., Murdoch, R.M., Stewart, G.T., 1975. Role of low level lead exposure in the aetiology of mental retardation. Lancet, I, 589-592.

Beevers, D.G., Erskine, E., Robertson, M., Beattie, A.D., Campbell, B.C., Goldberg, A., Moore M.R., Hawthornie, V.M. 1976. Blood-lead and hypertension. Lancet II, 1-3.

Beevers, D.G., Cruickshank, J.K, Yeoman, W.B., Carter, G.F., Goldberg, A., Moore, M.R. 1980. Blood lead and cadium in human hypertension. J Environ Pathol Toxicol. 4, 251-260.

Berlin, A., Amavis, R., Langevin, M. 1977. Research on lead in drinking water in Europe (in relation to the possible uptake of lead by man). WHO Working Group on health hazards from drinking water, London, 26-30 Sept.

Blair, J.A., Hillburn, M.E., Leeming, R.J., McIntosh, M.J., Moore, M.R. 1982. Lead and tetrahydrobiopterin metabolism possible effects on IQ. Lancet, I, 964.

Bryce-Smith, D., Desphande, R.R., Hughes, J., Waldron, H.A. 1977. Lead and cadmium levels in stillbirths. Lancet, I, 1159.

Burnet, J. 1869. History of the Water supply to Glasgow. Bell
    and Bain, Glasgow.
Campbell, B.C., Beattie, A.D., Moore, M.R., Goldberg, A., Reid,
    A.G. 1977. Renal insufficiency associated with excessive lead
    exposure. Br Med J, I, 482-485.
Campbell, B.C., Moore, M.R., Goldberg, A., Hernandez, L.A.,
    Carson, D.W. 1978. Subclinical lead exposure - a possible
    factor in the aetiology of gout. Br Med J, II, 1403-1404.
Christison, R. 1844. On the action of water upon lead. Trans.
    Roy Soc Edin, 15, 265-276.
Cutler, M.G., Moore, M.R., Ewart, F.G. 1979. Effects of
    delta-aminolaevulinic acid administration on social behaviour in
    the laboratory mouse. Psychopharmacology, 61, 131-135.
Department of the Environment, 1977 Pollution Paper No. 12.
    Lead in Drinking Water: A survey in Great Britain, 1976.
    HMSO,
Department of the Environment, 1981. Pollution Report No. 10
    European Community screening programme for lead - UK Results
    for 1979-80. HMSO.
Department of the Environment, 1982. Pollution Report No. 11.
    The Glasgow Duplicate Diet Study (1979/80). HMSO.
Donald, J.M., Cutler, M.G., Moore, M.R., Bradley, M. 1981.
    Developmental and social behaviour in mice after prenatal and
    postnatal   administration   of   low   levels   of   lead.
    Neuropharmacolgy, 20, 1097-1104.
Environmental Protection Agency 1980. Ambient water quality
    criteria for lead. USA Environmental Protection Agency CEPA
    440/5 - 80-057.
Forteath, B.J. 1981. Lead in drinking water - a report of an
    identification   programme   within   Renfrew   District   1980-81.
    Renfrew District Council, Oct.
Goldberg, A. 1972. Lead poisoning and haem biosynthesis. Br J
    Haematol, 23, 521.
Goldberg, A. 1974. Drinking water as a source of lead pollution.
    Environ Health Perspect, 2, 103-105.
Hamilton, D. 1981. The healers, a history of medicine in
    Scotland. Canongate, Edinburgh.
Hrdina, P.D., Hanin, I., Dubas, T.C. 1980. Neurochemical
    correlates of lead toxicity. In Lead Toxicity eds Singhal, R.A.,
    Thomas, J.A., Urban and Schwarzenberg pp 273-300.
Khan, M.Y., Buse, M., Louria, D.B. 1977. Lead cardiomyopathy
    in mice: A correlative ultrastructural and blood level study.
    Arch Patho Lab Med, 101, 89-94.
Kopp, S.J., Glonek, M., Erlanger, E.F., Perry Jr. M.B., Barany,
    M. 1980. Cadmium and lead effects on myocardial function and
    metabolism. J Environ Patho Toxicol, 4, 205-227.
McIntosh, M.J., Moore, M.R., Goldberg, A., Fell, G.S.,
    Cunningham, C., Halls, D.J. 1982. Studies of lead and
    cadmium exposure in Glasgow. Ecology of Disease (in press).
Meredith, P.A., Moore, M.R., Campbell, B.C., Thompson, G.G.,
    Goldberg, A. 1978. Delta-aminolaevulinic acid metabolism in
    normal and lead exposed humans. Toxicology, 9, 1-9.

Meredith, P.A., Petty, M.A., Reid, J.L., Moore, M.R., Donald, J.M., Cutler, M.G., Bradley, M.1981. Neurochemical and neurobehavioural aspects of lead exposure. Preceedings Heavy Meltas in the Environment, Amsterdam, pp 557-560.

Moore, M.R. 1973. Plumbosolvency of waters. Nature, 243, 222-223.

Moore, M.R. 1977. Lead in drinking water in soft water areas – health hazards. The Science of the Total Environment, 7, 109-115.

Moore, M.R. 1980. Exposure to lead in childhood: the persisting effects. Nature, 283, 334-335.

Moore, M.R., Bushnell, I.W.R. 1982. Lead and child development. Proceedings International Lead Conference, Cincinnati, (in press).

Moore, M.R., Meredith, P.A. 1976. The association of delta-aminolaevulinic acid with the neurological and behavioural effects of lead exposure. In Trace Substances in Environmental Health, ed. Hemphill, D.D., University of Missouri, Columbia, pp 363-371.

Moore, M.R., Meredith, P.A., Goldberg, A., Carr, K.E., Toner, P.G., Lawrie, T.D.V. 1975. Cardiac effects of lead in drinking water of rats. Clinical Science and Molecular Medicine, 49, 337-341.

Moore, M.R., Meredith, P.A., Campbell, B.C., Goldberg, A., Pocock, S.J. 1977. Contribution of lead in drinking water to blood lead. Lancet II, 661-662.

Moore, M.R., Meredith, P.A., Goldberg, A. 1977. A retrospective analysis of blood lead in mentally retarded children. Lancet, I, 717-719.

Moore, M.R., Campbell, B.C., Meredith, P.A., Beattie, A.D., Goldberg, A., Campbell, D. 1978. The association between lead concentrations in teeth and domestic water lead concentrations. Clin. Chim. Act, 87, 77-83.

Moore, M.R., Goldberg, A., Meredith, P.A., Lees, R., Low, R.A., Pocock, S.J. 1979a. The contribution of drinking water lead to maternal blood lead concentrations. Clin. Chim. Act, 95, 129-133.

Moore, M.R., Hughes, M.A., Goldberg, D.J. 1979b. Lead absorption in man from dietary sources. Int. Arch. Occup. Environ. Health, 44, 81-90.

Moore, M.R., Meredith, P.A., Goldberg, A. 1980. Lead and hame biosynthesis. In Lead Toxicity eds Singhal, R.L., Thomas, J.A., Urban and Schwartzenberg, Baltimore and Munich, pp 79-118.

Moore, M.R., Goldberg, A., Fyfe, W.M., Richards, W.N. 1981. Maternal lead levels after alterations to water supply. Lancet II, 203-204.

Moore, M.R., Goldberg, A., Pocock, S.J., Meredith, P.A., Stewart, I.M., McAnespie, H., Lees, R., Low, R.A. 1982. Some studies of maternal and infant lead exposure in Glasgow. Scott MJ, 27, 113-122.

Oliver, T. 1914. Lead poisoning: from the industrial medical and social points of view. Lewis, London.

Richards, W.N., Britton, A., Cochrane, A. 1980. Reducing plumbosolvency - the effect of added lime on the Loch Katrine supply to Glasgow. J. Inst. Wat. Engrs. Scis, 34, 315.

Richards, W.N., Moore, M.R. 1982. Plumbosolvency in Scotland - the problem remedial action taken and health benefits observed. J. Am. Water Works Assoc. (in press).

Sherlock, J., Smart, G., Forbes, G.I., Moore, M.R., Patterson, W.J., Richards, W.N., Wilson, T.S. 1982. Assessment of lead intakes and dose response for a population in Ayr Human Toxicology, 1, 115-122.

Smart, G.A., Warrington, M., Evans, W.H. 1981. The contribution of lead in water to dietary lead intakes. J. Sci. Food Agric, 32, 129-133.

WHO. Lead. Environmental Health Criteria No. 3, Geneva 1977.

Wibberley, D.G., Khera, A.K., Edwards, J.H., Rushton, D.I. 1977. Lead levels in human placentae from normal and malformed births. J. Med. Genet., 14, 339-345.

Lead Versus Health
Edited by M. Rutter and R. Russell Jones
© 1983 John Wiley & Sons Ltd.

AIR LEAD AND DUST IN THESSALONIKI

Professor Augustinos Anagnostopoulos

Chemical Engineering Department
Faculty of Technology
Thessaloniki University
Greece

INTRODUCTION

In recent years much research has been directed towards the toxic effects of lead on human health. This is now a subject of wide-spread concern since children are particularly susceptible to the influence of neurotoxins and absorb lead more readily than adults. (Bryce-Smith and Stephens 1980. Alexander et al, 1973). Furthermore, urban children are particularly at risk from the ingestion of lead-rich street dust. (Day et al, 1975; Day et al, 1979; Duggan, 1980).

Organlead petrol additives are mostly decomposed to inorganic lead during combustion and both organic and inorganic lead can be found in street dust. (De Jonghe et al, 1981). Our techniques do not distinguish between organic and inorganic lead compounds (Anagnostopoulos et al, 1981 a,b), but there are available methods to separate these two components and to quantify the amount of each present in particulate matter (Harrison and Laxen 1977 and 1978). The nature of this organic lead has not yet been established (it may consist of tri- or di-alkyl-lead). In this work we report findings for street dust as inorganic lead.

There are several means by which to assess the contribution of organic and inorganic compounds to atmospheric lead (Birch et al, 1980). It is important to know this ratio since organolead compounds would be expected to have a disproportionate impact on nerological dysfunction in the exposed population. The data presented here demonstrate that environmental lead pollution is a serious problem in Thessaloniki, as in many other Western cities.

METHODS

The lead content of the road dust has been estimated in main streets and in the playgrounds of seventeen elementary schools in the city. 220 urban samples were collected from street dust during the period May-July 1981. Four of these samples were taken from a nearby village, Retziki, twelve kilometres from the city. We also estimated the relative amounts of particulate lead and vapour tetra-alkyl-lead (TAL) in the atmosphere of Thessaloniki. Air samples were obtained during the period May-September 1981. Dust samples were collected by the use of a plastic spatula and a small plastic sweeper into polythene bags. In each location four samples were taken within a distance of about ten to twenty metres from the edge of the pavement. In schools, samples were taken from playgrounds near to the main entrance. The dust samples were put through a 60 mesh sieve, leached with concentrated nitric acid and left for twenty-four hours. After this time the solution was filtrated and the filtrate was diluted to a volume of 100 ml. The lead concentrations were determined by flameless atomic absorption spectrophotometer (PERKIN-ELMER 503 HGA Model 174). 24 and 48 hour air samples were analysed as described by Birch et al. (1980) using atomic absorption spectroscopy. Particulate lead was determined using techniques described by the U.S. Environmental Protection Agency (1978).

RESULTS AND DISCUSSION

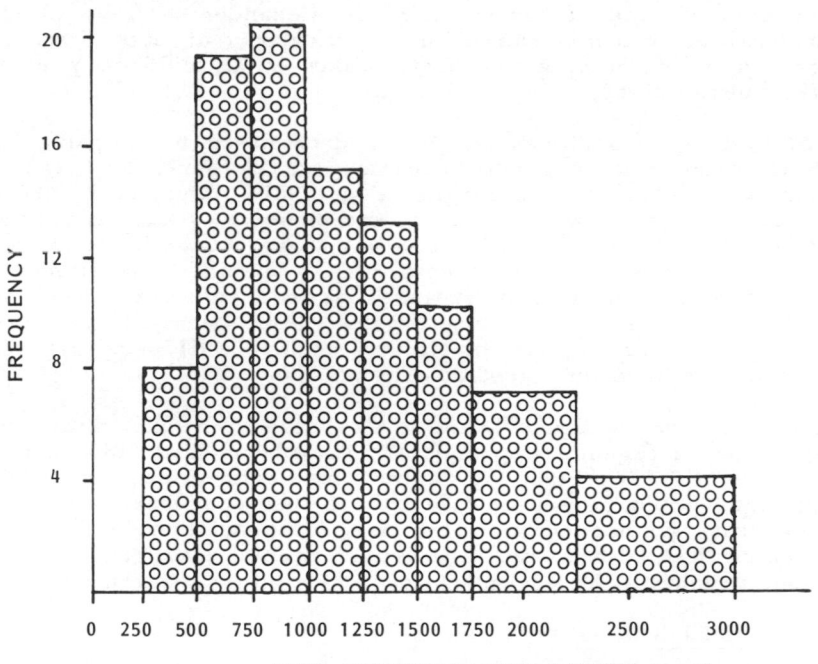

Fig. 1   Histogram of lead concentrations in street dust in the town centre of Thessaloniki

Lead values in the 96 samples taken from the town centre showed a range of 280 to 3000 µg/g with an average of 1150 µg/g and standard deviation of 550 µg/g (see Fig. 1). Values between 500-1000 µg/g comprised 41% of the samples - only 4% showed values of 2250-3000 µg/g. These results are not dissimilar to those recorded in London and Manchester with mean levels of 1530±600 and 1001±40 µg/g respectively. (Duggan and Williams, 1977; Day et al, 1975). Higher values with an average of 2130±960 µg/g have been recorded from Lancaster (Harrison, 1979).

TABLE 1. Levels of Lead in Thessaloniki's Street Dust

Number of samples	Range	Mean value and standard deviation	Mean Value of traffic per 24 h (cars)
28	496-2986	1296±633	50000
12	320-1468	723±318	40000
16	375-2287	1292±697	37000
20	477-2069	1207±431	37000
12	611-1743	942±299	36000
24	277-1697	791±318	31000
4	416-1040	723±325	30000
12	158-654	396±165	26500
8	102-600	288±164	18500

Values from all locations in Thessaloniki ranged from 30 to 3000 µg/g (see Table 1). Corresponding values are: Glasgow 150 to 2300 µg/g (Farmer and Lyon, 1977); and Birmingham 1000 to 2500 µg/g (Environmental Protection Unit, Birmingham, 1975). It should be emphasised, however, that the validity of such comparisons is limited by the sampling site, the sampling method and the sieving procedure, details of which are not provided in all of the above studies.

Table 2 shows the value of lead in street dust from districts with different traffic densities. The districts have been classified as A-D with decreasing 24 hour traffic flow, and type E corresponds to a rural area. It is evident that the level of lead in street dust relates directly to the volume of traffic and that a five-fold increase is observed between rural and urban locations. It is also apparent that the rural samples are themselves contaminated when compared with the lead concentrations of less than 20 ppm typically found in the earth's crust, (Swaine, 1955; Chow and Patterson, 1962).

TABLE 2. Lead values in relation to traffic flow in
different districts of Thessaloniki (4 samples
from each district)

Type	Range	Mean value and standard deviation
A	470-660	574±87
A	491-695	565±88
B	276-377	320±48
B	143-360	227±95
B	163-294	224±54
C	90-394	232±125
D	69-224	161±66
D	111-152	130±20
D	30-107	73±54
E	72-141	108±27

Type A : 27,000 - 50,000 cars per day
Type B : 5,000 - 27,000 cars per day
Type C : 1,500 - 5,000 cars per day
Type D :   100 - 1,500 cars per day
Type E : Less than 100 cars per day

Comparison of dust lead values (48 samples) at two fixed locations
in the town centre on two dates showed an increase from a mean
level of 873 µg/g on April 8 to a level of 1510 µg/g on June 27.
The increasing lead concentration probably reflects the decreasing
rainfall encountered after April 8. On average pre-rainfall values
(1820 µg/g) were approximately double the values found in
post-rainfall samples (990 µg/g).

Dust lead values obtained for seventeen playgrounds in Thessaloniki
were somewhat lower than the concentrations found in outside
streets with mean levels of 372 µg/g and 500 µg/g respectively.
Nevertheless, on the whole, the schools with a high level of lead in
the playground dust came from areas in which the street dust had a
high lead content. The association suggests that most of dust lead
in playgrounds stems from the fall-out of particulate lead emitted by
petrol-driven motor vehicles (Day et al, 1975; Day et al, 1979).
Although higher playground values have been recorded elsewhere,
fortuitous ingestion of lead-rich dust may still make a significant
contribution to the lead intake of children in Thessaloniki.

Total air lead concentrations (21 samples) at two locations, 4 and 5 metres above the streets with a mean traffic flow of 50,000 and 40,000 cars per day showed a mean level of 2.23 and 1.9 $\mu g/m^3$ with a range of 0.91-4.31 and 1.01-4.24 respectively.

Alkyl-lead concentrations ranged from 15-220 ng Pb m^{-3} which respresents an organic/inorganic lead ratio of 1.2 - 10%. This ratio is somewhat smaller than that found in London (Birch et al, 1980) and Copenhagen (Neilsen et al, 1978). This may be due to the fact that our samples were taken from points where the traffic was rather "free-flowing" and combustion was apparently more complete. Another possibility is that the very fine dust particles present in Thessaloniki's atmosphere may absorb TAL and hence lower its atmospheric concentration. Finally, sunshine may accelerate the decomposition of TAL to its degradation products. It is not possible to say which of these explanations is correct at the present time.

CONCLUSIONS

In conclusion it may be said that:

(1)   Like many other European cities, Thessaloniki is highly contaminated with lead in road dust.

(2)   The level of contamination relates directly to traffic density.

(3)   The ratio of organic and inorganic atmospheric lead is somewhat lower than other major cities and ranges from 1-10%. Our intention is to pursue these findings by doing blood lead measurements in the exposed population.

DISCUSSION

Duggan   The lead in dust values you quote for Thessaloniki are quite low compared with those for London. For example, you found values of some 400 ppm for playgrounds; a figure of 1000-1500 ppm would be more typical in London. The street values in Thessaloniki were about a 1000, whereas in central London levels of 2- to 3000 are reported. Similarly, your suburban values are equivalent to rural values in the UK. The findings emphasize the major differences according to geographical area. Does Greece have any national guidelines on the level at which dust lead values are regarded as unacceptably high because of the risks to health?

Anagnostopoulos   No, we do not have any official standards.

Duggan   Your lead in air values seem quite high when compared with the lead in dust figures. How long did you sample the air for these analyses?

Anagnostopoulos   About 24 to 48 hours.

Bryce-Smith   Were there any industrial sources of lead emissions in Thessaloniki?

Anagnostopoulos   There was a factory that produced tetraethyl lead. I cannot say whether it contaminated the city or not because we obtained only very few samples from the industrial area. Also, we were not able to measure organic lead levels in dust.

Grandjean   We have found organo-lead compounds in street dust in our own studies.

Laxen   I, too, have measured organic lead in street dusts (Harrison and Laxen, 1978). The percentage was around 1% but we do not know in what form the organic lead was present.

REFERENCES

Alexander, F.W., Delves, H.T., Clayton, B.E., (1973), The uptake and excretion by children of lead and other contaminants, Proceedings of the International Symposium Environmental Health Aspects of Lead, Amsterdam 1972, 319-331, Commission of the European Communities, Luxembourg.

Anagnostopoulos, A., Joannas, K., and Georgiou, E., (1981a), "Lead in dust in some streets of Thessaloniki", Proceedings of International Conference on Environmental Pollution, Ed. Anagnostopoulos, A., University of Thessaloniki, Greece.

Anagnostopoulos, A., Kyriakou, G., and Tzimou, R., (1981b), "Determination of lead in the atmosphere of Thessaloniki", Proceedings of International Conference on Environmental Pollution, Ed. Anagnostopoulos, A., University of Thessaloniki, Greece.

Birch, J., Harrison, R.M., Laxen, D.P.H., (1980), A specific method for 24-48 hour analysis of tetra-alkyl lead in air, Sci. Total Environ., 14: 31-42.

Bryce-Smith, D., Stephens, R., (1980), Lead or Health, Conservation Society, London.

Chow, T.J., Patterson, C.C., (1962), the occurrence and significance of lead isotopes in Pelagic sediments, Geochem. Cosmochim. Acta 26: 263-308.

Day, J.P., Ferguson, J.E., Chee, T.M., (1979), Solubility and potential toxicity of lead in urban street dust, Bull. Environ. Contam. Toxicol., 23: 497-502.

Day, J.P., Hart, M., Robinson, M.S., (1975), Lead in urban street dust, Nature, 253: 343-344.

De Jonghe, W., Jiang, S., Adams, F., (1981), Alkyl lead compounds in the environment, In "Proceedings of an international conference on environmental pollution", Ed. Anagnostopoulos, A., University of Thessaloniki, Greece.

Duggan, M.J., (1980), Lead in Urban Dust: an assessment, Water Air Soil Pollut., 14: 309-321.

Duggan, M.J., Williams, S., (1977), Lead in dust in city streets, Sci. Total Environ., 7: 91-97.

Environmental Protection Unit of the City of Birmingham, (1975), Lead in urban dust and on clothing, Environ. Health, 83: 267-268.

Farmer, J.G., Lyon, T.D.B., (1977), Lead in Glasgow street dust and soil, Sci. Total Environ., 8: 89-93.

Harrison, R.M., (1979), Toxic metals in street and household dusts, Sci. Total Environ., 11: 89-97.

Harrison, R.M., Laxen, D.P.H., (1977), Organolead compounds absorbed upon atmospheric particulates: A minor component of urban air, Atmos. Environ., 11: 201-203.

Harrison, R.M., Laxen, D.P.H., (1978), Sink processes for tetra-alkyllead compounds in the atmosphere, Environ. Sci. Tech., 12: 1348-1392.

Nielsen, T., Jensen, K.A., Grandjean, P., (1978), Organic lead in normal human brains, Nature, 274: 602-603.

Swain, D.J., (1955), Commonwealth Bureau of Soil Science, Technical Communication No. 48, York.

U.S. Environmental Protection Agency, (1978), Air quality criteria for lead, Federal Register, 43: 46246.

Lead Versus Health
Edited by M. Rutter and R. Russell Jones
© 1983 John Wiley & Sons Ltd.

LEAD IN DUST AS A SOURCE OF CHILDREN'S
BODY LEAD

M. J. Duggan

Environmental Sciences Division
Scientific Branch
Greater London Council

INTRODUCTION

Several authorities have set standards or guidelines for community
exposure to airborne lead. These imply, and in some cases have
been explicitly derived from maximum allowable increases in
blood-lead levels. For example, the standard of $2\mu g/m^3$ proposed
by the Commission of the European Communities (1975) was based
on the premise that the contribution made by inhaled lead to the
blood-lead level should not exceed $5\mu g/dl$. However, inhalation is
not the only route by which people take in lead derived from air
pollution. Many authors have suggested that the unwitting
ingestion of dust via dirty hands gives rise to a significant lead
intake, particularly for young children. If so, standards should be
defined in terms of any combination of airborne lead and
lead-in-dust that brings about some maximum allowable increase in
blood-lead level (Duggan, 1980; Greater London Council, 1981).

Not all agree with the view that lead-in-dust represents an
important source of lead for urban children. Most studies of the
variation of blood-lead level with age have shown a peak value at 2
to 3 years; Ter Haar (1979) attributed this to the gnawing of
paintwork by children in this age group. Chamberlain et al (1978)
pointed out that several surveys of blood-lead levels in children
and their mothers showed child/mother ratios in the region of 1.3.
Further, almost always blood-lead levels have been found to be
higher in adult males than females, with a male/female blood-level
ratio often rather more than 1.3. Thus, the blood-lead levels of
young children appear to be intermediate between those of their
parents. Chamberlain (Personal Communication) came to the conclusion that for urban areas, excluding the immediate vicinity of
smelters, there is no evidence of an important pathway of lead
uptake that affects children but not adults. The Lawther Committee
apparently reached the same conclusion, since they ignored any
uptake from dust and dirt in their estimates of the contribution of
various sources of lead to the body burden of inner-city children
(Department of Health and Social Security, 1980). However, there
are data from several types of study that suggest that lead in dust
makes a significant contribution to the blood-lead of urban children.

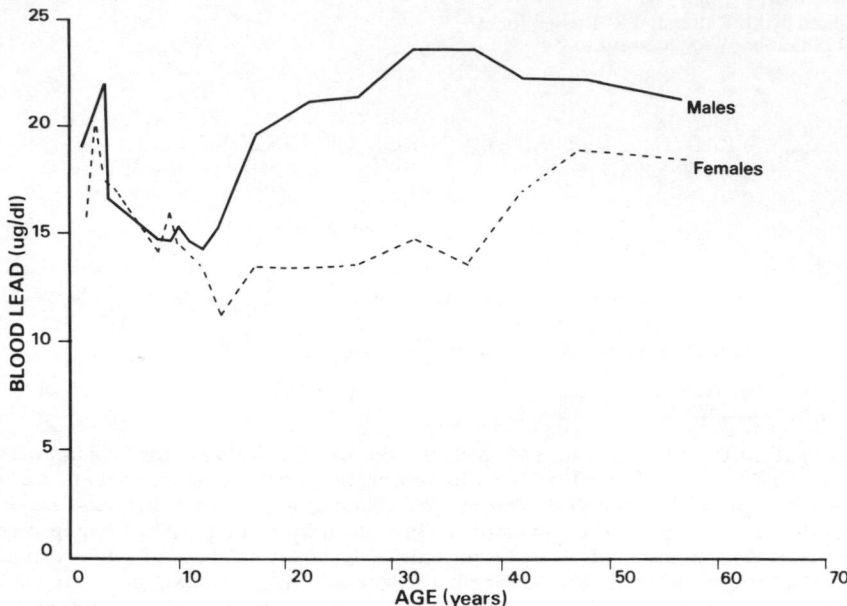

Fig. 1.   Blood lead levels in Birmingham UK;
Department of the Environment, 1978

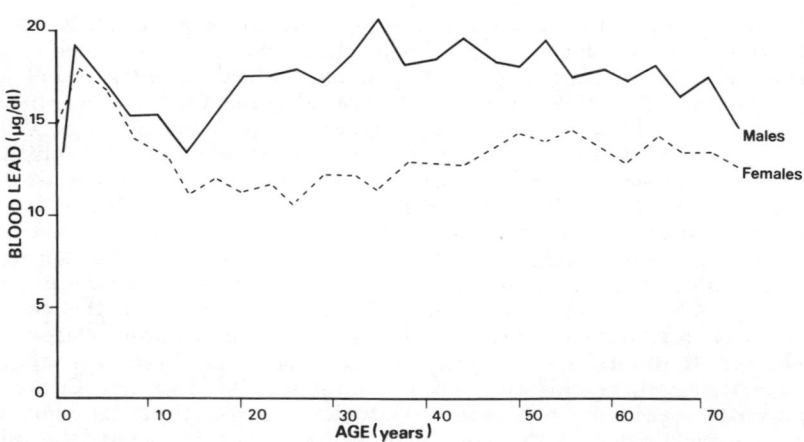

Fig. 2.   Blood lead levels in the United States;
Mahaffey et al, 1979

Changes in blood-lead level with age were recorded in two large
scale general population surveys; that in Birmingham U.K.
(Department of the Environment, 1978), and that undertaken as
part of the Second U.S. National Health and Nutrition Examination
Survey (Mahaffey et al, 1979). In spite of major differences
between the study populations, there are some similarities in the
two sets of results (see Figures 1 and 2). Both showed a peak
childhood value at 2 to 3 years, followed by a decline until early
adolescence; there was little or no variation with sex during this
period. During adolescence the blood-lead levels of the males, but
not the females, rose quite sharply. After adolescence there was a
slow rise until middle age, and then some suggestion of gently
declining levels throughout the rest of life. A male/female ratio
greater than unity persisted from adolescence onwards.

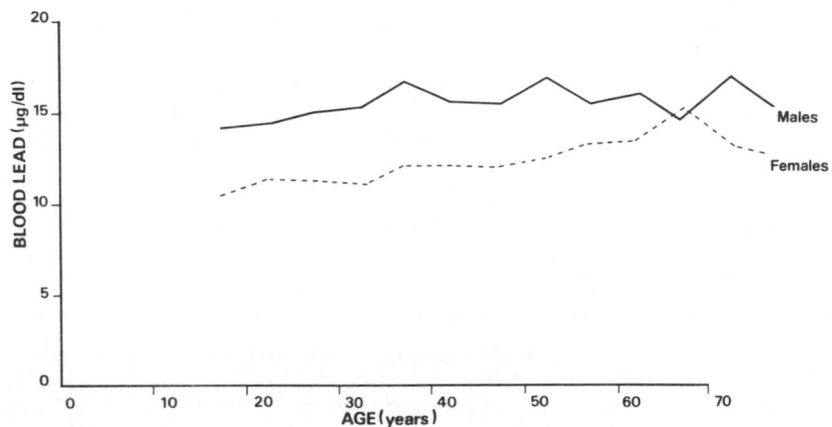

Fig. 3. Blood lead levels in the United Kingdom;
Department of the Environment, 1980

The blood-lead results from the most recent U.K. survey (Department of the Environment, 1981), (inner and outer city measurements
combined) give a rather similar pattern (see Fig. 3). The report
on this study does not give the basic data for children but it does
contain a graph of blood-lead level (controlled for a number of
variables) against age that shows a maximum value at 2 years.
Figs. 1 to 3 illustrate the need to define age when referring to the
blood-lead levels of a population. Some blood-lead ratios of interest
for adults in the age group 20 to 40 years, and for two years old
children, are given in Table 1.

It is not clear how the blood-lead level changes during the first
year or so of life. The concentration of lead in cord-blood is
usually slightly lower than that in the mother's blood and this

implies that the initial rise shown in Figs. 1 and 2 constitutes the
continuation of a rise that started at birth. However, it has been
suggested that the blood-lead level actually falls during the first
few months of life before beginning to rise. Haas and his
co-workers (1972) measured the blood-lead levels of several groups
of people in a German city: 294 mothers, their newly-born infants
(by cord-blood samples), 162 hospitalized children aged 8 days to 5
years (those with conditions likely to influence blood-lead levels
were excluded), and 201 healthy children aged 6 years to 8 years.
The mean blood-lead levels of mothers and their newly-born were
unremarkable - 16.9 µg/dl and 15.7 µg/dl respectively - but the
levels in the other children were unusual in their very low values
during the first year of life, and their steady rise in subsequent
years with no evidence of a peak value during the second and third
years. The results are summarised in Fig. 4. The ratio of
blood-lead levels in 2 year old children compared with women was
about 0.4.

TABLE 1. Blood-lead ratios from three surveys

Survey	No. of People examined	Blood-lead ratio	
		Man/Woman	Child/Woman
Birmingham (1978)	1607	1.56	1.38
NHANES (1979)	4635	1.54	1.55
UK Dept of Env. (1981)	4981	1.35	–

There are other studies that suggest that children isolated from a
normal environment show little or no evidence of peak blood-lead
levels at 2 to 3 years. Sartor and Rondia (1981) measured lead
concentrations in blood collected from adult blood donors in Liege,
and from 127 children (0 to 14 years) in a hospital in the same
city. Their results are summarised in Figure 5. It can be seen
that the ratio of blood-lead levels in 2 year old children compared
with women was about 0.9.

Nygaard et al (1977) looked at the blood-lead levels of 126 young
children from seven different areas in Denmark (see Table 2).
There were some significant differences between the mean blood-lead
concentrations of the groups but there was no obvious relationship
between age and blood-lead. The two groups (K and F) having the
lowest blood-lead values might have been expected to be among the
highest if there were a peak at 2 to 3 years. Both these groups
were isolated from the general environment insofar as group K were
children in hospital, and group F were from a day nursery - the
authors comment that 'Children of that age at day nursery are
protected from contact with the environment compared to the
kindergarten children in group G from the same place'.

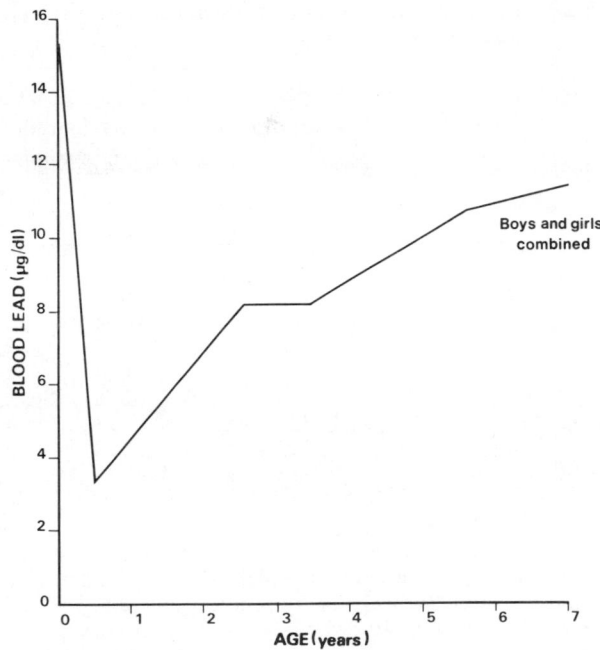

Fig. 4.   Blood lead levels in new born, hospitalised, and
school children in Nurnberg;
Haas et al, 1972

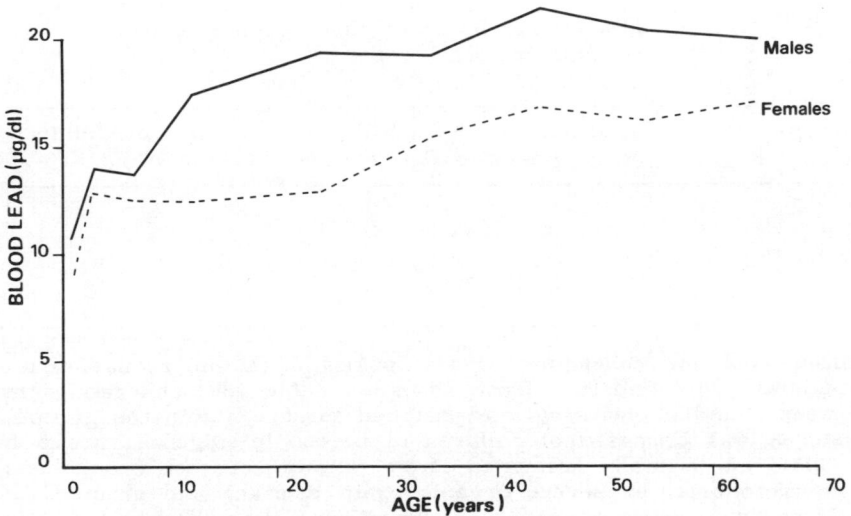

Fig. 5.   Blood   lead   levels   in   adults   and   hospitalised
children in Liege;
Sartor and Rondia, 1981

M. J. Duggan

TABLE 2. Blood-lead levels of Danish Children (Nygaard et al, 1977).

Group	No. of Children	Mean age (yrs)	Blood-lead level (µg/dl)	
			Mean	95% confidence interval
A	20	5.0	6.7	± 1.22
G	9	4.8	9.2	± 1.82
D	6	4.6	10.1	± 2.22
B	9	3.9	6.9	± 1.82
K	64	3.8	5.6	± 0.68
C	10	3.7	8.3	± 1.64
F	8	1.8	4.3	± 0.50

It is worth noting here that blood-lead surveys carried out in Scandinavian countries tend to give a different picture from that in the U.K. and U.S. surveys mentioned above. Thus, the survey made by Nygaard et al (which included adults as well as children) showed generally low blood-lead levels, and a steady increase in the level from birth to old age with no significant differences between males and females; the number of people (about 100) from whom samples were taken was rather small. Relatively low blood-levels in adults have also been reported by Nordman (1975) and in young children by Bach (1979) and by Taskinen et al (1981).

TABLE 3. Blood-lead levels of three groups of children (Gibson et al, 1967)

Group	Blood-lead level (µg/dl) Mean ± S.D.	No. of Children > 40 µg/dl
A	29.6 ± 18.6	3
B	16.4 ± 9.8	0
C	32.4 ± 30.3	6

Gibson and her colleagues (1967) looked at three groups, each containing 20 children, from Glasgow. All the children were between 3 and 11 years old and matched for age within the groups. Group A was composed of children of normal intelligence, group B of children mentally retarded from known causes (mongolism, phenylketonuria, or severe organic brain damage) and group C of children who were mentally retarded in the absence of any recognised cause. The results of this study are summarised in Table 3. The authors suggest that the relatively low blood-lead levels found in group B may have been due to these children being under closer supervision and being more restricted in their movements than the other two groups.

Zielhuis et al (1978) measured lead concentrations in blood from 48 patients (2 months to 6 years of age) in an Amsterdam hospital. They found a significant positive relationship between age and blood-lead. For example, the blood-lead level of the 0-3 year age group was 11.9 µg/dl, while that of 4-6 year age group was 15.5 µg/dl. In other words, no peak value at 2 to 3 years was observed.

It is of course quite possible that children in hospital eat less, and so take in less lead, than comparable healthy children. Presumably, this would tend simply to lower the blood-lead levels in all age groups. The peak value at 2 to 3 years would show up even in hospitalised children if it were a basic characteristic of this age. It does not. Moreover, in the two studies (Haas et al, 1972; Sartor and Rondia, 1981) where measurements were made on both hospitalised and normal individuals, there was a smooth transition between the blood-lead levels of the two groups (Figs. 4 and 5).

It is difficult to make theoretical estimates of the blood-lead levels of children. The ratio of the intakes of air and food per unit blood volume of young children compared with women is about 1.5 (International Commission on Radiological Protection, 1975). Nevertheless, it does not follow that the ratio of blood-lead concentrations (child : mother) to be expected is also 1.5, because there are other parameters - notably the fraction of ingested lead which is transferred to blood, and the clearance rate of lead from blood - which probably vary with age. There are no measured values of the half-life of lead in blood for children, and very few measurements of gut absorption. But even if calculations of blood-lead levels are made with assumed values of these and other parameters (food intake, air intake, concentrations of lead in food and in air, blood volume, etc) it requires curious assumptions to produce a curve of blood-lead versus age that shows a peak in early childhood. It is more likely that the occurrence of child/woman blood-lead ratios greater than unity (or more accurately, greater than some number less than unity) results from an important pathway of lead uptake affecting children and not adults.

One other study is of interest here. Elwood et al (1978) examined mother-and-child pairs (children 0-16 years) living in two housing estates in North Wales; one estate had lead water-piping, the other copper. The results are summarised in Table 4. The blood-lead levels and the child/mother blood-lead ratio in the copper-piped estate are typical for urban areas. The levels in the lead-piped estate are considerably higher, and the child/mother ratio is close to unity. This last result is at first sight surprising. Why should a larger than usual intake of ingested lead for both mothers and children result in an unusually low child/mother ratio? It could be simply that the elevated blood-lead level usual in the first few years of life is due to the intake of lead in dust, and this is relatively small (as a fraction of total intake) for the children living on the lead-piped estate.

TABLE 4. Blood-lead levels of mothers and children
(Elwood et al, 1978)

Piping	No. of pairs	Blood-lead level (μg/dl) mean ± S.D.		Ratio Child/Mother
		Children	Mothers	
Lead	38	41.6 ± 13.0	39.6 ± 13.7	1.05
Copper	19	19.3 ± 10.6	13.9 ± 4.8	1.39

CHILD/ADULT BLOOD-LEAD RATIOS IN AREAS OF HIGH AND LOW CONTAMINATION

Those studies in which investigators have compared two or more groups of people exposed to different levels of lead contamination are of interest. If the uptake of lead in dust is important for children, but less so for adults, then the child/adult blood-lead ratio might be expected to be higher in the more contaminated area. Elwood et al (1977) measured the blood-lead levels of mother and children (0-5 years) living in the vicinity of a large battery factory. They studied two groups - leadworkers' families, and randomly selected controls. Capillary-blood measurements showed that the child/mother blood-lead ratio was greater for the group exposed to the higher contamination.

TABLE 5. Blood-lead levels of mothers and children
(Elwood et al, 1977)

Group	Mean blood-lead levels (μg/dl)		Ratio Child/Mother
	Children	Mothers	
Leadworkers' families	33.1	23.6	1.40
Control families	27.0	27.0	1.23

Johnson et al (1975) studied two populations in California, one living near a Los Angeles freeway, the other at Lancaster in a desert area. The populations were divided into three age groups - group I (0-16 years), group II (17-34 years) and group III (35 years and over) - and males and females were considered separately. The authors expressed the measured blood-lead values in terms of both arithmetic and geometric means; the latter are used in this discussion. Some of their results are given in Table 6.

TABLE 6. Air and blood-lead levels in California
(Johnson et al, 1975)

Area	Air lead ($\mu g/m^3$)	Mean blood-lead level ($\mu g/dl$)					Ratio Child/Woman (M&F)
		Group I			Group II		
		M	F	M&F	M	F	
Los Angeles	6.3	20.8	14.9	18.0	15.1	11.8	1.53
Lancaster	0.64	10.4	9.6	10.7	10.9	8.0	1.34

The child/woman ratio was greater in the more exposed group; the effect was rather more pronounced when the arithmetic means were used. It is possible to make estimates of α from these data: is defined as the increase, Δ Pb B, in blood-lead level which arises from an increase Δ Pb A, in the concentration of airborne lead. If it is assumed that the difference in the Los Angeles and Lancaster blood-lead levels was due solely to the higher intakes of inhaled lead by the Los Angeles groups, then the value of α for male children is 1.8, for female children it is 0.9, and for adults (group II males and females combined), it is 0.6. It seems unlikely that such differences in α really exist, and the assumption that inhalation is the only important route for children could therefore be incorrect.

TABLE 7. Air and blood-lead levels near a Belgian smelter
(Roels et al, 1980)

Type of School	Air lead ($\mu g/m^3$)	Mean blood-lead level ($\mu g/dl$)		Ratio Child/Teacher
		Children	Teachers	
Near smelter	2.68	27.8	18.0	1.54
Control	0.46	11.7	12.8	0.91

In a study carried out around a lead smelter in Belgium, Roels et al (1980) measured the blood-lead levels of children (9-14 years) and some teachers at two schools within 1 km of the smelter, and also at two control schools. The relevant results are summarised in Table 7. The child/teacher ratio was greater for the schools nearer the smelter.   A possible explanation might be that the teachers at the 'near smelter' schools tended to live further away from the smelter than the children and so were exposed to lower average concentrations of airborne lead.   The value of α for the teachers (estimated from Table 7) was about 2 - the commonly accepted value - which suggests that they were exposed to the concentrations of airborne lead quoted in the Table for most of the time.   The value of α for the children (again, estimated from the Table) was about 7.   This is an unusually high value and suggests that, either the children were affected by an additional route of lead to the body, or their homes were much nearer the smelter than were the schools. This latter explanation seems unlikely from the authors' description of the study area.   (Roels et al, 1978).

TABLE 8. Blood-lead levels of mothers and children
(Barltrop et al, 1975)

Soil-lead content	Mean blood-lead level (μg/dl)		Ratio Child/Mother
	Children	Mothers	
High	29.0	14.2	2.0
Medium	13.8	18.7	1.3
Low	20.7	14.1	1.5

Baltrop et al (1975) measured the blood-lead levels of mothers and children exposed to lead contaminated soils and dusts in a rural area of Derbyshire with minimal atmospheric pollution.   The data were classified into three groups depending on the soil-lead content found at the child's home and are summarised in Table 8.   The child/mother ratios do not show a consistent trend with soil-lead content.

TABLE 9. Blood-lead levels of adults and children
(Yankel et al, 1977)

Region	Mean blood-lead level (μg/dl)		Ratio Child/Adult
	Children (2-3 yrs)	Adults	
I (near smelter)	73.5	37	2.0
II	53	33	1.6
III	36	30	1.2
IV	34.5	34	1.0
V (far from smelter)	32	32	1.0
VI Control	23.5	–	–
VII Control	29	32	0.9

Yankel et al (1977) carried out an extensive environmental survey around a large lead smelter in Idaho. They placed their study population into sub-groups according to age and distance from the smelter; the region was divided into five areas (area I nearest to and area V furthest from the smelter) and there were two control areas. Some of the results are given in Table 9; their figures for 2 year old and for 3 year old children have been pooled. The child/adult blood-lead ratio tended to decrease as the distance from the smelter increased, i.e., the ratio was enhanced for the more exposed groups.

TABLE 10. Blood-lead levels of mothers and children
(Lansdown et al, 1974)

Distance from factory	Mean blood-lead level (μg/dl)		Ratio Child/Mother
	Children (5 yrs)	Mothers	
Less than 400m	38	30	1.27
400 - 500m	31	26	1.19

In a study of environmental contamination around a lead smelter in London, Lansdown et al (1974) measured blood-lead levels in mothers and children, and grouped the results according to the distance of the homes from the factory. Their findings (Table 10) showed that the child/mother ratio was marginally higher for the group living nearer the factory.

TABLE 11. Blood-lead levels of community and leadworkers' children (Millar, 1978)

Group	Mean blood-lead level (μg/dl)		Ratio Young/Old
	Young Children	Old Children	
Leadworkers' children	27.4	17.5	1.57
Community children	21.1	15.6	1.35

Millar (1978), in a study of contamination around another lead works in London, measured the blood-lead levels of both leadworkers' children and community children. He reported no measurement on adults, but since he grouped the children by age it is possible to compare the blood-lead levels of young (0-4 years) and older (6-11 years) children. His results for workers' children and for community children showed that in each case, the young child/old child blood-lead ratio was higher for the more exposed group.

TABLE 12. Blood-lead levels of community children according to distance from factory (Millar, 1978)

Distance of home from factory	Mean blood-lead level (µg/dl)		Ratio Young/Old
	Young Children	Old Children	
Less than 280m	22.4	15.6	1.44
280 - 400m	19.7	15.6	1.26

Differences between the blood-lead levels of young and older children (but not adults) were also reported in a study carried out by Schmitt and his co-workers (1979) around a smelter in Canada. Their results (see Table 13) showed a consistent pattern, in which the young child/old child blood-lead ratio increased both with increasing contamination and with the gap between the two age groups.

TABLE 13. Soil and blood-lead levels near a Canadian smelter (Schmitt et al, 1979)

Distance from smelter (km)	Soil lead (ppm)	Mean blood-lead level (µg/dl) of children			Ratio Youngest/ Oldest
		1-3 yrs	about 6 yrs	about 15 yrs	
Less than 1.6	1662	28.8	25.1	10.4	2.8
1.6 - 3.2	1341	26.6	24.6	11.8	2.3
More than 3.2	354	18.7	17.8	11.5	1.6

In another Canadian study, Roberts et al (1974) also measured the blood-lead levels of people living in the neighbourhood of smelters. They did not report the data for children and adults separately but they noted that 'although there was no significant trend for adults, the blood-lead concentrations of the children increased with proximity to both smelters'. It follows that the child/adult blood-lead ratio was higher for the more exposed groups.

TABLE 14. Blood-levels of women and children near a
motorway (Day et al, 1977)

Time of measurements	Mean Blood-lead level (µg/dl)		Ratio Child/Woman
	Children (0-10 yrs)	Women	
Before opening	16.3	14.0	1.16
6 mths after opening	15.4	13.9	1.11
1 yr after opening	16.5	14.7	1.12

Day et al (1977) looked at blood-lead levels in a group of people
living close to a motorway immediately before, and at two intervals
after its opening.   Neither the absolute blood-lead levels, nor the
child/woman ratios, showed any trend over time.   The traffic flows
on this motorway (about 20,000 vehicles per 24 hr.) were not
particularly high, and their growth was to some extent balanced by
falls in traffic flows on already existing roads.

TABLE 15. Blood-lead levels of adults near a motorway
(Waldron, 1975)

Time of Measurements	Mean blood-lead level (µg/dl)	
	Men	Women
Before opening	14.41	10.93
about 9 mths after opening	18.95	14.93
about 15 mths after opening	23.73	19.21

In another motorway study, Waldron (1975) reported marked
increases in the blood-lead levels of a group of adults living near a
motorway interchange in Birmingham U.K.   He made no measurements of children's blood-lead levels so that no child/woman ratios
are available from this study.   Waldron commented that the
increases in blood-lead levels observed (Table 15) were greater
than would be expected from airborne lead alone.

Worth and her colleagues (1977) measured the blood-lead levels of
several hundred people in Massachusetts in an investigation
designed to find the contributions made by tap water, and by other
sources, to lead intake.   A minority of the study population were
'referrals from the neighbourhood health centres'; the authors do

not indicate why referrals were made but presumably increased exposure to environmental lead was suspected. The child/adult blood-lead ratio was somewhat greater in the more exposed group.

TABLE 16. Blood-lead levels of adults and children in Massachusetts (Worth et al, 1978)

Type of case	Mean blood-lead level (µg/dl)		Ratio
	Children (2-6 yrs)	Adults (20-50 yrs)	Child/Adult
Referred	32.85	21.91	1.50
Non-referred	23.99	18.99	1.26

TABLE 17. Blood-lead levels of adults and children, all races, from urban and rural areas (Annest et al, 1982)

Type of area	Mean blood-lead level (µg/dl)		Ratio
	Children (0.5-5 yrs)	Adults (18-74 yrs)	Child/Adult
Urban (10^6 or more persons)	18.0	15.2	1.18
Rural	13.9	13.4	1.04

Data from the second National Health and Nutrition Examination Survey (Annest et al, 1982) allow a comparison of the child/adult blood-lead ratio in urban populations with that in rural populations (see Table 17 for data on all races combined). The child/adult blood-lead ratio was marginally greater in the more exposed urban group.

Annest et al (1982) also compared 'central city' with 'non-central city' populations (Table 18). The child/adult blood-lead ratio was greater in the more exposed central city group. However, although the blood-lead levels of inner city children were higher than those from non-central city areas, the difference was not statistically significant at the 5% level.

TABLE 18. Blood-lead levels of adults and children, all races, from central city and non-central city areas (Annest et al, 1982)

Type of area	Mean blood-lead level (μg/dl)		Ratio
	Children (0.5-5 yrs)	Adults (18-74 yrs)	Child/Adult
Central City	20.0	14.7	1.36
Non-central city	16.5	15.6	1.06

In almost all the other studies discussed in this section the difference between the blood-lead levels of the more highly exposed children and the less exposed children was shown by the authors to be statistically significant. In those studies where the authors tested the difference between the blood-lead levels of children and mothers - or young children and old children - in the same exposure group, statistically significant differences were found (Elwood et al, 1977; Barltrop et al, 1975; Millar, 1978). The two population surveys mentioned above also showed statistically significant differences between young children and women (Department of the Environment 1978 - Mahaffey et al, 1979). None of the authors calculated the errors associated with the individual ratios given in Tables 5 to 18 above (not surprisingly, because they did not calculate the ratios) and no attempt is made to calculate them here - indeed it is not always possible to do so from the published data. However, in almost all the studies the result was the same: the child/adult (or young child/old child) blood-lead ratio appeared to increase as the level of contamination increased. It is unlikely that chance alone is responsible for the similar pattern of so many diverse studies, and a pathway to the body that is more important for children than for adults is therefore indicated.

One possibility that should be mentioned here is the effect of sampling capillary blood (usually by finger prick) rather than venous blood. Most comparisons that have been made between the two types of sample show that a higher lead concentration is found in capillary blood. A possible explanation is skin contamination. Since young children are more likely than adults to have dirty hands one might expect the effect of skin contamination to be greater for children than for adults, as well as being greater in more contaminated areas. If the studies mentioned above had all been done by capillary sampling (or if the children had been done by capillary and the adults by venous sampling) then skin contamination might provide an explanation for the apparently higher blood-lead levels seen in children compared with adults, and for the apparent enhancement of the child/adult blood-lead ratio in

contaminated areas.   However in all the studies described in this
section - except those of Schmitt et al (1979) and Yankel et al
(1977) in which the sampling method was not described - either all
capillary or all venous sampling was used.   Those studies in which
use was made of venous sampling (and from which Tables 6, 7, 8,
11 and 12 are derived) did not show any different pattern from the
others.   Finally, of the two large blood-lead surveys mentioned
earlier, one was carried out by venous sampling of the adults and
capillary sampling of the under 5 year olds, (Department of the
Environment, 1978) the other by venous sampling for all age
groups; (Mahaffey et al, 1979) in spite of these differences, the
results from the two surveys are very similar.

For all these reasons it seems unlikely that some artifact of
sampling accounts for the pattern found in these studies.

POSSIBLE ROUTES FROM THE ENVIRONMENT TO THE BODY

As was noted in the Introduction, since the turn of the century
(Gibson, 1904) the ingestion of lead-in-dust via the hands has
frequently been suggested as an important pathway for young
children.   The most casual observation of young children's
behaviour suggests the likelihood of this occurrence.   However,
other possible reasons for a high uptake of lead during early
childhood have been put forward.

The value of α may be larger for young children than for adults.
Children inhale more air relative to their body weight than do
adults.   If the fraction of inhaled lead transferred to blood, and
the half-life of lead in blood, are assumed to be the same for the
child as for the adult then α for a 2 year old child would be about
4 (Duggan 1975, Ratcliffe 1981).   However, such estimates are of
limited value because there is no reason to believe that these two
parameters are the same for child and adult; further, it seems
unlikely that α would peak at 2 to 3 years of age.   The results
from some of the environmental studies make it difficult to accept
that the enhanced blood-lead levels found in children are a
consequence of a high value of α.   For example, if the differences
in blood-lead reported by Schmitt et al (1979) were used solely to
inhalation, a value of α equal to zero would have to be assumed for
15 year old children, together with a very high value (probably
about 7) for the youngest children.   Again, high blood-lead values
of leadworkers' children, which correlate well with lead in housedust, have been reported by some authors.   The levels of airborne
lead are not usually given but are probably quite low.   An explanation of the results based on inhalation would require the assumption
of very large differences, Δ Pb A, in the concentrations of airborne
lead at different workers' houses, and/or very large values of α.
For example, in the study reported by Baker et al (1977) the
difference, Δ Ph B, between the highest and lowest blood-lead
groups was 43 μg/dl.   Any combination of Δ Pb A and α which
would give this variable of Δ Pb B is scarcely tenable.   Finally,

Walter et al (1980) in an examination of the data from their Silver Valley study carried out an analysis to identify the important variables (in the prediction of children's blood-lead levels) and how these changed with age. They concluded that the effect of air-borne lead was virtually constant for all age groups (1 year to 9 years) while the effect of household dustiness declined with age.

Some airborne lead is deposited onto food and kitchen utensils. This entry route may well be responsible for a significant fraction of some people's total intake (Stephens, 1978), but it is probably equally important for both children and adults and it is unlikely to account for an enhanced child/adult ratio. It could however be partly responsible for an enhanced urban/rural ratio.

The resuspension of deposited lead and its subsequent inhalation has been mentioned as a factor which may be more important for young children than for adults (Roels et al 1978, Schmitt et al 1979). It is difficult to judge the relative importance of this pathway, but there are some pointers. Thus, Lepow et al (1975), in an attempt to resolve this problem, measured the concentration of airborne lead at two heights (2ft and 5ft) at each of four sites where their study children played. The differences between the concentrations at the heights were not significant at any of the sites. Again, during the study mentioned earlier, Roels et al (1980) measured not only airborne lead, and blood-lead levels, but also the amount of lead, PbH, on the hands of the children. The authors found that the multiple regression coefficient of PbB.PbA.log PbH calculated for the four groups of children combined was highly significant. Standardisation of PbA resulted in a still significant partial correlation between PbB and log PbH, whereas the partial correlation between PbB and PbA became insignificant when standardised for log PbH. The authors concluded that the ingestion of lead via dirty hands was a much more important factor contribution to PbB than was PbA. A further finding of interest was that the boys had significantly higher PbH levels and - like the boys in the study of Johnson et al (1975) - significantly higher PbB levels, than did the girls. The average boy/girl ratios for these two parameters were about 2 and 1.2 respectively.

Several workers have shown that measured values of the lead present on children's hands, combined with quite modest assumptions about the frequency of hand mouthing, suggest that many children are likely to ingest substantial quantities of lead (comparable with the amount taken in via diet) by the hand-to-mouth route. (Lepow et al 1975, Day et al 1975, Duggan and Williams 1977, Sayre et al 1974). A study by Charney et al (1980) is of interest. About 50 children with high blood-lead levels (40-79 µg/dl) were matched with 50 children with low levels (less than 29 µg/dl), and housedust lead, lead on hands, and several other variables noted for each child. Children in the high blood-lead group showed significant differences from the low lead children in a number of ways: for example, they had higher hand-lead levels, their homes had high dust-lead levels, they played more often in outside soil and their soil had a higher lead content, they mouthed objects more often and they sucked their fingers more often.

There are, then, some grounds for believing that the ingestion of lead in dust, sometimes soil, via the hands is the pathway mainly responsible for the enhanced child/adult blood-lead ratio so frequently observed.

QUANTITATIVE RELATIONSHIPS

A review of those published studies from which a quantitative relationship between children's blood-lead levels and the concentration of lead in dust or soil can be inferred has been carried out (Duggan 1980). It was concluded that the factor δ - defined as the increment, Δ PbB, in blood-lead level associated with an increment, Δ PbD, in the concentration of lead in dust or soil - varied from about 1 to 10 $\mu g/dl$ per 1000 ppm, with a median value of about 5 $\mu g/dl$ per 1000 ppm. The increase in blood-lead level indicated by this relationship is additional to any increase due to airborne lead.

Since that review, the U.K. results for the first campaign of the E.E.C. screening programme for lead have become available (Department of the Environment, 1981). The report detailed blood-lead measurements for children living in the vicinity of smelters and for those living near busy main roads. A report on measurements of environmental lead near some of these works and roads has also been published (Turner and Carroll, 1980). It was therefore anticipated that estimates of δ could be derived from all these data, but this has not proved possible. There is not sufficient cross referencing between the blood-lead and the air and dust lead measurements, and the dust sampling was confined to gutters of major roads, together with a very few house interiors. A possible exception is provided by the data from the Greenwich Survey. More children (400 in all) were examined here than at any of the other locations, and additional environmental measurements are available from another survey (Greater London Council, 1979). However, the two surveys were carried out at different times and the area around the lead works was sub-divided in different ways. It is therefore difficult to combine the dust and blood-lead data properly, but a low value of δ - probably about unity - is indicated.

The investigation carried out by Barltrop et al (1975) in Derbyshire is often cited as a study which shows that, although lead in soil and dust does have some effect upon blood-lead, the effect is a small one, (see Table 19).

The values of δ obtained from these data are about 0.6 and 4 $\mu g/dl$ per 1000 ppm for lead in soil and lead in dust respectively. Since 2 year old children spend more of their waking hours indoors than in the garden, the value of δ for housedust is the one of greater significance. This value of 4 µg/dl per 1000 ppm is close to the median value (5 µg/dl per 1000 ppm) obtained from the review.

TABLE 19. Soil, dust and blood-lead levels in three regions in Derbyshire (Barltrop et al, 1975)

Mean level of lead in:		
Soil (ppm)	Housedust (ppm)	Children's blood (µg/dl)
420	531	20.7
3390	1564	23.8
13969	2582	29.0

Some work by Rice and her colleagues (1978) was not used in the review because they measured zinc protoporphyrin (APP) rather than δ blood-lead levels. However, in one of the studies that was used – that by Watson et al (1978) – the authors measured both blood-lead and ZPP levels. Their blood-lead measurements gave a value for δ of about 7 µg/dl per 1000 ppm – fairly close to the median value; their ZPP measurements give a value for δ (ZPP) of about 9 µg/dl ZPP/dl per 1000 ppm. The value of δ (ZPP) estimated from the results of Rice et al (1978) is about the same – 11 µg/dl ZPP/dl per 1000 ppm. Erythrocyte protoporphyrin varies exponentially with blood-lead level and it may therefore be more appropriate to work in terms of the logarithm of the ZPP level. The values of δ (ln ZPP) obtained from these two studies are 0.26 and 0.23. Hence, the work of Rice et al suggests a quantitative relationship (between body-lead and lead in dust) similar to the one derived in the review.

DISCUSSION

There is a prima facie case for the hypothesis that the ingestion of urban dust via dirty hands gives rise to a significant intake of lead during early childhood. The peak level of blood-lead frequently observed at 2 to 3 years of age, the enhancement of the child/adult blood-lead ratio which occurs in contaminated areas, and the relationship between blood-lead and lead-in-dust seen in many studies, can all be accounted for by the hypothesis.

For most urban children it is likely that a greater intake of lead comes about from the ingestion of dust than from the inhalation of airborne material. It follows that there is a need for a lead-in-dust standard to be used in parallel with a lead-in-air one. It is sometimes said that a lead-in-dust standard is impractical because the monitoring required presents such difficulties – principally those arising from large spatial and temporal variations in the concentration of lead-in-dust. However, while it is true that the

taking of a few spot samples can give a very misleading picture,
the setting up of an effective monitoring programme is quite
practicable particularly if large area sampling is used (Duggan,
1981a). It should be noted here that analogous difficulties of
monitoring have not prevented the adoption of standards for
airborne lead (Duggan, 1981b).

Perhaps there is also the view that if δ were really as high as
5 µg/dl per 1000 ppm then one might expect a greater difference in
the blood-lead levels of urban and rural children than is actually
observed. But there are few studies comparing matched populations
of children from urban areas with those from rural (or suburban)
areas on which to base such a view. What studies there are do not
present a uniform picture. The measurements made by Taskinen et
al (1981) of blood-lead levels of Finnish preschool children show a
very low mean value (about 6 µg/dl), no correlation with age, and
no significant differences in the blood-lead levels of children from
three different types of area (urban, rural and smelter); the
authors mention an annual mean concentration of airborne lead of
0.94 µg/m³ at one of the busiest city-centre crossings in Helsinki,
but otherwise give no data on air and dust-lead in their survey
areas. A recent study by Elwood et al (1982) among pre-school
children in Wales showed no difference in the mean blood-lead level
of a group living adjacent to busy major roads compared with that
of a group living in a rural area. By contrast, some work from the
United States suggests that the blood-lead levels of urban children
may be about 10 µg/dl higher than those of rural children (such a
large difference could not be accounted for by the inhalation route
alone) although it must be noted that there were difficulties in
matching for race (Angle and McIntire, 1979; Joselow et al, 1974;
Cohen et al, 1973). The most recent data from the second National
Health and Nutrition Examination Survey (Annest et al, 1982)
suggests that, for both black and white children, those living in
large urban areas have blood-lead levels between 3 and 4 µg/dl
higher than those in rural areas (Chapter 3). Finally, in a study
of urban and suburban school children (aged 10-15 years) in
Tokyo, Okubo et al (1978) found significantly higher blood-lead
levels in the urban groups. The blood-lead levels of the urban
children decreased with age while those of the suburban were
roughly constant; the urban/suburban difference therefore
decreased with age (from about 5.5 µg/dl for the 10 year old to
about 1.5 µg/dl for the 15 year olds). The authors report similar
concentrations of airborne lead in the urban and suburban areas
(about 0.55 µg/m³ and 0.4 µg/m³ respectively) and speculate that
exposure to lead in street dust is probably responsible for the
differences in blood-lead levels.

There is a general paucity of data on lead-in-dust concentrations in
rural communities. Levels in outer suburbs or in medium-sized
towns are sometimes not much less than in inner-city areas (Day et
al, 1975; Little and Heard, 1978). It would be instructive to have
blood-lead data on children from urban and rural areas where

comprehensive measurements of environmental lead levels have shown a marked urban/rural difference.

When the lead content of petrol sold in the U.K. is reduced from 0.4 to 0.15 g/l at the end of 1985, there will presumably be a prompt, pro-rata drop in the concentration of airborne lead, and a gradual (but not necessarily pro-rata) decline in the concentration of lead in dust in urban areas. There is not sufficient data available to estimate the relevant rate constants, but one might expect most of the decline to take place in weeks or months rather than years (the rate of decline of lead-in-soil concentrations will of course be much slower - probably imperceptible). It will be of interest to see whether or not concentrations of lead in air and in dust fall sufficiently to meet a combined air/dust standard or guideline of the kind mentioned earlier (Duggan 1980; Greater London Council, 1981). It will be of even greater interest to observe the effect of the reduction in petrol-lead on the blood-lead levels of young urban children in this country.

SUMMARY

The importance of urban dust as a source of lead for young children is still disputed. Although blood-lead data from various population surveys usually show a peak concentration in early childhood, there is evidence that such a peak is small or absent altogether in children without much access to the general environment. An examination of those studies where groups of people in regions of low and high lead contamination have been compared shows that the child/adult blood-lead ratio is almost always enhanced in the more exposed groups. This implies a route of lead uptake that is important for children but less so for adults, and it is likely that this route is the dust-hand-mouth one. There is sufficient data to suggest a quantitative relationship between raised levels of blood-lead and lead-in-dust. There is a strong case for a lead-in-dust standard but some will probably remain unpersuaded unless or until there is reliable blood-lead and environmental-lead data involving matched groups of young people from urban and rural areas.

REFERENCES

Angle, C.R., McIntire M.S., (1979), Environmental lead and children: the Omaha Study, J. Toxicol. Environ. Health, 5,855-870.

Annest, J.L., Mahaffey, K.R., Cox, D.H., Roberts, J., (1982), Blood lead levels for persons aged 6 months to 74 years of age: United States, 1976-80. Advance Data from Vital and Health Statistics, No. 79 DHHS Pub. NO. (PHS) (82-125). Public Health Service, Hyattsville, Md, May 12, 1982.

Bach, E., (1979), Voksnes belastning med bly, Dansk Institute for Klinisk epidemiologi Copenhagen.

Baker, E.L., Folland, D.S., Taylor, T.A., Frank, M., Peterson, W., Lovejoy, G., Cox, D., Housworth, J., Landrigan, P.J.,

(1977), Lead poisoning in children of leadworkers, New Engl. J. Med., 296, 260-261.

Barltrop, D., Strehlow, C.D., Thornton, I., Webb, J.S., (1975), Absorption of lead from dust and soil, Postgrad. Med. J., 51, 801-804.

Chamberlain, A.C., Heard, M.J., Little, P., Newton, D., Wells, A.C., Wiffen, R.D., (1978), Investigations into lead from motor vehicles, Harwell Report AERE - R.9198, HMSO, London.

Charney, E., Sayre, J., Coulter, M., (1980), Increased lead absorption in inner city children: where does the lead come from?, Pediatrics, 65, 226-231.

Cohen, C.J., Bowers, G.N., Lepow, M.L., (1973), Epidemiology of lead poisoning, a comparison between urban and rural children, J.A.M.A. 226, 1430-1433.

Commission of the European Communities, (1975), Proposal for a Council Directive on Air Quality Standards for Lead, COM (75), 166.

Day, J.P., Hart, M., Robinson, M.S., (1975), Lead in urban street dust, Nature 253, 343-345.

Day, A.G., Evans, G., Robson, L.E., (1977), An environmental study of an urban motorway, City of Bristol Environmental Health Department.

Department of the Environment, (1978), Lead pollution in Birmingham, Pollution Paper No. 14, HMSO, London.

Department of the Environment (1981), European Community screening programme for lead: United Kingdom results for 1979-1980, Pollution Report No. 10, HMSO, London.

Department of Health and Social Security, (1980), Lead and Health - The Report of the DHSS Working Party on Lead in the Environment, HMSO, London.

Duggan, M.J., (1975), Inorganic lead in ambient air - how should its significance be assessed, Greater London Council Scientific Branch Report ESG/EA/R17A.

Duggan, M.J., Williams, S., (1977), Lead in dust in city street, Sci. Total Environ., 7, 91-97.

Duggan, M.J., (1980), Lead in urban dust: an assessment, Water, Air and Soil Pollution, 14, 309-321.

Duggan, M.J., (1981a), The concentration of lead in playground dust at Telferscot and Hyde Farm Schools, Greater London Scientific Branch Report ESD/R103.

Duggan, M.J., (1981b), Measurements of environmental lead - the problem of representative sampling, Clean Air, 11, 87-89.

Elwood, P.C., Thomas, H., Sheltawy, M., (1978), Blood-lead levels in mothers and their children, Lancet, (i), 1363-1364.

Elwood, P.C., Gallacher, J., Toothill, C., (1982), Lead in petrol, Br. Med. J., 284, 1189.

Elwood, W.J., Clayton, B.E., Cox, R.A., Delves, H.T., King, E., Malcom, D., Ratcliffe, J.M., Taylor, J.F., (1977), Lead in human blood and in the environment near a battery factory, Brit. J. Prev. Soc. Med., 31, 154-163.

Gibson, J.L., (1904), A plea for painted railings and painted walls of rooms as the source of lead poisoning amongst Queensland children, Australian Medical Gazette, April issue, p.149.

Gibson, S.L.M., Lam, C.N., McCrea, W.M., Goldberg, A., (1967), Blood-lead levels in normal and mentally deficient children, Arch. Dis. Childh., 42, 573-578.

Greater London Council, (1979), Lead pollution in Abbey Wood Thamesmead, Public Services and Safety Committee Report PS 252.

Greater London Council (1981), Guidelines for the assessment of lead pollution, Joint report of the Recreation and Community Services Policy Committee and the Planning and Communications Policy Committee, 16 February and 11 March.

Haas, T., Mache, K., Schaller, K., Wiek, A., Mache, W., Valentin, H., (1972), Untersuchungen uber die okologische bleibelastung im Kindersalter, Proceedings of an International symposium on Environmental Health Aspects of Lead, Amsterdam.

International Commission on Radiological Protection, (1975), Report of the Task Group on Reference Man, Pergamon Press.

Joselow, M.M., Banton, J.E., Fisher, W., Balentine, J., (1974), Environmental contrasts: blood lead levels of children in Honolulu and Newark, J. Environ. Health, 37, 10-12.

Johnson, D.E., Tillery, J.B., Prevost, R.J., (1975), Levels of platinum, palladium and lead in populations of Southern California, Environ. Health Perspect., 12, 27-33.

Lansdown, R.G., Clayton, B.E., Graham, P.J., Sheperd, J., Delves, H.T., Turner, W.C., (1974), Blood-lead levels, behaviour and intelligence; a population study, Lancet, (i), 538-541.

Lepow, M.L., Bruckman, L., Gillette, M., Markowitz, S., Robino, R., Kapish, J., (1975), Investigations into sources of lead in the environment of urban children, Environ. Res. 10, 415-426.

Little, P., Heard, M.J., (1978), An environmental lead survey near motorways in West London, Harwell Report AERE-R8354, HMSO, London.

Mahaffey, K.R., Annest, J.L., Barbano, H.E., Murphy, R.S., (1979), Preliminary analysis of blood-lead concentrations for children and adults: HANES II, 1976-1978, In: Trace Substances in Environmental Health - XIII, a symposium ed. D.D. Hemphill, University of Missouri, Columbia.

Millar, I.B., (1978), Monitoring of lead in the environment, J. of Epidemiol. and Commun. Health, 32, 111-116.

Nordman, C.H., (1975), Environmental lead exposure in Finland. A study of selected population groups, Academic dissertation, Institute of Occupational Health, Helsinki.

Nygaard, S-P., Ottosen, J., Hansen, J.C., (1977), Whole-blood lead concentrations in Danes: relation to age and environment, Danish Med. Bull., 24, 49-51.

Okubo, T., Tsachiya, K., Nagasake, M., Nakayima, T., Kamijyo, H., Mizoguchi, L., (1978), A further study of the biological effects of lead on urban and suburban Tokyo school children, Int. Arch. Occup. Environ. Hlth., 41, 17-23.

Ratcliffe, J.M., (1981), Lead in man and the environment, Ellis Horwood Limited, Chichester, England.

Rice, C., Fishbein, A., Lilis, R., Sarkozi, L., Steven, K., Selikoff, I.J., (1978), Lead contamination in the homes of employees of secondary lead smelters, Environ. Res., 15, 375-380.

Roels, H.A., Bucket, J.P., Lauwerys, R., Bruaux, P., Claeys-Thoreau, F., Lafontaine, A., Van Overschelde, J., Verduyn, G., (1978), Lead and cadmium absorption among children near a non-ferrous metal plant. A follow-up study of a test case, Environ. Res., 15, 290-308.

Roels, H.A., Buchet, J.P., Lauwerys, R., Bruaux, P., Claeys-Thoreau, F., Lafontaine, A., Verduyn, G., (1980), Exposure to lead by the oral and pulmonary routes of children living in the vicinity of a primary lead smelter, Environ. Res., 22, 81-94.

Roberts, T.M., Hutchinson, T.C., Paciga, J., Chattopadhyady, A., Jervis, R.E., Van Loon, J., Parkinson, D.K., (1974), Lead contamination around secondary smelters; estimation of dispersal and accumulation by humans, Science, 186, 1120-1123.

Sartor, F.A., Rondia, D., (1981), Setting legislative norms for environmental lead exposure: results of an epidemiological survey in the East of Belgium, Toxicology Letters, 7, 251-257.

Sayre, J.W., Charney, E., Vostal, J., Pless, I., (1974), House and hand dust as a potential source of childhood lead exposure, Am. J. Dis. Child., 127, 167-170.

Schmitt, N., Philion, J.J., Larsen, A.A., Harnadedk, M., Lynch, A.J., (1979), Surface soil as a potential source of lead exposure for young children, Canad. Med. J., 121, 1474-1478.

Stephens, R.A., (1978), The total relationship between airborne lead and body lead burdens, Proceedings of a Symposium on Lead Pollution, Health Effects, at University College London, 1978. The Conservation Society, London.

Taskinen, H., Nordman, H., Hernberg, S., (1981), Blood-lead levels in Finnish preschool children, Sci. Total Environ., 20, 117-129.

Ter Haar, G., (1979), In: Proceedings of an International Conference on Heavy Metals in the Environment, Imperial College, London.

Turner, A.C., Carroll, J.D., (1980), The determination of environmental lead near works and roads in conjunction with the EC blood-lead survey 1978-9, Warren Spring Laboratory Report LR 189 (AP), Stevenage, U.K.

Waldron, H.A., (1975), Lead levels in blood of residents near the M6-A38 (M) interchange, Birmingham, Nature, 253, 345-346.

Walter, S.D., Yankel, A.J., von Lindern, I.H., (1980), Age-specific risk factors for lead absorption in children, Arch. Environ. Health, 35, 53-58.

Watson, W.W., Witherell, L.E., Giguerre, G.C., (1978), Increased lead absorption in children of workers in a lead storage battery plant, J. Occup. Med., 20, 759-761.

Worth, D., Craum, G., Karelekas, P., De Vos, E., Liberman, M., Matrange, A., Ryan, C., (1978), The contribution of household tap water to blood lead levels. Proceedings of Second International Symposium on Environmental Lead Research, Cincinatti, Academic Press.

Yankel, A.J., von Lindern, I.H., Walter, D.S., (1977), The Silver Valley Study: the relationship between childhood blood lead levels and environmental exposure, J. Air Pollut. Control Assoc., 27, 763-767.

Zielhuis, R.L., del Castilho, P., Herber, R.F.M., Wibowo, A.A.E., (1978), Levels of lead and other metals in human blood: suggestive relationships, determining factors, Environ. Health Perspect., 25, 103-109.

Lead Versus Health
Edited by M. Rutter and R. Russell Jones
© 1983 John Wiley & Sons Ltd.

THE CONTRIBUTION OF LEAD IN PETROL TO HUMAN
LEAD INTAKE

Dr. Robin Russell Jones, MRCP,
Deputy Chairman, CLEAR,
2 Northdown Street
London, N1.

Dr. Robert Stephens, Ph.D., D.Sc.,
University of Birmingham,
PO Box 363
Birmingham, B15 2TT.

ENVIRONMENTAL STUDIES

Introduction. The input from lead in petrol to humans is a controversial issue. Many different methods have been used to quantify this contribution and the subject is complicated by the multiplicity of routes by which lead in air gains access to the human system. This review attempts to resolve some of the confusion existing in the literature by a critical analysis of the methods which have been used to investigate the problem.

The alimentary and respiratory tracts are the main portals of entry of lead into man and animals. Consequently most lead gains access to the human system as a result of man's basic biological functions ... eating, drinking and breathing. However, lead in food, water and air is derived from both natural and industrial sources. In order to quantify the contribution of lead in petrol to lead in humans it is necessary to know the relative contribution of each source to each pathway. In addition, fortuitous ingestion of lead-rich dust, dirt, soil, or paint pose additional hazards, especially in young children in whom hand to mouth activities are common. Of these various types of exposure only paint can be identified with certainty as a source. The remainder represent pathways of exposure to man from sources of lead which may be either industrial or natural.

These preliminary considerations are crucial since much of the literature (and most of the confusion) is concerned with the relative contribution of lead in food, air and water to man's total lead intake. Using this type of analysis appears deceptively simple since the relative uptake of lead by the pulmonary and gastro-intestinal routes can be measured with some precision in human volunteers by means of stable lead isotopes. (Chamberlain et al., 1975; Rabinowitz et al., 1977). What cannot be measured with such precision, however, is the relative contribution that lead in petrol makes to each pathway. Although it is generally agreed that lead

Dr. Robin Russell Jones, MRCP
Dr. Robert Stephens, Ph.D., D.Sc.

in petrol accounts for over 90 per cent of atmospheric lead, the contribution of airborne lead to lead in food and lead in dust is still a controversial subject. Yet, unless some estimate is derived for these two pathways, any subsequent analysis is meaningless for the assessment of the contribution of lead in petrol to human lead intake. These problems are well illustrated by the report of the DHSS Working Party on lead in the environment. (Department of Health and Social Security, 1980). In Table 13 of that report the relative input from food (45-90%), water (0-45%) and air (10-20%) are quantified for urban adults. There is room for disagreement on the precise figures that should be attached to each of these three pathways and on their applicability to children, but the general message is not in dispute. The problem, however, arises when an attempt is made to identify sources of lead in food. Natural and man-made varieties are mentioned, and three types of contamination resulting from human activities are itemised: lead solder in canned foods; uptake of lead by food from tap water during cooking; and contamination of soil crops and food by lead in air and lead in dust. Canned foods are calculated to contribute approximately 15% of dietary intake and the contribution from cooking water is shown to vary from 0-55%, depending upon the lead concentration and hardness of the tap water. It is clear, however, that these calculations leave a substantial residue unaccounted for. Indeed, the origin of 85% of lead in food prior to cooking remains unexplained. It is not clear from the published document whether this should be attributed to natural or industrial sources, but unless some attempt is made to quantify the relative contribution from each, any subsequent conclusions about the contribution of lead in petrol to human lead intake are liable to be in serious error.

Another aspect of this problem that requires close attention is the analytical procedures used for the measurement of dietary lead. These relate both to the sensitivity of the method and the precautions taken to exclude sample contamination. Both require particular attention if accurate measurements are to be obtained at lead concentrations below one part per million. Many dietary surveys have been undertaken over the last three or four decades, and many different estimates for dietary lead intake from food have been offered. Yet, the degree of variation may reflect nothing more than the sensitivity of the method used and the skill with which these measures were carried out. This problem has been highlighted by recent studies in Australia where improved methods of chemical analysis have shown that lead in a range of 'dust-free' Australian foods is seven to ten times lower than those previously reported. (Kacprzak, 1982). Indeed, it has been estimated that the daily lead absorption for a three year old child from food and drink is only 9.5 μg rather than the 62.5 μg used in the Australian Academy of Science Report (1981). Clearly, such claims require verification. At the same time, they raise the possibility that the lead content of typical diets may have increased over the past few decades, without this being reflected in official surveys.

Such considerations are even more crucial when dealing with material that derives its lead content from natural, as opposed to industrial, sources. According to Patterson (Chapter 2), it is possible to measure the lead content of fish muscle, ancient trees, prehistoric snow strata, and oceanic depths only by the use of ultra-clean laboratory conditions and an appropriately sensitive method of quantitative analysis (isotopic dilution mass spectrometry). Over the past two decades, these techniques have been applied by scientists at the California Institute of Technology to the measurement of lead at concentrations which conventional methods are unable to verify. Despite the availability of these data, however, official documents continue to rely on estimates for natural levels of lead that are known to be in error by one to three orders of magnitude. This tendency is unfortunate since it encourages the belief that much of man's lead intake is derived from natural rather than industrial sources.

SOURCES OF LEAD IN AIR

Although considerable data exist on the relative contribution from natural and industrial sources to lead in air, a scientific consensus has proved harder to achieve. Data for natural emissions in Table 1 were obtained by measuring lead/silicate ratios in fumarolic gases from high and low halogen emitting volcanoes under ultra-clean laboratory conditions. (Patterson, 1980). Such phenomena account for less than 1 per cent of total lead emissions to the atmosphere and the data identify natural sources as insignificant contributors to atmospheric lead levels. At the other extreme, estimates of up to 210,000 tons have been derived from data not obtained under ultra-clean laboratory conditions (Goldberg and Gross, 1971); these figures were used by the DHSS Working Party in their report "Lead and Health" (DHSS 1980). By contrast, the National Academy of Science report (1980) relied on data that identified a contribution of less than 5 per cent from natural sources to lead in air (Nriagu, 1979), and accepted that the figure may well be less than 1 per cent (Settle and Patterson, 1980). Clearly, some attempt should be made to rationalise this situation since two official reports produced in the same year differed in their assessment of the natural input of lead to air by a factor of one hundred. Normally, values obtained using improved techniques replace data obtained by earlier, less precise measurement. Alternatively, if the more recent data are to be rejected, then the reasons for doing so should be stated. Until normal scientific procedures are followed, the debate about the contribution from natural sources of lead will probably remain unresolved.

The input from industrial sources to lead in air is not in serious dispute. Of the 450,000 tons emitted annually, approximately 273,000 tons derives from the combustion of petrol and sump oil. However, the contribution to ambient air lead levels from motor vehicles is disproportionately high since most of the industrial lead processes are associated with the production of large lead particulates which fall out close to the emission source (Roberts 1974).

Dr. Robin Russell Jones, MRCP
          Dr. Robert Stephens, Ph.D., D.Sc.

By contrast, the internal combustion engine represents a mobile
source which emits lead as a fine aerosol with over 90 per cent of
the particles less than 0.1 μm in diameter. Particles in this size
distribution remain airborne for long periods, they are carried large
distances by the prevailing winds (Facchetti, 1979), they are
readily respired and they are easily absorbed (Morrow et al.,
1980). The addition of lead to petrol has therefore created a
source of lead that is unique in terms of its capacity to penetrate
the environment and the human system.

TABLE 1.   Air lead emissions (worldwide)

NATURAL*   tonnes per year

Volcanic and windblown dust	2,000
Forest fires 500	
Vegetation	1,000
Sea spray	20
TOTAL	3,520

INDUSTRIAL**

Petrol and oil burning	273,000
Non ferrous metal processes	85,500
Iron smelting	50,000
Industrial lead processes	7,400
Coal burning	14,000
Wood burning	4,500
Waste burning	8,900
Miscellaneous	6,000
TOTAL	449,300

NATURAL	:	INDUSTRIAL
0.8		99.2

* Data from National Academy of Science (1980)

** Data from Nriagu, J.O. (1979)

Over 90 per cent of atmospheric lead is derived from motor vehicle
emissions (DHSS 1980). Although air lead values in rural sites are
considerably lower than those found in urban areas, the global
impact of petrol lead technology is not apparent until deposition
rates at rural sites are compared with levels that existed in
prehistoric times.

The estimated natural concentration of lead in air is about 0.04 ng/m³ and it is interesting that levels of this order have been recorded recently in the westerly winds of the North Atlantic (Chester et al., 1974). Overland the lowest recorded air lead concentration is 0.23 ng/m³. Ambient air lead levels in rural areas of Britain range between 50 and 500 ng/m³ (Cawse, 1974-77), whilst average air lead levels in major European cities range from 400 to 8000 ng/m³ (World Health Organisation), 1977). In urban areas, atmospheric lead levels therefore exceed rural levels by a factor of only ten, whereas rural levels exceed natural levels by a factor of one thousand. These calculations are borne out by comparing air/soil ratios of lead with non-industrial elements such as scandium, which gave rise to an enrichment factor for lead of 1100 at Plymlimon, a remote mountain area in North Wales (Peirson et al., 1973).

These measurements support the early observations of Patterson (1965). As long ago as 1963 it was reported that lead concentrations in snow 800 km east of Los Angeles were elevated ten thousand times above natural concentrations (Tatusomoto and Patterson, 1963); this input of industrial lead to snow has also been demonstrated in remote areas of Norway and elsewhere (Elgmork et al., 1973; Ashmead, 1972). Later it was shown that over 97 per cent of the lead entering the Thomson Canyon, a remote site in the high Sierra crest, was derived from industrial sources (Hirano and Patterson, 1974). Again, these observations were supported by more recent studies which document the transfer of industrial lead into a remote alpine basin (Schinner, 1980) and a north American deciduous forest (Lindberg et al., 1981). One aspect of this process which gives cause for concern is the cumulative effect of lead emissions in the environment. Thus, the doubling time of lead in the humus of a northern hardwood forest is about 50 years (Siccama and Smith, 1978), while the total lead content of the organic matter of the forest floors in central Massachusetts have increased by 70 per cent between 1962 and 1978 (Siccama et al., 1980). The contribution that lead in petrol has made to this situation can best be assessed from studies which document lead levels in the northern ice cap over the past 3,000 years (Murozomi et al., 1969). Lead silicate dust ratios remained virtually constant until the onset of the industrial revolution in 1750. After this time lead levels rose gradually until about 1940, since when the rise has been exponential (Chapter 2, figure 2). A similar chronological sequence is documented in pond sediments from the Thompson Canyon (Chapter 2, figure 3). Organo-lead compounds were first used as petrol additives in 1923 and world-wide exploitation of this technology coincided with the upsurge of lead concentrations recorded at the above sites. In toto, the current flux of lead to the earth's surface is about 300 times its natural value (O'Brien et al., 1980). These data demonstrate that atmospheric lead is equivalent to industrial lead; that lead found in rural air derives mainly from urban emissions; and that the proposition that air lead contains a substantial contribution from natural sources is no longer consistent with the available evidence.

Dr. Robin Russell Jones, MRCP
Dr. Robert Stephens, Ph.D., D.Sc.

SOURCES OF LEAD IN FOOD

Soil Lead. As mentioned previously, it is the inability of most analytical procedures to differentiate between natural and industrial lead, combined with official statements that people derive most of their lead from food, that has generated the impression that most people derive their lead from natural sources (Department of the Environment, 1974; Department of Health and Social Security, 1980). Improved analytical methods have modified these attitudes, and it is now conceded by legislative advisers that lead ingested via food and drink has a significant industrial input (Australian Academy of Science, 1981). Considerable controversy still exists, however, on the relative contribution of industrial lead and natural lead to the lead content of soil and its subsequent uptake by plants and crops. Thus, a recent study in Toulouse found a high "natural" blood lead concentration attributed to the high levels of "soluble" lead in the soils of south-west France (4.5 ppm) (Servant and Delapart, 1981), and it has been suggested that the lead content of UK food may be elevated because its base rocks are richer in lead than some other countries (Tolan and Elton, 1972). There are several reasons why such claims should be treated with caution. First, there are a number of barriers which diminish the movement of lead from soil to animals and man (Kahn, 1980) including chemical speciation of lead in the soil by interaction with inorganic and organic species like phosphates and humates (Miller et al., 1975; Pauli, 1975), plant root binding by pectates (Ramamoorthy and Leppard, 1977) and accumulation of lead in xylem sites within plants (Tanton and Crowdy, 1971). All combine to protect the new vegetation and the fruiting and flowering of plants from lead. As a general guide, a ten-fold reduction from roots to foliage and a similar reduction from foliage to fruit means that 100 ppm of lead taken up by the roots would result in grain containing about 1 ppm (O'Brien, 1979). Extraordinary fluctuations in the "natural" lead content of soil would therefore be required to explain the observation that remote civilisations have blood lead levels one tenth of those found in modern industrial societies (Poole and Smythe, 1980; Hecker et al., 1974; Piomelli et al., 1980). In fact the lead content of agricultural soil in the U.K. (30 ppm) is only twice the average lead content of the earth's crust (16 ppm) (Swaine, 1955). Furthermore, analogues of lead such as barium do not show significant fluctuations in human subjects despite geographic variation in the barium contents of soil-bearing substrates (Ericson et al., 1979).

It seems more likely that the fluctuations occurring in the lead content of soils result mainly from industrial sources: either airborne fallout onto agricultural land, or from the direct disposal of lead-containing wastes, such as fertilisers made from lead-rich sewage sludge. In one instance, 35 years of sludge application raised the soil lead concentration from 61 to 1015 ppm, a level sufficient to cause illness and death of cattle (DeJonghe, 1981). Although not so dramatic, the impact of airborne fallout of industrial lead is equally important because of its ubiquitous nature.   As mentioned previously, the Thompson Canyon studies were successful in accurately quantifying the impact of industrial lead on remote ecosystems and an enrichment factor of ten was calculated for the lead content in the humus fraction of the upper five centimetres of soil in remote watersheds (Elias et al., 1975). For agricultural sites, the input to soil from industrial conurbations is considerably greater and has been documented in several major European countries (Ronneau and Hallet, 1981; Rohbock et al., 1981).

TABLE 2.   Mean lead deposition rates at different locations

	$\mu g/m^2/day$
Rural (UK)	70
Rural (France)	40
Urban (Swansea, London, Birmingham) (1974)	100
Birmingham 'Spaghetti Junction' (M6-A 38 M)	966
A446/M1 Junction	330
Chelsea Embankment	630
Chelsea Physic Garden	98
London (representative value)	148
Greenland	0.08
Antarctica	0.01

Data from Bryce-Smith and Stephens (1980)

Table 2 shows the mean lead deposition rates for different locations in Europe, Greenland and Antarctica.   Although urban exceeds rural tenfold, the most significant difference is that rural deposition rate in the UK are one thousand times greater than in Greenland and almost ten thousand times greater than in Antartica.

It is important to maintain this perspective when assessing the contribution of lead in petrol to dietary lead.   It is known from studies of naturally occurring lead isotopes that airborne lead will penetrate the upper five to ten centimetres of soil (Moore and Poet, 1976; Robbins, 1978; Servant and Delapart, 1979), and that this process will be accelerated by agricultural processes such as ploughing.   Since root crops derive most of their lead content from the upper few centimetres of soil, it cannot be assumed that they are protected from airborne pollution simply because they grow underground.   In highly contaminated areas these effects are readily apparent.   For example, the lead content of London soil ensures that root crops (radishes) grown within ten kilometres of Marble Arch are statutorily unfit for human consumption (Davies et al., 1979).   In rural areas, the relative input from industrial

Dr. Robin Russell Jones, MRCP
Dr. Robert Stephens, Ph.D., D.Sc.

sources to the lead content of root crops is more difficult to quantify. It should be emphasised, however, that this difficulty stems from a lack of precise data in this area, rather than from any evidence to the contrary. It seems highly probable that the lead content of arable soils is increasing and will continue to increase as a result of man's industrial activities. As O'Brien has pointed out, the present inputs of lead to agricultural land will commit man to increase lead burdens for several generations into the future (O'Brien, 1979).

Airborne Lead. Although airborne fallout can contribute significantly to the uptake of lead by plants from soil, its main impact is direct deposition on the leafy parts of vegetables and crops. This route is of particular concern from a biological point of view since it by-passes the barriers to the translocation of lead developed in natural ecosystems. These effects were clearly demonstrated in the Thompson Canyon studies where the translocation of a non-essential element, barium, through a natural ecosystem was compared with that of lead (Patterson, 1980; Elias et al., 1982). Although barium has industrial uses, these do not involve the production of barium aerosols. The biopurification of calcium with respect to barium during the transfer of calcium from rock to carnivore is shown in figure 4, Chapter 2. It will be observed that natural barriers for the translocation of barium cause the barium/calcium ratio to fall by a factor of one thousand. The biopurification of calcium with respect to lead is shown in figure 5, Chapter 2. It will be observed that the fall in the Pb/Ca ratio is decelerated by the input of airborne lead to soil and is further slowed by direct deposition of lead onto the surface of vegetation and is then reversed by the additional input to the carnivore from the deposition of lead onto fur. This means that the observed Pb/ca ratio in carnivores is increased fifty fold above the ratio anticipated from studies of the lead analogue barium.

For agricultural crops grown in close proximity to urban areas the impact of direct fallout of airborne lead will be correspondingly greater (deposition rates shown in Table 2 will apply). Furthermore the road network ensures that many more acres of agricultural land are in close proximity to vehicle emissions. It has been pointed out, for example, that in the United States there are approximately 3×10^6 kilometres of road with an average weekday traffic flow of greater tan 1,000 vehicles hourly. Since the largest particulates are confined to a 50 metre zone on either side of the roadway, the size of the roadside ecosystem in the US with grossly elevated lead levels may approximate 118 square miles (Smith, 1976). Considerable evidence for such contamination has been published (Chow, 1970; Everett et al., 1967; Motto et al., 1940; Page et al., 1971; Williamson and Evans, 1972; Rabinowitz, 1972; Graham and Kalman, 1974; Ward et al., 1977; Little and Wiffen, 1977; Ward et al., 1978; Farmer, 1979; Wheeler and Rolfe, 1979; Flanagan et al., 1980; Koslow et al., 1977; Healy and Aslam, 1980), and the lead content of crops grown in such locations often renders them statutorily unfit for human consumption.

It is, therefore, unfortunate that no attempts are made to limit the use of such land for agricultural purposes. Statements that such contamination can be removed by normal washing procedures are factually incorrect. Even thorough laboratory washing procedures only removes 50 per cent of deposited lead due to the inclusion of lead in stomata, retention by cuticularwax, and possibly electro-static sources depending on the type of leaf (Arvik and Zimdahl, 1974; Lagerwerff et al., 1973; Gange and Joshi, 1971).

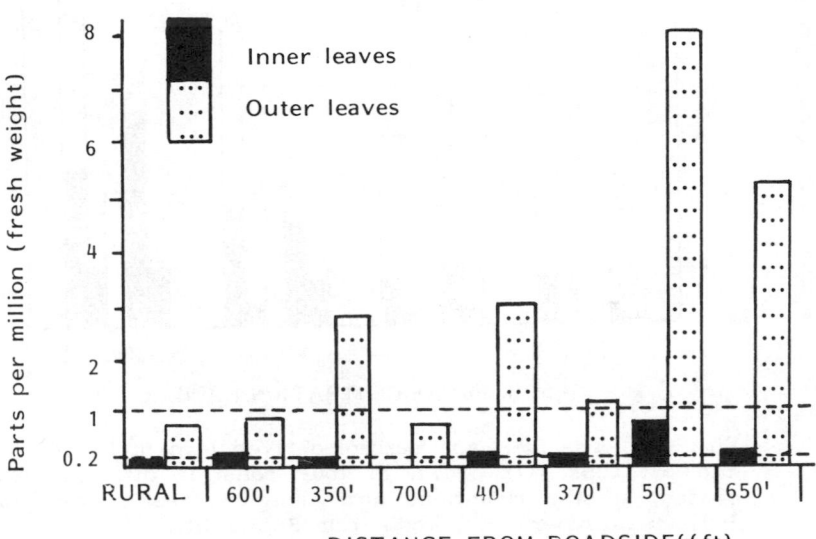

Fig. 1.   Lead levels in cabbages. Data from Bryce-Smith and Stephens, 1980.

One method of assessing the relative impact of lead in air and lead in soil on plants is to measure the lead content of outer leaves (which are exposed directly to airborne pollution) with the lead content of inner leaves (whose lead uptake is mainly from soil). Studies on cabbages have shown a ratio of approximately 10:1. Absolute values are lower in rural areas but the same ratio still applies. It is of interest that even in rural areas the lead content of outer cabbage leaves renders them statutorily unfit for use in canned infant food (See Fig. 1).

Similar results are obtained by comparing the relative inputs of aerosol and soil lead to lettuce and oat crops grown in soils of different lead content in mountains and along a heavily trafficked main road (Rabinowitz, 1972).

Dr. Robin Russell Jones, MRCP
           Dr. Robert Stephens, Ph.D., D.Sc.

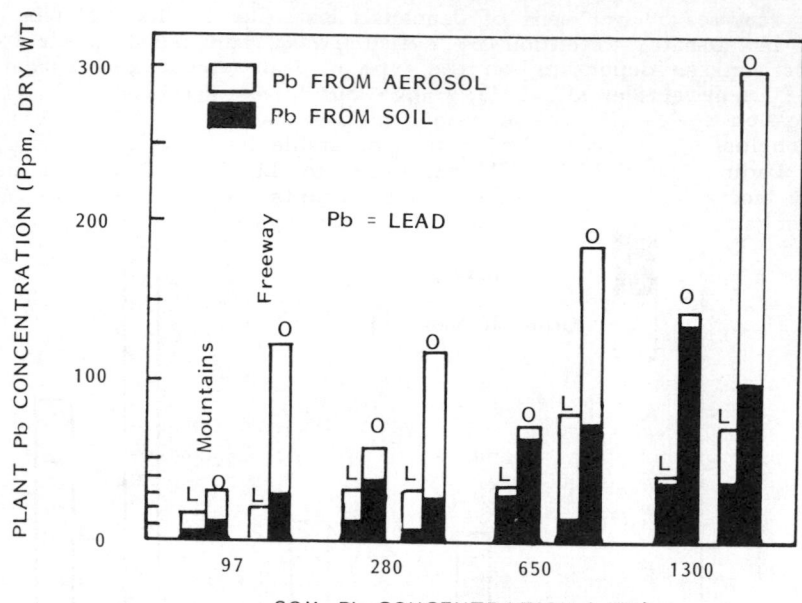

Fig. 2.   The soil- and aerosol-derived lead in lettuce (L)
and oat tops (O) grown in four soils of different lead
content in the mountains and along a freeway carrying
360,000 cars per day. Data from Rabinowitz, 1972.

Very high levels of lead in soil are necessary before uptake of lead
from soil even approximates to direct fallout of airborne lead.   The
average lead content of U.K. soil (30 ppm) means that most above
ground crops derive most of their input from airborne fallout even
in remote country areas.   Thus, a Danish study found that grass
grown in a rural area derived 90-99 per cent of its lead content
from airborne sources (Tjell, 1979).   Such studies also identified
airborne lead as the main lead source for grazing livestock.
Although this view has been challenged by others (Crump and
Barlow, 1982) it is supported by studies of radioactive ^{210}Pb.

^{210}Pb is a natural source of airborne lead produced in the
atmosphere by the radioactive decay of the noble gas ^{222}Rn.   It
has a half life of 22 years and can therefore be used as a
radioactive tracer for the pathways through marine and terrestrial
ecosystems which link lead in air to lead in man.   The fact that
such studies have proved successful is testimony to the exquisite
sensitivity of the methods available since total global fallout of
^{210}Pb is only 5 kilograms per year (Robbins, 1978).   Since the

contribution from the decay of ^{222}Rn in soil is negligible, ^{210}Pb in the upper 20 centimetres of soil is derived almost exclusively from airborne fallout (Robbins, 1978; Moore and Poet, 1976; Servant and Delapart, 1979). In consequence, the concentration of ^{210}Pb found in human teeth does not vary appreciably even though soil ^{222}Rn concentrations vary considerably according to the type of base rock found locally (Holtzman, 1978).

Studies on the relative uptake of ^{210}Pb from soil and air confirm the conclusions derived from studies of stable lead (Berger et al., 1965; Ladinskaya et al., 1973; Aarkrog and Lippert, 1971). Thus barley accumulated only very small amounts of ^{210}Pb from soil (Wilson and Cline, 1966) while cabbages again show substantial quantities of ^{210}Po (a decay product of ^{210}Pb) in outer leaves but not in inner leaves (Francis et al. 1968). One review concluded that both direct deposition and root absorption occurs but that the former is ten to a hundred times greater than the latter (Parfenov, 1974).

^{210}Pb has also been used to identify the contribution of air lead to lead in animals and humans. An early study showed that the ^{210}Pb content of ox bone was higher than that of human bone and this may reflect direct uptake of ^{210}Pb from soil by grazing livestock (Hill and Jaworowski, 1961). More recently, ^{210}Pb and stable lead concentrations in the liver and kidneys of cattle grazing in a rural area were shown to be significantly correlated (Bunzl et al., 1979). However, when cattle were grazed on old mining land with a lead content of 7,000 ppm in soil and 6.8 ppm in fresh grass, no correlation was found (Bunzl et al., 1980).

About two dozen studies of ^{210}Pb in man have involved analysis of bones and teeth and ^{210}Pb concentrations have been related to the level of ^{210}Pb in air (Holtzman, 1965). The significance of these findings can be assessed by comparing the total global fallout of ^{210}Pb (5 kilograms per year) with the total fallout of exhaust lead (4×10^8 kg per year). It is difficult to deny that anthropogenic lead contributes significantly to dietary lead through airborne fallout when confronted with the pathways mapped out by ^{210}Pb.

(c) Processing and Preparation. Major contamination of foodstuffs results from the use of lead soldered cans and these are now banned as containers for infant food. For other children and for adults, diets with an average proportion of canned foods contain 15 per cent more lead than diets which exclude such foods (Department of Health and Social Security, 1980; Australian National Health and Medical Research Council, 1979).

Contamination of foodstuffs by airborne lead may also occur after harvesting. It is unfortunate that food processing factories and air drying procedures tend to be carried out in urban locations where contamination by lead-rich dust can provide an additional input of industrial lead to the diet. Similar considerations apply in the home where foodstuffs may become further contaminated by lead-rich dust

Dr. Robin Russell Jones, MRCP
Dr. Robert Stephens, Ph.D., D.Sc.

during preparation and at meal times. These ubiquitous forms of dietary lead are seldom acknowledged in official estimates. Since 1974, annual total dietary surveys in the U.K. have indicated an average mean lead intake of 113 μg based on a food intake of 1.34 kg per day, but it is not clear what percentage of this intake can be attributed to contamination of the dietary samples after harvesting.

The impact of industrial sources on relatively uncontaminated nutrients was demonstrated by Settle and Patterson (1980) who showed a lead content of 0.03 ng/g in tuna fish from relatively unpolluted waters, 7 ng/g in a dye-punched unsoldered can, and 1400 ng/g in a lead-soldered can. Technologies routinely used in the handling and processing of foodstuffs may therefore elevate their lead content some 5,000 times. Obviously with more highly contaminated samples such as land based food crops the enrichment factor is considerably less, but stringent precautions are still necessary if large positive errors are to be avoided in the laboratory analysis of dietary lead at concentrations below 1 ppm.

SOURCES OF LEAD IN WATER

Without the benefit of ultra-clean laboratories the lead content of marine water and fresh water is difficult to determine and little confidence can be placed in published data. The natural lead content of marine water must be estimated from past inputs to the sediments and residence times in surface waters. By such procedures it has been estimated that the prehistoric natural lead content in the surface waters of the North Pacific was about 5 ng lead per kilogram of water (Schaule and Patterson, 1979; Patterson, 1980). Industrial lead input to surface waters in the Northern Hemisphere have raised the lead content of the upper 1,000 metres, and depth profiles of lead indicate an input about 40 times greater than that due to the natural weathering of the earth (Chapter 2, Table 1). Thus, even in coastal waters with relatively low levels of lead (25 ng per kilogram), it can be shown by the use of stable lead isotopes that most of the lead is derived from motor vehicle emissions (Stukas and Wong, 1981). Similarly, a recent Government survey of North Sea pollution came to the conclusion that 58 per cent of the industrial input derives from atmospheric fallout (Monitor, 1982). The major contributor to lead in marine ecosystems is therefore identified as lead in petrol.

The natural level of lead in fresh water is estimated to be less than 20 ng/kg but background levels are commonly elevated one hundred fold, even in remote watersheds (Patterson, 1980). Although such levels are still low by comparison with the lead content of tap water, there is no justification for assuming that the lead content of fresh water represents a natural level prior to its entry into the distribution system. The lead content of tap water varies markedly according to the plumbosolvency of the water supply and the amount of lead in the distribution system which may be present in the form of lead-lined tanks, lead pipes or lead solder. The widespread use of lead stabilisers in PVC piping represents a more modern type of exposure.

Adult lead intake from water commonly ranges from 15-30 µg per day but lead taken up by foodstuffs from water during cooking can be an additional source of ingested lead. Vegetables and rice cooked in water containing lead may absorb up to 80 per cent of the lead in the water (Little et al., 1981).

SOURCES OF LEAD IN DUST

The literature which identifies lead in dust as an important route of exposure for pre-school children is summarised by Duggan (Chapter 7) and may be itemised as follows:

1. Children of lead workers show elevated lead burdens and this must result from contamination of the home environment by lead-rich dust brought home on clothing.

2. Blood lead levels in children (but not adults) are correlated with levels of lead in soil.

3. A peak in blood lead levels is seen in the early years of life. Although this has been attributed to higher gastro-intestinal uptake of lead, the child/mother blood lead ratios are higher in urban areas than in rural areas.

4. Values for alpha (the factor which relates air lead and blood lead) derived from clinical studies on children are higher than corresponding studies in adults. This suggests an important route of exposure to airborne lead that is independent of the pulmonary route.

Although the importance of lead in dust to children's intake has been a subject of some controversy, there is little doubt that the hand to mouth activities commonly observed in young children, combined with a high rate of gastrointestinal absorption, could make a significant contribution to their lead intake. Thus, Vostal et al., (1974) found 20 µg of lead per hand for city children and 5 µg per hand for suburban children. Assuming a sucking frequency of ten times per day, Duggan and Williams (1977) derived an intake of 50 µg of lead per day and a gut absorption of 12 µg per day. Duggan calculated that urban dust containing 1,000 ppm of lead would raise a two year old's blood lead level by 5 µg/dl (Duggan, 1980). Similar figures have been derived by Day et al., (1975) who calculated that between 5 and 50 µg of lead can be transferred via sticky sweets.

Urban dust might also contain particles of leaded paint, but as a general rule such particles are not so easily absorbed as petrol-derived compounds by virtue of their chemical composition and larger particle size, (Barltrop and Meek, 1979). There is good evidence that car exhaust particulates are the main contributors to lead in roadway dust (Linton et al., 1980; Biggins and Harrison, 1980), and that they also contribute substantially to dusts collected in the vicinity of buildings, even those bearing high lead paint and situated some distance from a road. Unfortunately the same techniques have not been used on household dust, and it is more difficult to assess precisely the relative contribution of airborne lead and paint to exposure within the home (Jaworski, 1978). It is known, however, that concentrations of airborne lead within houses are directly related to concentrations outdoors and that "the home offers little if any protection from atmospheric particulate lead", (Butler and Macmurdo, 1974). Furthermore, internal dust lead levels of 600-680 ppm are typically found in small urban communities even in well-kept homes with low lead paintwork (Solomon and Hartford, 1976).

Undoubtedly the deterioration of leaded paintwork can raise internal dust concentrations to alarmingly high levels, but evidence that this is of significance to general population exposure is lacking. No study has managed to resolve this problem totally but such data as are available suggest a very weak correlation between blood lead in children and their exposure to leaded paint (Chapter 4, figure 8). Another general population study concluded that lead in paint is not a significant route of exposure except for individuals who display pica (Walter, 1980). Until more data are available it is difficult to quantify precisely the relative contribution of airborne lead and paint lead to lead in dust. At the same time, this lack of information should not be used to obscure the general impact of airborne lead in urban areas. There is a direct relationship between levels of lead in street dust and traffic flow (See Chapter 6, Table 2), and street dust will be carried into urban households on shoes and clothing. A rise in household dust concentrations from 500 to 1,000 ppm was documented by the Environmental Health Department, Bristol, following the opening of a nearby traffic system (Personal Communication). It would be difficult to account for such changes in terms of lead in paint.

CONCLUSIONS

As mentioned previously, the contribution of lead in petrol to lead in humans can be quantified only if the relative contribution of each source to each pathway is known. Patterson has calculated that for a typical urban dweller the enrichment factors for food, water and air are 100, 750 and 21,000 times respectively (see Table 3). If Patterson's calculations are correct, it means that less than 1 per cent of lead in each compartment is derived from natural sources. That is a crucial figure which requires verification. Perhaps the most reliable method for testing the validity of these data is the direct measurement of the lead burdens in skeletal remains from pre-technological societies. Thus, Ericson et al., (1979) found a total lead burden of 3×10^{-4} grams in the skeletal remains of ancient Peruvians living 1600 years ago, and values of the same order have been obtained by other workers analysing bones and teeth from ancient Nubia and Egypt (Grandjean et al., 1979;

TABLE 3.   Relative lead absorptions of urban dwellers
(ng per day)

	Natural*	Contemporary Urban**	Enrichment Factor
Water	2.0	1,500	750
Air	0.3	6,400	21,333
Food	210	21,000	100

Adapted from: National Academy of Science (1980)

* Natural:
$$Air = 0.04 \text{ ng m}^{-3} \times 20 \text{ m}^3 \times 0.4;$$
$$Water = < 20 \text{ ng kg}^{-1} \times 1.0 \text{ kg d}^{-1} \times 0.1;$$
$$Food = < 2.0 \text{ ng g}^{-1} \times 1.5 \text{ kg d}^{-1} \times 0.07$$

** Urban:
$$Air = 800 \text{ ng m}^{-3} \times 20 \text{ m}^3 \times 0.4;$$
$$Water = 15,000 \text{ ng kg}^{-1} \times 1.0 \text{ kgd}^{-1} \times 0.1;$$
$$Food = 200 \text{ ng g}^{-1} \times 1.5 \text{ kg g}^{-1} \times 0.07$$

Shapiro et al., 1978). Lead burdens found in industrialised man today are typically elevated five hundred times above these levels (Chapter 2, figure 1). The identification of extremely low pre-technological body lead burdens therefore demonstrates that natural levels of dietary lead were also extremely low, and indicate a natural blood lead level of less than 0.2 µg/dl. By contrast, blood lead levels of non-technological civilisations living in remote areas of the world today are in the 1-5 µg/dl range (Poole and Smythe, 1980; Hecker et al., 1974; Piomelli et al., 1980). Although this is almost ten times less than those found in industrialised societies, it is still ten times greater than that which existed in prehistoric times.

Table 4 identifies the four main pathways that comprise the lead intake of a two year old urban child and the relative contribution that lead in petrol makes to each. Gastrointestinal absorption has not been precisely measured in this age group; but since this is known to fall from 50 per cent in infancy to 10 per cent in adult life, a figure of 25 per cent is used for the gastrointestinal uptake of lead in food (Alexander et al., 1973).

The absorption rate for lead particulates in urban dust is probably higher and a gastrointestinal uptake of 40 per cent is used to calculate the daily intake via this route. A figure of 40 per cent is used also for the pulmonary absorption of airborne lead (Chamberlain et al., 1975).

It will be observed from Table 4 that the high rate of gastrointestinal absorption in children reduces the relative input via the pulmonary route to 7.5 per cent. However, neurotoxins tend to be more potent when inhaled than when swallowed and urban air contains a significant proportion of organolead compounds (Grandjean,

Dr. Robin Russell Jones, MRCP
Dr. Robert Stephens, Ph.D., D.Sc.

Chapter 9). Consequently, the pulmonary route may be toxicologically important even though inhalation accounts for only a small percentage of total lead intake. In this context it is particularly unfortunate that Western toxicologists have explored only the effects of ingested lead in biological systems.

TABLE 4. Contribution of lead in petrol to the lead intake of a 2 year old urban child.

	Route	Input (µg/day)	Percentage of Total	Contribution from lead in petrol to each route	Contribution from lead in petrol to human lead intake
1.	AIR	3^a	7.5	0.9*	6.75
2.	DUST	14^b	35.0	0.9** x 0.9*	28.35
3.	FOOD	20^c	50.0	0.75^+ x 0.9*	33.75
4.	WATER	3^d	7.5	0.1^{++}	0.75

TOTAL 69.60 %

Input

(a) 3 µg of lead by 40% lung absorption from 7.5 m³ of air containing lead at 1 µg/m³.

(b) 14 µg of lead by a 40% gut absorption from 35 mgm of dust containing lead at 1,000 ppm.

(c) 20 µg of lead by a 25% gut absorption from 0.8 kg of food containing 0.1 ppm of lead.

(d) 3 ug of lead by a 25% gut absorption from 1.2 litres of water containing lead at 10 µg/L.

Conversion Factors

* 0.9 represents a 90% contribution from petrol lead to lead in air containing 1 µg/m³.

** 0.9 represents a 90% contribution from airborne lead to dust containing 1,000 ppm of lead.

+ 0.75 represents an overall contribution of 75% from airborne lead to the lead content of foodstuffs.

++ 0.1 represents a contribution of 10% from airborne lead to tap water containing lead at 10 µg/L.

The second route of exposure for urban children is the fortuitous ingestion of lead-rich dust and this is calculated to contribute approximately 35 per cent of lead intake. This figure includes the transfer of lead-rich dust via fingers and food, and should be distinguished from the contamination of foodstuffs by dust which occurs during cultivation and processing. This latter contribution is reflected in the lead content of food and will be equivalent for both rural and urban populations. By contrast, the contamination of food during preparation and at mealtimes will be higher in urban than in rural households and is therefore included under route 2 in Table 4.

The second part of the analysis deals with the contribution that lead in petrol makes to each of the four routes identified in Table 4. This is almost total for air (greater than 90%) and probably negligible for water (less than 10%). For urban dust containing 1,000 ppm of lead, a contribution from airborne sources of 90 per cent produces a figure of approximately 28 per cent for the contribution of lead in petrol to children's lead intake via the lead in dust route. This figure may need to be revised when more precise information is available but it is certainly consistent with the urban/rural differences identified in the NHANES II Study (Chapter 3).

Perhaps the part of the analysis that is most difficult to verify, however, concerns the contribution of lead in petrol to lead in food since this will depend upon the type of food (fish, animal, plant), the type of plant (root crop or surface crop), and the input from other sources during handling and processing. However if one accepts that the contribution of natural sources to lead in food is only 1 per cent (see Table 3) then 99 per cent of lead in food has to be accounted for in terms of industrial contamination. 15 per cent can be attributed to the use of lead solders and a further percentage can be attributed to industrial practices, such as sewerage disposal and old mine tailings which can raise the lead content of soil locally. However, the impact of these processes is probably limited (less than 10%), particularly since uptake of lead from soil by plants is generally inefficient. This means that the remaining 75 per cent of dietary lead may result from direct of indirect deposition of airborne lead. Since 90 per cent of airborne lead is derived from motor vehicle emissions, the contribution of lead in petrol to dietary intake is considerable. The fact that it cannot be quantified precisely should not allow the general impact of petrol lead on terrestrial and marine ecosystems to be obscured. Without a reliable method of labelling petrol lead on a worldwide basis, these calculations will be difficult to verify and will remain open to dispute. Nevertheless, a substantial contribution from lead in petrol to the food chain remains the most likely explanation for the substantial reductions in blood lead levels observed in rural populations following the introduction of unleaded fuel to the United States (Chapter 3, figure 11).

In conclusion, Table 4 identifies a total contribution from lead in petrol to the lead intake of a two year old urban child of almost 70 per cent. Clearly this figure is based on several assumptions that may need modification in the light of new data. However, Smythe (1982) has used similar calculations to derive a contribution of 80 per cent from lead in air to the lead intake of an urban child. Certainly these percentages would be reduced in situations where the contribution from water or some other adventitious source was excessive. A water lead content of 10 μg/L was used in Table 4 but the percentage contribution from this route would be much higher in plumbosolvent areas (Moore, Chapter 5). However, as far as ubiquitous or unavoidable exposure is concerned, lead in petrol is probably contributing at least two thirds of human intake during the early years of life. Clearly, this analysis is very different from the figure of 10 per cent calculated by the Lawther committee (Department of Health and Social Security, 1980). On the other hand, the NHANES II Study produces a correlation coefficient of 0.95 for the relationship between blood lead levels and the amount of lead used in gasoline production (Chapter 3, figure 13) and this is not consistent with a contribution from lead in petrol of 10 per cent. Furthermore, rural populations probably derive a similar percentage of their intake from lead in petrol. Clearly, the absolute input via lead in air and lead in dust will be lower in rural areas, but since lead in petrol is identified as the main contributor to lead in food, the percentage contribution of petrol lead will vary much less than the absolute contribution. Again these observations are reinforced by the NHANES II Study which documented an equivalent fall in blood lead levels for rural and urban populations.

HUMAN STUDIES

INTRODUCTION   The preceding section on environmental lead has identified three major pathways from lead in petrol to lead in man: direct inhalation (route 1), fortuitous ingestion of lead-rich dust (route 2), and contamination of food supplies (route 3), either by direct deposition of airborne lead or by uptake of lead in air via soil. Fig. 3. represents a simplified version of what is undoubtedly an immensely complex process. Unfortunately studies that are supposed to assess the contribution of lead in petrol to lead in humans seldom recognise even this degree of complexity. Three methods have been used and, although none can identify with certainty the total input from lead in petrol to humans, they differ markedly in their ability to identify a minimum contribution.

Group Comparisons   Without doubt the least satisfactory approach is to examine blood lead levels in specifically exposed groups such as taxi drivers, traffic policemen etc (Zettner et al, 1977; Gothe et al, 1973; Aggarwal et al, 1979; Flindt et al, 1976). Such studies have often failed to detect significant differences from "control" groups but this is scarcely surprising since the "control" groups usually comprised urban residents who differed only in their degree of exposure via route 1. Since place of residence is probably similar, all three routes would have been identical for most of the week (during non-working hours).

Another approach has been to compare blood lead levels in rural and urban communities. Such studies have found significant differences (Hofreuter et al, 1961; Thomas et al, 1967; Rabinowitz et al, 1975), small differences (Nordman, 1975; Tsuchiya et al, 1975), or no differences (Elwood et al, 1982; Barltrop, 1982). However, such urban/rural comparisons are independent of route 3 and are an accurate reflection of routes 1 and 2 only if the two populations are equivalent in all other respects. The inability of investigators to provide details on the nutritional status and adventitious exposure of each population makes their results difficult to interpret.

Urban/rural comparisons are of considerable value however when the population sample is sufficiently large to exclude such effects. Thus the urban/rural differences identified in the NHANES II data present a valid method of quantifying the contribution of routes 1 and 2 to human lead intake. Thus children aged 6 months to 5 years showed a decrease in blood lead gradient according to degree of urbanisation ......22.2, 20.3 and 18.3 for black children, 16.6, 15.4 and 13.5 µg/dl for white children residing in large urban, smaller urban, and rural communities respectively (Chapter 3, Fig. 4). A mean difference of 3-4 µg/dl represents a difference in percentage terms of approximately 22 per cent. However, to calculate the real contribution it is necessary to make allowance for the non-linear relationship between lead intake and blood lead level. although no specific data exists for lead in dust, curvilinear relationships have been derived for lead in water (Moore, Chapter 5, Fig. 4) and dietary lead (Moore, Chapter 5, Fig. 8), and there is no particular reason why lead in dust should be handled differently. Similar considerations apply to the relationship between lead in blood and lead in air where alpha (defined as the elevation of blood lead in µg/dl/average exposure to air in lead µg/m³) tends to decrease as air lead and blood lead increase (Hammond et al, 1981, see Fig.4)

The figure of 22 per cent, being the percentage difference between rural and urban paediatric populations, therefore requires modification. This cannot be accomplished with any precision since the shape of the relationship between dust lead and blood lead has yet to be delineated. Nevertheless, the NHANES II data probably indicates a real contribution to urban children's intake of 30-40 per cent via routes 1 and 2. These estimates are approzimations, but they are consistent with percentage contribution from air lead and dust lead obtained in Table 4 and are supported by studies using stable lead isotopes (Facchetti 1979).

BLOOD LEAD CORRELATIONS

Air Lead. The relationship between air lead and blood lead has been used in two ways to estimate the contribution of lead in petrol

Dr. Robin Russell Jones, MRCP
          Dr. Robert Stephens, Ph.D., D.Sc.

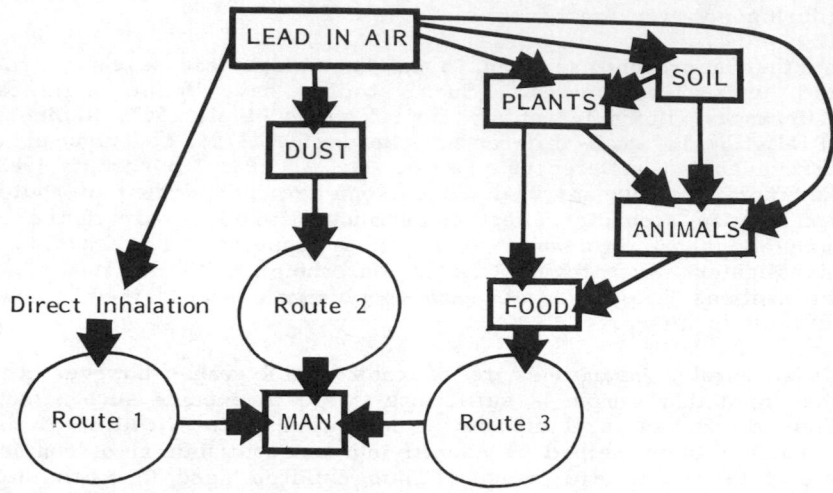

Fig. 3.   Pathways from lead in air to lead in man.

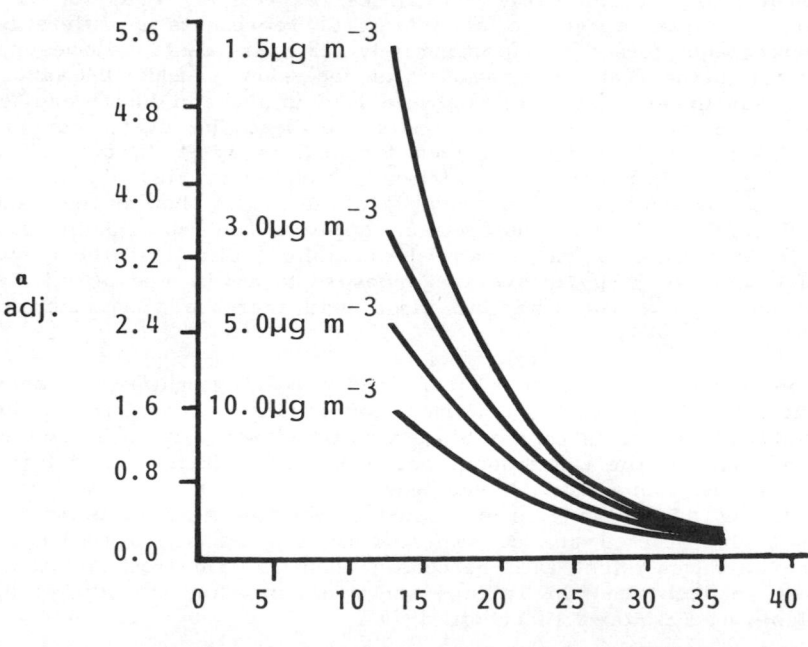

Baseline blood lead concentration μg/dl

Fig. 4.   Variation of alpha with air lead and baseline blood
lead concentration.   Adapted from Hammond et al, 1981.

to human intake.   In experimental studies volunteers are exposed to
different levels of lead in air, and the value of α so derived is
used to calculate daily intakes of lead at different ambient air lead
concentrations (Griffin et al, 1975).   A complementary method is to
use a stable lead isotope in the air mixture to quantify the transfer
of lead in air to lead in blood (Chamberlain et al., 1975).   Such
procedures represent a legitimate method of calculating the
contribution of air lead to human intake via route 1, and were used
in Table 4 but they have no value in assessing the total
contribution of lead in petrol to human lead intake.

Another approach has been to examine air lead/blood lead
correlations in the general population.   Such studies are commonly
cited in support of the thesis that lead in air accounts for only a
small proportion of lead intake (Lynman et al., 1981; Snee 1981).
Again, however, such studies are of limited value since local air
lead concentrations do not provide a direct measure of intake via
route 2 and are largely independant of route 3.   Furthermore, no
account is taken of the curvilinear relationship between air lead and
blood lead.   Nevertheless, such studies do identify air lead as a
weak predictor of blood lead.   Furthermore, values of α derived
from population studies in children are generally higher than
equivalent studies in adults (Snee 1981).   This suggests either that
pulmonary absorption is higher in early life or more likely that
airborne lead is contributing significantly to children's intake via
lead in dust.   Thus, Azar et al. (1973) used personal air samplers
to measure air lead exposure in male adults at five different
locations in the United States.   Although statistically significant
correlations were not found within groups, when the data from all
five groups were combined (149 subjects), a statistically significant
regression was found between air lead and blood lead.
Approximately 44% of the variance in blood lead was explained by
air lead (Azar et al, 1973).

Similarly, Tepper and Levin (1975) carried out population study
involving approximately 2,000 adult females using fixed air monitors
in eleven different communities across the United States.   Although
there was no consistent relationship between air lead and blood lead
levels across geographical areas, residents in urban areas had blood
lead levels that were consistently higher than those of residents of
suburban areas (range 0.9-4.5 µg/dl).   Closer correlations between
air lead and blood lead have been identified in children though it is
of interest that again air lead accounts for only a proportion of the
variance.   Thus, in a study of Sydney school children 'r' values of
0.35 and 0.36 were derived from the air lead/blood lead data
(Garnys et al, 1979).   Interestingly, a value for α greater than
five was obtained in this study over an air lead range of 0.16-1.16
µg/m^3.   If pulmonary absorption in children and adults is
equivalent, this high alpha value indicates a significant intake from
air lead via routes other than direct inhalation.

An even more dramatic assocation between air lead and blood lead of
paediatric populations was found in a study of 176,000 New York

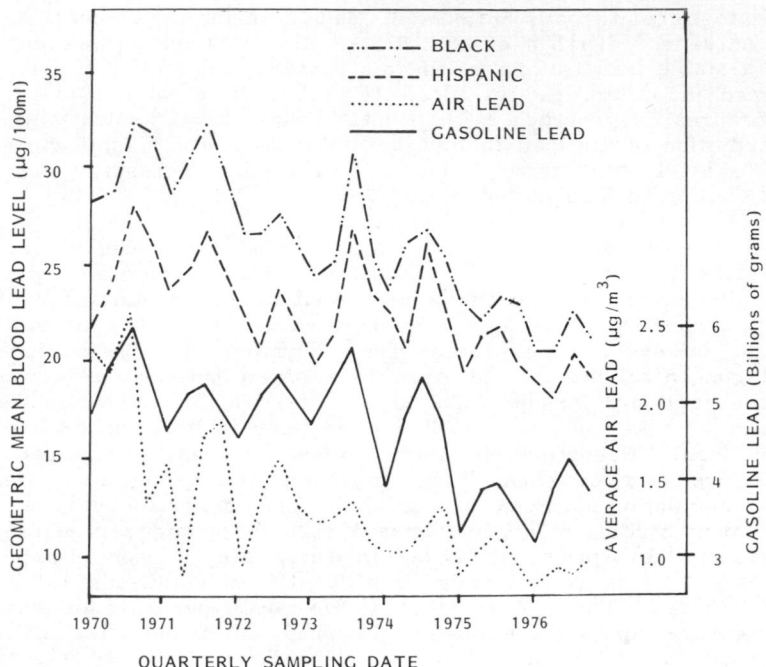

Fig. 5. Variation of blood lead in New York children with air lead and gasoline lead. Data adapted from Billick et al, 1979, 1980.

school children from 1970-1976, in which seasonal fluctuations in air lead correlated closely with seasonal fluctuations in blood lead (Billick et al, 1979, 1980). Certainly, air lead must be regarded as the most important dynamic source of lead in the environment and this might account for the remarkable correlation obtained form the seasonal data (p<0.0001).

Petrol Lead. Billick's New York data is also important because of the close association between blood lead and sales of leaded petrol in the New York ares (see Figure 5). When viewed annually, blood lead correlates more closely with petrol lead than with air lead - an observation which again argues that lead in dust is an important route of exposure in children. It might be said that the relatively weak association with air lead results from the use of only one air sampling site in the New York studies, but this criticism has less force than it might since similar effects were observed in Chicago where data from five air sampling sites were available (Billick, Chapter 4). Again, blood lead correlates more closely with petrol lead than with air lead (compare figures 10 and 11 in Chapter 4).

However, for the assessment of the total contribution of lead in petrol to human lead intake, perhaps the most useful studies to date are those which correlate changes in petrol lead nationally with changes in blood lead, since this is the only method of assessing changes via route 3. Only two such studies are available. One was a small scale study carried out in Frankfurt two years after a reduction in lead content of West German petrol form 0.4 to 0.15 g/L (Sinn, 1980 and 1981). Although only adults were sampled, the results are quoted sufficiently often to merit careful consideration (Barry, 1981; Barry, 1982a). the other study involved a representative cross-sectional sample of the United States population and monitored lead levels in both paediatric and adult sections of the community during the first four years that lead-free gasoline was being introduced to the United States. The results of this study are reported in Chapter 3.

At first sight the two sets of results appear to conflict. In both studies a reduction in petrol lead of over 50 per cent occured but in Frankfurt the associated fall in blood lead levels was only 10 per cent whereas in the States the observed fall was 37 per cent. Many explanations for this discrepancy have been advanced and each needs to be examined carefully. One approach has been to suggest that the fall in the NHANES II data was due to factors other than the changes in petrol lead (Barry, 1982a; Barry, 1982b). It is certainly true that the reduction in the lead content of canned foods over the same period may have made a contribution (Annest, Chapter 3). However, from the data already presented canned foods contribute 15 per cent of the lead in a typical diet so a reduction from 0.38 to 0.21 ppm would only reduce dietary intake by 6.7 per cent (and total lead intake by less than 5 per cent). Even if the higher FDA estimate of 30 per cent is used, this still leaves 27 per cent unaccounted for in the general population and 32 per cent unaccounted for in the 6-17 year old age group where a 42 per cent fall was recorded (Chapter 3, Figure 10). Consequently, changes in the lead content of canned foods may have made a contribution to the fall in blood lead levels but they can account for at most only a quarter of the observed reduction.

It has also been suggested that the reduction in the NHANES II Study may relate to educational programmes of the Federal programmes designed to reduce adventitious lead exposure in high risk groups. Again, this explanation is not supported by the available data since equivalent reductions were observed in all sections of the population (Chapter 3, Figure 10). Indeed, some of the smallest reductions were seen in populations such as urban blacks who might be expected to benefit most if the changes recorded were due to reduce exposure to lead in paint. Furthermore, a seasonal variation was noted in the NHANES II data, except for one summer where blood lead levels fell (1979). That was also the summer of the American fuel crisis. By contrast, exposure to adventitious lead is not known to fluctuate seasonally.

Another way of reconciling the American and German data is to

identify reasons for the relatively small reductions in the Frankfurt
studies. One criticism is that the study relied on measurements in
adults and not children, but this objection does not necessarily
invalidate the findings since in the NHANES II data the percentage
reduction in adults was only 5 per cent lower than the observed
reduction in children. Another objection to the Frankfurt studies
is the relatively short follow-up period of only two years. It is
important to realise that the speed with which reductions in the
lead content of petrol take effect will be different for each pathway
mapped out in Figure 3. Thus, input of lead in air to humans by
direct inahaltion will change immediately, whereas the input from
dust and food will alter more slowly depending upon the life cycle
of the crops and the speed with which urban dust is replaced. By
contrast, lead in soil represents andμ almost permanent sink whose
lead content will remain unaltered for decades. The changes
documented in each study will therefore depend upon the length of
the follow-up period and it might be argued that the NHANES II
Study supercedes the Frankfurt studies because the followup period
was four years instead of two. This is and objection which can be
answered only when further data from Frankfurt are available. One
other factor which has been invoked to explain the Frankfurt
findings relates to the effect of reducing the lead content of petrol
on the size of the exhaust aerosol particles (Ganley and Springer,
1974). It had been shown experimentally that a reduction from 0.4
to 0.15 g/L will lower the mass median diameter of exhaust particles
from 0.03 μm to 0.025 μm and it has been pointed out that this will
increase pulmonary deposition by only 10 per cent (Heard, Wiffen
and Reed, 1981). As far as general population exposure is
concerned, however, a reduction in particle size will also mean that
particles remain airborne for longer periods, and this may explain
why ambient air lead concentrations in Frankfurt fell by only 46 per
cent. If this analysis is correct then substantial reductions in
population exposure may not be achieved by the proposed
reductions in the lead content of U.K. petrol to 0.15 g/L in 1985.

However, there are two further aspects of the Frankfurt study that
probably are of greater importance. First, the geographical area
affected by the petrol lead legislation was much smaller in Europe
than in North America, so that West Germany will be subject to
considerable contamination from neighbouring countries. This may
not be a significant factor in urban areas, but in rural areas it
means that the reduction in the lead content of West German petrol
is not reflected in the lead content of West German food. This
effect will be further exaggerated by food imports from countries
not controlled by the low-lead legislation. Finally, the populations
studied in Frankfurt were selected because of their exposure to
high levels of urban pollution. Although this is where maximum
reductions might be expected, the curvilinear relationship between
lead intake and blood lead ensures that this is the population where
the smallest reductions are observed in percentage terms. These
effects were also seen in the NHANES II Study where the reduction
in large urban areas (population greater than 10^6 persons) was less
than the reduction in small urban areas (population less that 10^6

persons), (Annest, Chapter 3, Figure 11). When these factors are
taken into consideration it is hardly surprising that a reduction of
only 10 per cent was observed in the Frankfurt residents.   The
NHANES II data and the Frankfurt studies have been discussed in
some detail because most of the current debate about the
contribution of lead in petrol to human lead intake revolves around
these two sets of data.   In assessing both these studies, however,
it is important to realise that a new equilibrium between blood lead
and lead intake is achieved only slowly.   It has been shown
experimentally, for example, that sheep grazed next to motorways
show elevated lead burdens six months after being moved to a rural
environment (Ward et al, 1978).   For this reason the percentage fall
in blood lead levels associated with a 55 per cent reduction in the
amount of lead used at American refineries documented in the
NHANES II Study has even greater significance.   If one allows for
a reduction in the lead content of canned foods by subtracting 10
per cent from the percentage reduction in paediatric populations of
42 per cent, then the total contribution from lead in petrol to
human lead intake can be calculated as 32/55 x 100 = 58%.   The
difference between this figure and the figure of 70 per cent
calculated from environmental data (see Table 4) is then accounted
for by the fact that reductions in petrol lead are not immediately
reflected in the blood lead of exposed populations.

Like any set of scientific observations, the NHANES II Study should
not be viewed in isolation.   Nevertheless, the accuracy of the
results and the reliability of the findings are not in serious dispute
since an appropriate method of quality control was employed
throughout.   Furthermore, another recent study of 11,837 cord
blood samples which documented a decline in lead concentrations of
11 per cent annually from 1979-1981, confirms that lead levels in
the United States population are continuing to fall (Rabinowitz and
Needleman, 1982).

Traffic Density.   Several studies have examined the effects of
residence near roadways on blood lead levels and these data have
been extensively reviewed by Bridbord, 1977.   the investigations
that included children provide a useful method of assessing the
impact of high exposures via routes 1 and 2.   Thus, Johnson et al
(1975) found an average mean blood lead level of 23.5 μg/dl in boys
aged one to sixteen resident near the San Diego freeway in Los
Angeles (traffic density 250,000 cars per day) compared with a
mean blood lead level of 11.1 μg/dl in a control population.   For
girls the corresponding values were 16.7 and 10.2 respectively.   It
has been argued that residence in heavily trafficked areas is
associated with increased exposures to adventitious sources of lead
but in this study participants were recruited from a student
housing area with low lead paint and the control population was
selected with equal care.   However, an even better method of
circumventing the effects of adventitious exposure is to measure
blood lead levels in the same population before and after increased
exposure to motor vehicle emissions.   The opening of a major
motorway interchange in Birmingham in 1972 provided an

opportunity for such a study (Waldron 1975). Blood lead levels in males rose from 14.4 to 23.7 µg/dl and a similar change was observed in females (10.9 to 19.21 µg/dl) over a period of seventeen months, with approximately half the increase occurring in the first six months after the interchange was opened to traffic. Both the traffic density (greater than 100,000 cars per day) and the blood lead levels are comparable to the Los Angeles study. The data demonstrate that increasing input via routes 1 and 2 can increase blood lead levels in children and adults by 60-80 per cent, and in these circumstances these routes will exceed the input from route 3.

ISOTOPIC LEAD EXPERIMENTS

Experiments in which isotopic tracers are used to identify the contribution of different sources (pathways) avoids many of the pitfalls identified in the human studies reviewed so far. In particular no allowance is necessary for the curvilinear relationship between lead intake and blood lead. In one such experiment long-term lead balance studies combined with a stable isotope lead tracer in the diet were used to identify a major non-dietary lead intake from respired air (Rabinowitz et al, 1977). By observing changes in the blood lead of subjects exposed to filtered low lead air, a mean lung absorption of 14±4 µg of lead per day were derived at an ambient air lead concentration of 2 µg/m³. When set against an intake of 28 µg per day from food and water this represents a pulmonary intake of almost one third for urban adults. Similar findings were obtained in a study of ten urban residnets from Dallas (Manton, 1977). By following changes in the isotopic composition of air and blood a contribution of lead in air was derived with a range of 7-41 per cent. Interestingly, when portable cascade impactors were used to measure the actual 24 hour lead exposures in three of these subjects, it was necessary to invoke direct contamination of food by airborne lead as a method of reconciling the two sets of measurements (Manton et al, 1976). Both these studies identify a local contribution from lead in air of between 30 and 40 per cent and are consistent with the urban/rural differences derived in the NHANES II data. Unfortunately, the calculations necessary to estimate the contribution from airborne lead are complex, and the investigators had no direct control over the isotopic composition of petrol.

A more direct approach is offered by the Isotopic Lead Experiment which has been carried out since 1975 in North-West Italy. In this project, lead from the Broken Hill mine in Australia, (isotopic ratio 1.04), differing significantly from lead found locally, (isotopic ratio 1.18), was added to petrol sold in Turin and the surrounding countryside (Facchetti, 1979). Observed changes in isotopic ratios allowed estimates for the contribution of recent vehicle emissions to lead in the environment and lead in humans. Thus it was possible to show that 95 per cent of air lead in Turin is derived from petrol. (see Figure 6). Human blood samples demonstrated a fall in the isotopic ratio which was less in Turin adults (1.1628 to 1.1325), than that observed in children, where the isotopic ratio fell to around 1.125. A percentage change of about 25 per cent can be calculates for the adult population of Turin, but this figure should be seen as a minimum since recycling of skeletal lead deposits will tend to dilute the contribution of recent vehicle emissions to blood lead. This effect could have been minimised by including infants and preschool children in the study. Unfortunately the only samples available for this group were obtained in 1980, during phase 3, but it is significant that these showed the lowest isotopic ratio of any blood sample in the study (1.1100). Assuming that the 1975 ratio in adults and children were similar, a percentage change of at least 40 per cent can be calculated forthe youngest members of the population. It is also probable that further reductions would have been observed if phase 2 of the experiment had been continued for longer than two years. Despite these limitations, the study is useful in identifying a minimum contribution for lead in petrol of around 30 to 40 per cent, and the results are broadly similar to those obtained by other workers (Manton et al, 1976; Rabinowitz et al, 1977).

The Isotopic Lead Experiment is continuing, and when final results are available it should be possible to quantify the extent to which local food supplies have been contaminated by local vehicle emissions. However such measurements cannot provide an accurate assessment of the total contribution via route 3, since local food supplies will also be contaminates by airbourne lead from outside the test area, and second because food grown outside the test area will be contributing substantially to the dietary intake of the population under scrutiny. The figures obtained in such studies should therefore be seen as minimum values, and cannot be used to assess the total contribution of lead in petrol to human lead intake.

CONCLUSIONS

There is little doubt that many members of the British medical profession are sceptical about the hazard to children from the use of lead in petrol (Waldron, 1981; Barltrop, 1982). One of the factors that may have contributed to this attitude is that the input from lead in petrol decreases with increasing blood lead levels, so that ubiquitous sources of exposure are seldom relevant in cases of clinical lead poisoning. Thus blood lead concentrations which may be lethal in children ($>$ 80 µg/dl) usually reflect greatly elevated lead intake from the deliberate or fortuitous ingestion of a high-lead source such as chewing leaded paint, licking or sucking lead-containing cosmetics etc. In the 30–80 µg/dl range an overlap situation exists between the above types of exposure and more general exposure such as heavily lead-contaminated dust in homes from nearby lead emitters, or from lead carried home by parents using lead at their place of employment. In addition, high levels of lead in drinking water can produce blood lead levels of this magnitude. Occasionally, moderately elevated blood leads are associated with high levels of lead in dust where the above situations do not apply. It is not clear, however, whether these

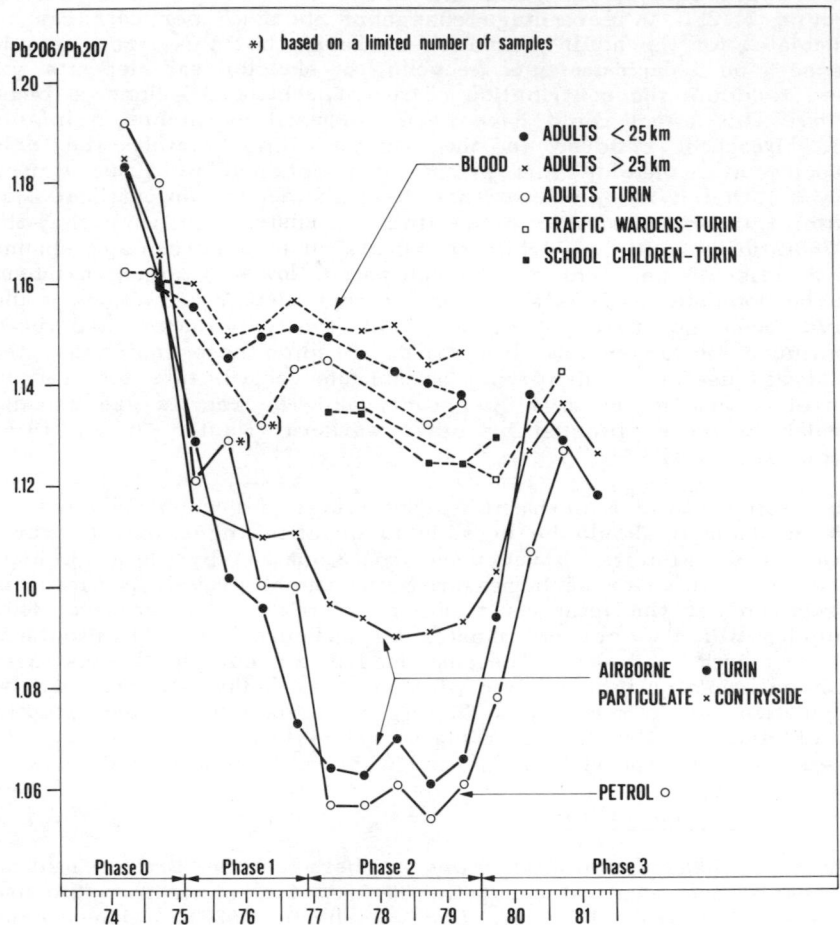

Phase "0" Identification of background values. July 1974 – July 1975.

Phase "1" Transition period to petrol lead of a new isotopic composition. August 1975 – April 1977.

Phase "2" Steady state period during which the new lead was used exclusively in local petrol. May 1977 – December 1979.

Phase "3" Gradual reversion to lead used previously. January 1980.

Fig. 6. The Isotopic Lead Experiment, Italy.

high lead in dust levels result from airborne pollution or some other source, and it is unfortunate that the analytical methods used do not distinguish petrol lead and paint lead. It is however in the blood lead range below 30 µg/dl that the ubiquitous forms of pollution outlined in this review have their maximal impact. Since over 95 per cent of the population have blood lead levels below this figure it is by attention to these generalised sources of exposure that maximal benefits will accrue to the population as a whole. These benefits should not be regarded as trivial since major neuropsychological deficits have been consistently associated with lead levels below 30 µg/dl and replicated in animal models (See this volume, Parts III and IV). Furthermore, lowering the blood lead distribution of a population will also have a significant effect on the percentage of people with levels above 30 µg/dl, even though lead in petrol may not be their main source of exposure (Billick, Chapter 4, Fig. 5). These considerations do not apply with very high levels of exposure (greater than 80 µg/dl) where the distribution curve is bimodal.

One other factor that requires attention is individual metabolism. Ten-fold differences in lead burden have been noted even in long-term stable populations (Radford, 1975) and this must reflect large variations in the absorption, distribution and excretion of lead by individuals. A major determinant is nutritional status so that children with associated deficiencies of iron or calcium may develop moderately elevated lead burdens even as a result of levels of exposure that are conventionally regarded as 'normal'. The realisation that identical levels of exposure are reflected in a range of blood lead levels is important if fruitless searches for adventitious sources are to be avoided.

In conclusion, the environmental data indicates an insignificant contribution from natural sources to human lead burdens, and lead in petrol is identified as the major contributor to children's lead intake. In urban areas the contribution may be as high as 70 per cent, and this analysis is consistent with the data available from human studies. The isotopic studies identify a minimum contribution of one third and the NHANES II data indicate a real contribution approaching two thirds. It follows that the most effective method of achieving a significant reduction in lead intake for the general population is by legislating to prohibit the addition of lead to petrol. The proposed reduction in the lead content of U.K. petrol to 0.15 g/L does not represent an adequate response to the scientific and medical data currently available.

REFERENCES

Aarkrog, A., and Lippert, J., (1971), Direct contamination of barley with ^{51}Cr, ^{59}Fe, ^{58}Co, ^{65}Zn, ^{203}Hg, ^{210}Pb. Rad. Bot., 11, 463-472.

Aggarwal, A.L., Patel, T.S., Rayani, C.V., Chatterjee, S.K., (1979). Biologic effects of airborne lead on occupationally exposed traffic policemen and permanent shopkeepers stationed at Ahmedabad City, Indian J. Med. Res., 70, 650-656.

Alexander, F.W., Delves, H.T., Clayton, B.E., (1973). The uptake and excretion by children of lead and other contaminants, Proceedings of the International Symposium, Environmental Health Aspects of Lead, Amsterdam 1972, 319-331, Commission of the European Communities Luxembourg.

Arvik, J.H., Zimdahl, R.L., (1974). Barriers to the foliar uptake of lead, J. Environ. Qual., 3:369-373.

Ashmead, H., (1972). Ecology, chelation and animal experimentation, J. Appl. Nutr., 24:8-17.

Australian Academy of Science, (1981). Health and environmental lead in Australia, Canberra.

Australian National Health and Medical Research Council, (1979). Report of the 87th Session.

Azar, A., Habibi, K., Snee, R., (1973). Relationship of community levels of air lead and indices of lead absorption. Proceedings of an International Symposium on Environmental Health aspects of lead, Luxembourg, 581-594.

Barltrop, D., Meek, F., (1979). Effect of particle size on lead absorption from the gut, Arch. Env. Health, 280-285.

Barltrop, D., (1982). Radio Interview, BBC Radio 4, May 1.

Barry, P.S.I., (1981). Letter, Lancet, 2:1264.

Barry, P.S.I., (1982a). Letter, B.M.J., 284:1877-1878.

Barry, P.S.I., (1982b). Letter, Lancet, 2:94.

Berger, K.C., Ernhardt and Francis, C.W., (1965). Polonium-210 analyses of vegetables, cured and uncured tobacco and associated soils, Science, 150, 1738-1739.

Biggins, P.D.E., Harrison, R.M., (1980). Chemical speciation of lead compounds in street dusts, Environ. Sci. Tech., 14:336-339.

Billick, I.H., Curran, A.S., Shier, D.R., (1979). Analysis of pediatric blood lead levels in New York City for 1970-1976, Environ. Hlth. Perspect. 31:183-190.

Billick, I.H., Curran, A.S., Shiers, D.R., (1980). Relation of pediatric blood lead levels to lead in gasoline, Environ. Hlth. Perspect., 34, 213-217.

Bridboard, K., (1977). Human exposure to lead from motor vehicle emissions, U.S. Department of Health, Education and Welfare.

Bryce-Smith, D., Stephens, R., (1980). Lead or Health, Conservation Society, London.

Bunzl, K., Kracker, W., Kreuzer, W., (1979). ^{210}Pb and ^{210}Po in liver and kidneys of cattle - 1. Animals from an area with little traffic or industry, Hlth. Phys., 37, 323-330.

Bunzl, K., Kracker, W., Kreuzer, W., (1980). Stable lead, ^{210}Pb and ^{210}Po in the liver and kidneys of cattle - 11. Animals from an area near an abandoned lead mine, Fd. Cosmet. Toxicol., 18:133-137.

Butler, J.D., Macmurdo, S.D., (1974). Interior and exterior atmospheric lead concentrations of a house situated near an urban motorway, Int. J. Env. Stud., 6:181-184.

Cawse, P.A., (1974-1977). A survey of atmospheric trace elements in the UK, AERE publ. No. R-7669, R-8038, R-8393, R-8869, HMSO, London.

Chamberlain, A.C., Heard, M.J., Stott, A.N.B., Clough, W.S., Newton, D., Wells, A.C., (1975). Uptake of inhales lead from motor exhausts, Postgrad. Med. J., 51:790-794.

Chester, R., Aston, S.R., Stoner, J.H., Bruty, D., (1974). Trace metals in soil-sized particles from the lower troposphere over the world ocean, J. Res. Atmosph., 8:777-789.

Chow, T.J., (1970). Lead accumulation in roadside soil and grass, Nature, 225:295-296.

Crump, D.R., and Barlow, P.J., (1982). Factors controlling the lead content of a pasture grass, Environ. Pollut. (B), 3:181-192

Davies, B.E., Conway, D., Holt, S., (1979). Lead pollution of London soils; a potential restriction of their use for growing vegetables, J. Agricul. Sci., 93:749-752.

Day, J.P., Hart, M., Robinson, M.S., (1975). Lead in urban street dusts, Nature, 253:343-345.

DeJonge, W.R.A., Chakraborti, D., Adams, F.C., (1981). Identification and determination of individual tetraalkyl lead species in air, Environ. Sci. Tech., 15:1217-1222.

Department of Environment, (1974). Lead in the environment and its significance to Man, Pollution Paper No. 2, HMSO, London.

Department of Health and Social Security (1980). Lead and Health, HMSO, London.

Duggan, M.J., (1980). Lead in urban dust: an assessment, Water Air Soil Pollut., 14:309-321.

Duggan, M.J., and Williams, S., (1977). Lead in dust in city streets, Sci. Total Environ., 7:91-97.

Elgmork, K., Hagen, A., Langeland, A., (1973). Polluted snow in Southern Norway during the winters 1968-1971, Environ. Pollut., 4:41-48.

Elias, R., Hirao, Y., Patterson, C.C., (1975). Impact of present levels of aerosol Pb concentrations on both natural ecosystems and humans, International conference on heavy metals in the environment, Toronto, Canada, 257-272.

Elias, R., Hirao, Y., Patterson, C.C., (1982). The circumvention of the natural biopurification of calcium along nutrient pathways by atmospheric inputs of industrial lead, Geochimica et Cosmo. Acta. (In Press).

Elwood, P.C., Gallagher, J., Toothill, C., (1982). Lead in petrol, B.M.J., 284:1189-1190.

Ericson, J.E., Shirahata, H., Patterson, C.C., (1970). Skeletal concentrations of lead in ancient Peruvians, New Eng. J. Med., 300:946-951.

Everett, J.C., Day, C.L., Reynolds, D., (1967). Comparative survey of lead at selected sites in the British Isles in relation to air pollution, Food Cosmet. Toxicol., 5:29-35.

Facchetti, S., (1979). Isotope study of lead in petrol, International conference on management and control of heavy metals in the environment, London, 95-102.

Farmer, J.G., (1979). Lead in wild blackberries from suburban roadsides, J. Sci. Food Agric., 30:816-818.

Flanagan, J.T., Wade, K.J., Currie, A., Curtis, D.J., (1980). The deposition of lead and zinc from traffic pollution on two roadside shrubs, Environ. Pollut., 1:(B) 71-78.

Dr. Robin Russell Jones, MRCP
          Dr. Robert Stephens, Ph.D., D.Sc.

Flindt, M.L.H., King, E., Walsh, D.W., (1976). Blood lead and
    erythrocyte aminolevulinic acid dehydratase levels in Manchester
    taxi drivers, Brit. J. Ind. Med. 33:79-84.
Francis, C.W., Chesters, G., Erhardt, W.H., (1968). ^{210}Fo entry
    into plants, Environ. Sci. Tech., S:690-695.
Ganley, J.T., Springer, G.S., (1974). Physical and chemical
    characteristics of particulates in spark ignition engine exhaust,
    Environ. Sci. Tech., 8:340-347.
Gange, P.J., Joshi, M.S., (1971). Lead quantities in plants, soil
    and air near some major highways in Southern California,
    Hilgardia, 41:1-30.
Garnys, V.P., Freemand, R., Smythe, L.E., (1979). Lead burden
    of Sydney school children, Department of Analytical Chemistry,
    University of New South Wales.
Goldbery, E.D., Gross, M.G., (1971). Man's impact on terrestrial
    and oceanic ecosystems, Ed. Matthews, W.H., Smith, F.E.,
    Goldbery, E.D., Massachusetts Institute of Technology Press,
    Cambridge, 371.
Gothe, C.J., Ohman, H., Lindstedt, G., (1973). Exposure to
    airborne lead in city atmospheres, Work Environ. Hlth.,
    10:13-18.
Graham, D.L., Kalman, S.M., (1974). Lead in forage grass from a
    suburban area in Northern California, Environ. Pollut., 7:209.
Grandjean, P., Neilsen, O.V., Shapiro, I.M., (1979). Lead
    retention in ancient Nubian and contemporary populations, J.
    Environ. Pathol. Toxicol., 2:781.
Griffin, T.D., Coulston, F., Goldberg, L., Wills, H., Russell,
    J.C., Knelson, J.H., (1975). Chemical studies on men
    continuously exposed to airborne particular lead, In Lead
    Supplement Volume II, Eds. F. Coulston and F. Korte, 221-240,
    Academic Press, New York.
Hammond, P.B., O'Flaherty, E.J., Gartside, P.S., (1981). The
    impact of air lead on blood lead in Man - a critique of the recent
    literature. Fd. Cosmet. Toxicol., 19:631-637.
Healy, M.A., Aslam, M., (1980). the distribution of lead in a
    roadside environment and its consequences for health, Publ.
    Hlth. (London), 94:78-88.
Heard, M.J., Wiffen, R.D., Reed, S., (1981). The variation of
    automobile exhaust particle size (at diameters <0.1 μm) with the
    concentration of lead in fuel. AERE G 2163.
Hecker, L.H., Allen, H.E., Dinman, B.D., Neel, J., (1974).
    Heavy metals levels in acculturated and unacculturated
    populations, Arch. Anviron. Hlth., 29:181-185.
Hill, C.R., Jaworowski, Z.S., (1961), Pb^{210} in some human and
    animal tissues, Nature, 190:353-354.
Hirano, Y., Patterson, C.C., (1974). Lead aerosol pollution in the
    High Sierra over-rides natural mechanisms which exclude lead
    from a food chain, Science, 184:989-992.
Hofreuter, D.H., Catcott, E.J., Keenan, R.G., Xintaras, C.,
    (1961). The public health significance of atmospheric lead,
    Arch. Environ. Hlth., 3:568-574.
Holtzman, R.B., (1965). ^{210}Pb (RaD) in inhabitants of a
    Caribbean island, Hlth. Phys., 11:477-480.

Jaworski, Z.S., (1978).   Effect of lead in the environment - 1978 Quantitative Aspects, National Research Council of Canada Division of Biological Science NRCC No. 16736, 595.

Johnson, D.E., Tillery, J.B., Prevost, R.J., (1975).   Levels of platinum, palladium and lead in populations of Southern California, Environ. Hlth. Perspect., 12:27-33.

Kacprzak, J.L., (1982).   Determination of lead in food by flameless AAS after dry ashing and chelation-solvent extraction, Report by Division of Analytical Laboratories, Health Commission of New South Wales, PO Box 162, Lidcombe, NSW (In Press).

Kahn, D.H., (1980).   Lead in the soil environment, Monitoring and Assessment Research Centre Report No. 21, London.

Koslow, E.E., Smith, W.H., Staskawicz, B.J., (1977). Lead-containing particles of urban lead surfaces, Environ. Sci. Tech. 11:1019-1021.

Ladinskaya, L.A., Parfenov, Y.D., Popov, D.J., Fedorova, A.V., (1973). ^{210}Pb and ^{210}Po content in air, water, foodstuffs and the human body, Arch. Environ. Hlth. 27:254-258.

Lagerwerff, J.V., Armiger, W.H., Specht, A.W., (1973).   Uptake of lead by alfalfa and corn from soil and air, Soil Sci. 115:455-460.

Lindberg, S.E., Turner, R.R., Shriner, D.S., Huff, D.D., (1981).   Atmospheric deposition of heavy metals and their interaction with acid precipitations in a North American deciduous forest, International Conference: Heavy metals in the environment, Amsterdam, 306-309.

Linton, R.W., Natusch, D.F.S., Solomon, R.L., Evans, C.A., (1980).   Physicochemical characterisation of lead in urban dusts. A microanalytical approach to lead tracing, Environ. Sci. Tech., 14:159-164.

Little, P., Fleming, R.G., Heard, M.J., (1981).   Uptake of lead by vegetable foodstuffs during cooking, Sci. Tot. Environ. 17:111.

Little, P., Whiffen, R.D., (1977).   Emission and deposition of petrol engine exhaust Pb-1. Deposition of exhaust Pb to plant and soil surfaces, Atmos. Environ., 11:437-447.

Lynman, D.R., Ter Haar, G.L., Hall, C.A., (1981).   The impact of environmental lead on children and adults, International Conference on Environmental Pollution, Thessaloniki, September 1981.

Manton, W.I., (1977).   Sources of lead in blood, Arch. Environ. Hlth., 32:149-159.

Manton, W.I., McSweeney, M., Wilkins, J.B., (1976).   Blood lead isotope ratios of individuals exposed to airborne lead changing linearaly in isotope ratio, 7th Internat. Mass Spec. Conf., Florence, Italy.

Miller, J.E., Hassett, J.J., Koeppe, D.E., (1975).   Effect of soil properties and extractable lead levels on lead uptake by soybeans, Commun. Soil. Sci. Plant Anal., 6:339-347.

Monitor, (1982).   How the North Sea copes with metal pollution, New Scientist, July 22:222.

Moore, H.E., Poet, S.E., (1976). ^{210}Pb fluxes determined from ^{210}Pb and ^{226}Ra soil profiles, J. Geophys. Res., 81, 1056-1058.

Morrow, P.E., Beiter, H., Amato, F., Gibb, F.R., (1980).
    Pulmonary retention of lead: An experimental study in Man,
    Environ. Red., 21:373-384.
Motto, H.L., Daines, R.H., Chilko, D.M., Motto, C.K., (1940).
    Lead in soils and plants: its relationship to traffic volume and
    proximity to highways, Environ. Sci. Technol., 4:231-237.
Murozomi, M., Chow, T.J., Patterson, C.C., (1969). Chemical
    concentrations of pollutant lead aerosols, terrestial dusts, and
    sea salt in Greenland and Antartic snow strata, Gwochemica et
    Cosmochemica acta, 33:1247-1294.
National Academy of Science, (1980). Lead in human environment
    National Academy of Science, Washington D.C.
Nordman, C.H., (1975). Environmental lead exposure in Finland.
    A study on selected population groups. Inst. Occup. Hlth.,
    Helsinki, Finland. Acas. Diss. Univ. Helsinki, May.
Nriagu, J.O., (1979). Global inventory of natural and
    anthropogenic emissions to trace metals to the atmosphere,
    Nature, 79, 409-411.
O'Brien, B.J., (1979). The exposure commitment method with
    application to exposure of Man to lead pollution, Monitoring and
    Assessment Research Centre, Report No. 13.
O'Brien, B.J., Smith, S., Coleman, D.O. (1980). Lead pollution of
    the global environment, Monitoring and Assessment Research
    Centre, London, Report No. 16:1-41.
Page, A.L., Ganje, T.J., Joshi, M.S., (1971). Lead quantities in
    plants, soil and sir near some major highways in Southern
    California, Hilgardia, 41:1-31.
Parfenov, Y.D., (1974), Polpmium-210 in the environment and in
    the human organism, Atom, Energy Rev., 12:75-143.
Patterosn, C.C., (1965). Contaminated and natural environments of
    man, Arch. Environ. Health, 11:344-360.
Patterson, C.C., (1980). An alternative perspective, U.S. National
    Academy of Science report on Lead in the Human Environment,
    265-349, National Academy of Science, Washington D.C.
Pauli, F.W., (1975). Heavy metal humates and their behaviour
    against hydrogen sulphide, Soil Sci., 119:98-105.
Peirson, D.H., Cawse, P.A., Salmon, L., Cambray, R.S., (1973).
    Trace elements in the atmospheric environment, Nature,
    241:252-256.
Piomelli, S., Corash, L. Corash, M.B., Seaman, C., Mushak, P.,
    Glover, B., Padgett, R., (1980). Blood lead concentrations in a
    remote Himalayan population, Science, 210:1135-1137.
Poole, C., Smythe, L.E., (1980). Blood lead levels in Papua New
    Guinea children living in remote area, Sci. Tot. Environ.,
    15:17-24.
Rabinowitz, M., (1972). Plant uptake of soil and stmospheric lead
    in Southern California, Chemosphere, 4:175-180.
Rabinowitz, M.B., Wetherill, G.W., Kopple, J.D., (1977).
    Magnitude of lead from respiration by normal man, J. Lab. Clin.
    Med., 90, No. 2, 238-248.
Rabinowitz, M.B., Needleman, H.L., (1982). Temporal trends in
    the lead concentrations of umbilical cord blood. Science,
    216:1429-1431.

Radford, E.P., (1975).   Biomedical aspects of trace metals, Am. Inst. Chem. Eng. Symp. Ser. 71, No. 149:39-46.

Ramamoorthy, S., Leppard, G.G., (1977).   Root surfaces and accretion of lead - I Physiocochemical analysis, J. Inorg. Nucl. Chem., 39, 1283; idem ibid, (1977), Root surfaces and accretion of lead - II A structural analysis of the mechanism, 39:1285-1286.

Robbins, J.A., (1978).   Geochemical and geophysical applications of radioactive lead, In: J. Nriagu (ed.), The biogeochemistry of lead in the environment, North Holland Biomedical Press, 285-393.

Roberts, T.M., Hutchinson, T.C., Paciga, J., Chattopadhyay, A., Jervis, R.E., Vanloon, J., Parkinson, D.K., (1974).   Lead contamination around secondary smelters: estimation of disposal and accumulation by humans, Science, 186:1120-1123.

Rohbock, E., Georgii, H. W., Perseke, C., Kins, L., (1981).   Wet and dry deposition of heavy metal aerosols in the Fedral Republic of Germany, International conference: Heavy metals in the environment, Amsterdam, 310-313.

Ronneau, C., Hallet, J. -Ph., (1981).   Sulphur and heavy metal deposition rates on agricultural soils of Belgium - extrapolation to Europe, International conference: Heavy metals in the environment, Amsterdam, 314-317.

Schaule, B., Patterson, C.C., (1979).   The occurence of lead in the Northeast Pacific and effects of anthropogenic inputs, Proceedings of an International experts discussion on lead: occurrence, fate and pollution in the marine environment, ed. Branica, Pergamon Press, Oxford.

Schinner, M., (1980).   The distribution of lead emissions over a wide area in an east Alpine basin, Environ. Pollut. (A), 22:247-258.

Servant, J., Delapart, M., (1981).   Blood lead and lead-210 origins in residents of Toulouse, Health Physics, 41:483-487.

Servant, J., Delapart, M., (1979).   Lead and lead-210 in some river waters of the southwestern part of France. Importance of the atmospheric contribution, Environ. Sci. Tech., 13:105-107.

Settle, D.M., Patterson, C.C., (1980).   Lead in Albacore: guide to lead pollution in Americans, Science, 207:1167-1176.

Shaprio, I.M., Mitchell, G., Davidson, I., Katz, S.H., (1975).   The lead content of teeth, Arch. Environ. Health, 30: 483-486.

Siccama, T.G., Smith, W.H., (1978).   Lead accumulation in a Northern hardwood forest, Environ. Sci. Tech., 12:593-594.

Siccama, T.G., Smith, W.H., Mader, D.L., (1980).   Changes in lead, zinc, copper, dry weight and organic matter content of the forest floor of white pine stands in Central Massachusetts over sixteen years, Environ. Sci. Tech., 14:54-56.

Sinn, W., (1980).   Relationship between lead concentrations in the air and blood lead levels of people living and working in the centre of a city (Frankfurt blood lead study) - I. Experimental method and examination of differences, Int. Arch. Occup. Environ. Hlth., 47:93-118.

Sinn, W., (1981). Relationship between lead concentrations in the air and blood lead levels of people living and working in the centre of a city (Frankfurt blood lead survey) – II. Correlations and conclusions, Int. Arch. Environ. Hlth. 48:1-23.

Smith, W.H., (1976). Lead concentration of the roadside ecosystem, J. Air Pollut. Control Assoc., 26:753-766.

Smythe, L.E., (1982). Lead burden of Sydney school children: An overview. Paper presented to 52nd Anzaas Congress May 11, 1982. Macquarie University, Australia.

Snee, R.O., (1981). Evaluation of studies of the relationship between blood lead and air lead, Int. Arch. Occup. Environ. Hlth., 48:219-242.

Solomon, R.L., Hartford, J.W., (1976). Lead and cadmium in dusts and soils in a small urban community, Env. Science Tech., 10:773-777.

Stukas, V.J., Wong, C.S., (1981). Stable lead isotopes as a tracer in coastal waters, Science, 211; 1424-1427.

Swaine, D.J., (1955). Commonwealth Bureau of Soil Science Technical Communication No 48, York.

Tanton, T.W., Crowdy, S.H., (1971). The distribution of lead chelate in the transpiration stream of higher plants, Pestic. Sci. 2:211-213.

Tatsumoto, M., Patterson, C.C., (1963). Concentrations of common lead in some Atlantic and Mediterranean waters and in snow, Nature, 199:350-352.

Tepper, L.B., Levin, L.S., (1975). A survey of air and population lead levels in selected American communities, In Lead, Eds. Coulston, F., Kork, F., Supplement, Vol. II, p. 152-196, Academic Press, New York.

Thomas, H.V., Milmore, B.K., Heidbreder, G.A., Kogan, B.A., (1967). Blood lead of persons living near freeways, Arch. Environ. Hlth., 15:695-702.

Tjell, J.C., Hovmand, M.F., Mosbaek, H., (1979). Atmospheric lead pollution of grass grown in a background area in Denmark, Nature, 280:425-426.

Tolan, A., Elton, G., (1972). Lead intake from food, International symposium on the environmental health aspects of lead, Amsterdam, p. 77-84.

Tsuchiya, K., Sugita, M., Seki, Y., Kobayashi, Y., Hori, M., Park, C.B., (1975). Study of lead concentration in atmosphere and population of Japan, Environ. Qual. Saf. (Suppl. II) Lead, 95-147.

Vostal, J., Taves, E., Sayre, J.W., (1974). Lead analysis of house dust. Method for the detection of another source of lead exposure in inner city children, Environ. Hlth. Perspect., 7:91-97.

Waldron, T., (1981). Occupational health expert hits out at antilead campaigners, Medical News, June 25, 1981, p. 3 and 6.

Waldron, H.A., (1975). Lead levels in blood of residents near the M6-A38 (M) interchange, Birmingham, Nature, 253, 345-346.

Walter, S.D., Yankel, A.J., Lindern, I.H., (1980). Age specific risk factors for lead absorption in children, Arch. Environ. Hlth. 35:53-58.

Ward, N.I., Brooks, R.R., Roberts, E., (1978). Blood lead levels in sheep exposed to automotive emissions, Bull, Environ. Contam. Tox., 20:44-51.

Ward, N.I., Brooks, R.R., Roberts, E., (1978). Heavy-metal pollution from automative emissions and its effects on roadside soil and pasture species in New Zealand, Environ. Sci. Technol., 11, 917-920.

Wheeler, G.L., Rolfe, G.L., (1979). The relationship between daily traffic volume and the distribution of lead in roadside soil and vegetation, Environ. Pollut., 18:265-274.

Williamson, P., Evans, P.R., (1972). Lead: levels in roadside invertebrates and small mammals, Bull. Environ. Contam. Toxicol., 280-288.

Wilson, D.O., Cline, J.F., (1966). Removal of plutonium-239, tungsten-185 and lead-210 from soil, Nature, 209, 941-942.

W.H.O., (1977). Environmental Health Criteria, 3. Lead, World Health Organisation, Geneva.

Zettner, A., Josselson, A.R., Ramras, D.G., Askew, J.B., (1975). Blood lead levels in San Diego policemen, Ann. Clin. Lab. Sci., 7, No. 3, 352-356.

PART 3
Toxicity of Lead

Lead Versus Health
Edited by M. Rutter and R. Russell Jones
© 1983 John Wiley & Sons Ltd.

HEALTH SIGNIFICANCE OF ORGANOLEAD COMPOUNDS

Philippe Grandjean, M.D.

Director, Department of Occupational Medicine
Danish National Institute of Occupational Health
Baunegaardsvej 73
DK-2900 Hellerup

HISTORY

The first organolead compound, hexaethyldilead, $Et_3Pb-PbEt_3$, was synthesized in 1853 (Shapiro and Frye, 1968). Almost 70 years later, on December 9, 1921, Kettering and his co-workers in the Research Laboratories of General Motors discovered the effect of Et_4Pb as an antiknock agent. In 1922 production of Et_4Pb was started, and on February 2, 1923, the first gallon of petrol containing Et_4Pb was sold to a motorist in Dayton, Ohio (Nickerson, 1954). Tetra and tri-alkyl-lead compounds were already known to be highly toxic (Grandjean and Nielsen, 1979). Nevertheless, in the course of 17 months, 139 cases of severe intoxication with 13 deaths occurred in connection with the increasing production and handling of Et_4Pb (Hunter, 1975). A violent public dispute about the addition of lead to petrol resulted, and production had to be stopped in 1925 for more than a year, until the occupational risk had been assessed and hygienic measures to protect workers instituted. A committee of seven experts appointed by the U.S. Surgeon General concluded that it was not necessary to ban ethyl gasoline, provided that manufacture, distribution and sale were properly regulated.

When leaded petrol was used, deposits of lead oxide in the exhaust pipe and combustion engine shortened the durability of the motor components. From 1928 onwards, therefore, dichloroethane (EDC) and dibromoethane (EDB) were added as scavengers to the antiknock fluid, so that the lead oxide formed during combustion was converted to the more volatile lead halogenides (Nickerson, 1954).

From 1960, Me_4Pb and mixtures of Me_4Pb and Et_4Pb were manufactured commercially and marketed (Shapiro and Frey, 1968). Me_4Pb is superior to Et_4Pb in high-aromatic fuel and has proven to be more effective when driving at low speeds. Since 1960, Me_4Pb has gained a greater share of the market as a lead additive to petrol.

From a modesr start in 1922, the production of tetra-alkyl-lead has increased to such an extent that few organic chemicals are produced in greater quantities than is R_4Pb. During recent years, its use has decreased slightly. Since 1975, new automobiles in the U.S. have been equipped with a catalytic converter which precludes the use of leaded petrol, and many countries have decreased the permissible lead content of petrol to limit pollution with inorganic lead. Due to increasing use of lead additives in other parts of the world, where no regulations prevail, the total world production seems to be less affected by these regulations than might have been expected.

As suggested by this historical background, a health evaluation of lead additives was carried out in 1926 and, with some additional information, again in 1960 when Me_4Pb was introduced. Most attention was focused on the risk of acute organolead poisoning and, later, on environmental pollution with lead exhausts. The current production rate is of a magnitude that could not have been forseen in 1926, or, perhaps, even in 1960. It is only 10 years since Laveskog (1971) established the occurence of organolead compounds in urban air. During the last few years much has been learnt about the environmental fate of organolead pollution and its biological effects. This information should be taken into account when evaluating the health significance of lead additives.

EXPOSURE SOURCES

The early cases of Et_4Pb intoxication occurred among both laboratory chemists and production workers (Hunter, 1975). More recently, most fatal intoxications have been associated with heavy exposures during the cleaning of storage tanks. Deaths have also occured as a result of inadvertent use as a stain remover or solvent (Grandjean and Nielsen, 1979). Accidental ingestion has rarely caused intoxication, but petrol sniffing, mostly among children, has resulted in a large number of organolead poisonings (Grandjean and Nielsen, 1979). The hydrocarbon content of petrol may cause neurotoxicity and induction of liver enzymes (Harman et al. 1981) and thereby act synergistically on the effects of organic lead. As a safety measure, orange or blue dye is usually added to leaded petrol, and containers as well as filling stations display warnings to prevent accidents. During the production, mixing and transport of M_4Pb and Et_4Pb, there is risk of contamination, but only a relatively small number of cases of poisoning have been reported (Grandjean and Nielsen, 1979). Motor mechanics and others who use leaded petrol to clean their hands may increase their body burden of lead in this way. Other particularly exposed groups are filling-station attendents and staff in garages and underground parking lots. Due to the diagnostic and analytical difficulties, however, the literature only gives descriptions of severe poisonings, while the general exposure levels have not been elucidated in detail.

During transport of antiknock fluids or leaded petrol, there may be accidents that result in escape of organolead compounds into the environment. In July, 1974, a Yugoslavian ship carrying 900 drums containing 200 tons of tetra-methyl-lead and tetra-ethyl-lead sank in the straits between the Mediterranean and the Adriatic, off the south Italian fishing village of Otranto (Tiravanti and Boari, 1979). Most of the drums were later recovered, and little environmental impact was seen. Last December, a vessel carrying about twice as much antiknock fluid collided with another ship in the Great Belt, Denmark. Fortunately, damage was limited, and no escape of organic lead was documented.

The uptake of R_4Pb by urban populations is associated mainly with inhalation of R_4Pb vapors. Some pollution may occur from organolead production plants, but the major air pollution sources are filling stations and automobiles. During filling operations and through spills, R_4Pb compounds evaporate due to their relatively high vapour pressure (0.3-30mm Hg at 20°C) (Grandjean and Nielsen, 1979). The total loss of antiknock fluid during transportation and transfer of petrol has been estimated at 1.4% (Huntzicker, 1975). Me_4Pb has a higher vapour pressure than has Et_4Pb, and higher air levels of Me_4Pb at filling stations must be expected. Studies by Nielsen and his colleagues (1981) in Denmark have indicated that 90% of organolead vapours at filling stations may be Me_4Pb, and that total organolead levels may exceed $1\mu g/m^3$. Other studies have found levels of the same magnitude or higher, up to $6.7\mu g/m^3$ (Grandjean and Nielsen, 1979).

Extensive experiments performed by Laveskog (1971) have shown that the highest organolead levels in automobile exhausts occur during cold starts: Laveskog found averages about 2,000 $\mu g/m^3$, while idling caused about one-tenth of that level, and even lower amounts were found when driving at a constant speed with a warm engine. Most studies suggest that about 0.2-0.4% of the organolead additives will be exhausted uncombusted when driving at constant speed. Under city driving conditions, higher R_4Pb levels would be expected due to frequent idling and starts, probably at 1.4-1.9% of the R_4Pb consumption (Grandjean and Nielsen, 1979). In addition, evaporation from fuel tank and caburetor and contributions from so-called blow-by gases, particularly from older cars may add to pollution levels.

As might have been expected, both particulate lead and organic lead levels in the city fluctuate with traffic intensity. In Europe, the organolead contribution is usually between 5 and 10% of the total lead level in city air pollution, but somewhat lower levels have been documented in the U.S. due to improved engine designs (Grandjean and Nielsen, 1979). Near highways, organic lead constitutes only a few percent of the total lead. On the other hand, very high concentrations have been documented in underground parking lots (Nielsen et al., 1981). Thus, long-term averages up to $4.7\mu g/m^3$ have been recorded, with organolead exhausts higher from cars leaving the garage than from those entering.

Considerable amounts of fuel may escape uncombusted from mopeds, chain saws, lawn mowers, and other two-stroke engines. Thus, an unpublished study from the Swedish Labour Inspectorate in Umeå has recently shown organolead levels about the occupational exposure limit (75 µg/m³) caused by chain saw fumes. Thus, we need to widen our perspective of potential exposure sources.

Toxicokinetics   Both Me_4Pb and Et_4Pb are lipophilic substances which may be absorbed through the skin. When pure Et_4Pb is applied to the naked skin of rabbits, they absorb lethal quantities in the course of about an hour (Kehoe and Thamann, 1931). The absorption increases with the area of the skin involved and decreases when the Et_4Pb has been diluted with gasoline. Absorbed Et_4Pb is distributed within a few hours to the entire organism. In the case of Me_4Pb, absorption through the skin seems somewhat slower than that of Et_4Pb (Davis et al., 1963).

Both Et_4Pb and Me_4Pb are also relatively rapidly absorbed through the alveoli and the gastrointestinal tract. Experiments by Heard et al. (1979) with radioactively-tagged R_4Pb have shown that humans absorb about 40 and 50% of inhaled Et_4Pb and Me_4Pb, respectively. Some of the organolead was later exhaled, resulting in final depositions of 30 and 40%, respectively. After absorption into the blood, R_4Pb is taken up by soft organs, especially the liver. A dealkylation then takes place, and Et_3Pb^+ and Me_3Pb^+ may be identified in the body.

The tri-alkyl-lead compounds are relatively stable and are responsible for the toxic actions (Grandjean and Nielsen, 1979). The highest concentrations of R_3Pb^+ occur in the liver and kidneys, but high concentrations have also been found in the brain. Unfortunately, very little information is available concerning the fate of organolead compounds in the human organism. A significant part of the amount absorbed appears to be excreted within several hours in urine and faeces. Some studies, however, have shown the existence of organolead compartments with half-lives of up to 100 days, and longer-term retention may be a possibility. Thus, at chronic exposures, organic lead may be accumulated in the body.

One organ of particular interest is the brain because the central nervous system is the critical organ in organolead intoxication. In fatal cases of Et_4Pb poisoning, organolead levels of about 10 mg/g wet weight or 50 µmol/kg have been found in the brain. One small study which we conducted in Copenhagen suggested that adults without occupational exposures may retain about 0.1 µmol/kg in the brain, with a tendency of higher levels in the city, especially among residents on lower floors (Nielsen et al., 1978). While this result suggests a safety margin of 500, several laboratory studies indicate that toxic effects could occur at levels of about 0.1 µmol/kg (see below).

Human Intoxication   Perhaps it is remarkable that only about 100 fatal cases of Et_4Pb poisoning have been reported in the literature, and none with Me_4Pb (Grandjean and Nielsen, 1979). Neurological signs and symptoms dominate the picture. The latency period between acute exposure to Et_4Pb and the onset of symptoms varies from a few hours in the most serious cases to as much as ten days. The initial effects are anorexia, vomiting, insomnia, tremor, weakness, fatigue, nausea, headache, aggression, depression, irritability, body pains, restlessness, hyperactivity, difficulties in concentrating, confusion, impairment of memory and strange sensations (e.g., of insects creeping all over the body or hairs in the mouth). According to Russian authors (Razsudov, 1976), Et_4Pb poisoning is associated with the so-called Et_4Pb triad of hypotension, bradycardia and hypothermia, perhaps due to hypothalmic changes. These observations have, to some degree, be substantiated by experiences in other parts of the world. From the onset of the first symptoms and signs, hours or even days may pass before a serious exacerbation occurs in the form of acute mania, convulsions, delirium, fever and coma, perhaps related to the continued conversion of Et_4Pb to Et_3Pb^+. In serious cases, death has followed in 36 hours or after several days. The longer the period until symptoms set in or become aggravated, the better the prognosis. Even after acute, toxic psychosis, however, apparently complete recovery has been observed in two to six months, although minor symptoms and signs may persist for some time. In some cases, however, intellectual impairment and decreased working ability have remained as long-term sequelae (Grandjean and Nielsen, 1979).

Less attention has been paid to chronic, nonfatal exposures. However, a number of reports from the USSR, Italy and Japan have focused on this aspect of organolead toxicity. Again, central nervous system complaints and signs of dysfunction are associated with organolead or leaded petrol exposures. Frequent symptoms in exposed workers included increased fatigability, sensation of weakness, loss of appetite, lack of concentration, memory loss, sleep disturbance, headache and dizziness. Signs of CNS abnormalities include changes in EEG recordings, changes in the automatic nervous system (such as hypotension) and psychological dysfunction in cognitive test performance. Some evidence suggests an increased prevalence of vague, nonspecific neuropsychological symptomatology in men exposed to leaded petrol. In this regard, the possible interaction between various neurotoxic components of leaded petrol deserves a thorough examination.

Only one study has described the variations in some general health indicators and sickness absence between long-term Et_4Pb production workers and a reference group (Robinson, 1976). Unfortunately, the health indicators were rather general, such as height, weight, blood pressure, haemoglobin and electrocardiogram readings, so that any occurence of neurotoxicity was not ruled out. A mortality study at the same production plant indicated that no excess occurred over a period of 20 years (Robinson, 1974). Again, because of the limited sensitivity (only 51 deaths were recorded in this young population), any excess morality due to neurological disease or cancer cannot be ruled out. On the contrary, a more complete follow-up study in U.S. organolead production workers is underway, and preliminary data suggests an excess mortality due to multiple myeloma (Haring, 1980). Thus, with regard to the long-term health significance of organolead exposures, we need to learn much more before we can define the safety of these operations. In passing, the fact should be noted that the two scavengers, 1,2-dichloroethane and 1,2-dibromoethane, have shown carcinogenic effects in bioassays carried out at the U.S. National Cancer Institute (1978, 1982). These compounds occur in urban air pollution, the concentrations being of similar magnitude as those of organolead.

Mutagenic effects   While studies of mice exposed to Et_4Pb by the dominant lethal method have shown negative results (Kennedy et al., 1975), other investigations have suggested a mutagenic potential of organolead compounds. Thus, in various in vitro systems, both Me_3Pb^+ and Et_3Pb^+ have caused disturbance of the mitotic spindle, leading to arrested metaphases ("C-mitosis") and shortened chromosome lengths (Ahlberg et al., 1972); in some studies, polyploid cells could be detected (Roderer and Schnepf, 1977). In general, these findings have been confirmed by recent, unpublished experiments with human lymphocytes by Ole Andersen. Also, a clastogenic effect is indicated by a slight increase of sister chromatid exchange rates in human lymphocytes exposed to tri-alkyl-lead compounds in vitro; these studies have been carried out by my colleagues Erik Niebuhr and Hans C.Wulf (unpublished findings). The earliest in vitro effects have occured at tri-alkyl-lead concentrations of about 10^{-7} mol/l, Et_3Pb^+ being more toxic than Me_3Pb^+. In the absence of sufficient animal experiments and epidemiological experience, the health significance of such data may be a matter of controversy. The results reviewed strongly suggest, however, that the organolead compounds may have important toxic potentials in humans.

Biochemical mechanisms   The neurotoxic effects of organolead exposures appear to be related to the biochemical effects on membranes of the R_3Pb^+ molecule. For some years, the related organotin compounds have been known to concentrate in cell membranes and induce an exchange of anions. Bjerrum (unpublished findings) has now shown that both Me_3Pb^+ and Et_3Pb^+ induce an exchange of extracellular chloride with intracellular hydroxyl ions. Et_3Pb^+ appears to be 10-fold as effective as is Me_3Pb^+. In mitochondria, this transport obliterates the normal "pH gradient" across the membrane, and Aldridge et al. (1977) have demonstrated that the oxidative phosphorylation is the uncoupled. In nerve cells, the transport induced could lead to intracellular accumulation of chloride. Under such conditions, a nerve cell may need more energy. Because the energy production by oxidative phosphorylation is, at the same time, inhibited or blocked, the nerve cell may ultimately die (Cremer, 1981). Indeed, experiments carried out at Aldridge's laboratory in Carshalton by Seawright and co-workers (1980), have shown nuronal death in specific areas of the brain: primiarily the hippocampus, the amygdala and the pyriform cortex. Thus, recent discoveries in this area may lead us to believe that we understand the general outline of the toxic mechanisms. Also, mention should be made of the occurence of enzyme inhibitions at Et_2Pb^+ concentrations at $10^{-7}M$ and above (Grandjean and Nielsen, 1979).

CONCLUSIONS

Organolead production world-wide is currently about 300,000 metric tons per year. A total of about 7,000 tons of organolead is emitted to the atmosphere, especially from filling stations and automobiles. In urban air, 24-hour mean levels are often about 0.3 $\mu g/m^3$, but much higher concentrations have been detected at filling stations, garages, etc. Organolead compounds are readily absorbed through the respiratory and gastrointestinal tracts and through the skin. They are metabolized in the body into tri-alkyl-lead compounds which are responsible for the toxic effects . The brain is the organ most sensitive to intoxication. Symptoms of poisoning include insomnia, anorexia, nausea, tremor, restlessness, cramps, delirium and coma. Low concentrations of Et_3Pb and Me_3Pb^+ have been shown to induce an exchange of chloride and hydroxide over biological membranes, to uncouple oxidative phosphorylation and to inhibit some enzymes in vitro. In one investigation, organolead concentrations of about $10-^7M$ were found in samples of brain tissue from people of the general population, levels which are about 1% of concentrations found in the brain after fatal intoxications but of a magnitude which may cause subtle biochemical changes. Some evidence might suggest the occurence of slight, nonspecific neuropsychological dysfunction related to occupational exposures to leaded petrol, but the neurotoxic potential at low-level exposures remains uncertain. In addition, mutagenic effects have been demonstrated in vitro at organolead levels of $10^{-7}M$ and above, particularly inhibition of spindle formation and induction of C-mitosis, but also a slight induction of sister chromatid exchange. Although these effects have now been demonstrated in human cells, the health implications are uncertain in the absence of sufficient animal experiments or epidemiological data. Current occupational exposure limits to inorganic and organic lead compounds are of the same magnitude, despite the high acute toxicity of organolead compounds and their potentials for long-term health effects. Indeed, inorganic lead appears to be a product of the slow detoxification of tri-alkyl-lead compounds in the body. The limited attention paid to organolead compounds may be due to the fact that they behave very differently from inorganic lead and that only sophisticated research has revealed important information on their environmental occurence and biological effects. Perhaps the time is near for a thorough consideration of occupational and environmental health implications of tetra-alkyl-lead emissions.

ACKNOWLEDGEMENT

This review has been based on extensive cooperation with Torben

Nielsen, Department of Chemistry, Riso National Laboratory, and
our joint review paper from 1979. A full account including more
recent data will appear in a monograph to be published by CRC
Press in early 1983.

DISCUSSION

Russell Jones: The lethal dose of tetraethyl lead in humans is
                  about a quarter of a gram, so that every gallon
                  of petrol sold in the UK contains sufficient lead
                  to kill five adult males. If, instead of being a
                  technological reality, it was suggested that lead
                  should be added to petrol in order to reduce its
                  price by two to three pence a gallon, how do
                  you think that proposal would be received?

Grandjean: In my view, if you had discovered today that
                  organic lead is a useful anti-knock compound, I
                  do not think its addition to petrol would be
                  allowed. The only reason we are continuing
                  this practice is that we have done it for years.
                  The introduction of tetraethyl lead in 1925 was
                  based on a series of experiments which would
                  be regarded as wholly inadequate by current
                  standards.

Silbergeld: Would you care to comment on recent reports
                  that organic lead compounds can be formed by
                  various organisms that occur naturally?

Grandjean: Arne Jernelöv in Sweden, who first identified
                  methylation of mercury, told me that there is a
                  lack of evidence that lead is actually methylated
                  from inorganic lead to tetraethyl lead. In their
                  recent review of the evidence, Chau and Wong
                  (1982) were also very cautious in drawing
                  conclusions. It seems that some methylation
                  does occur, but it is not known whether it is
                  mediated by micro-organisms or whether it is a
                  chemical methylation in sediments. Neverthe-
                  less, it is clear that trimethyl lead from auto
                  exhausts can be chemically or microbially
                  methylated to the tetra compound.

Question: Would you like to comment on the American
                  Conference of Governmental Industrial
                  Hygienists and the current proposed reduction
                  in lead?

Grandjean: The ACGIH recommendations for exposure limits
                  to triethyl lead and tetramethyl lead are about
                  0.1 and 0.15 milligrams per cubic metre respec-
                  tively. The Occupational Safety and Health

Administration, of the Department of Labour in the United States, has a somewhat different limit of 0.07 or 0.075 for these two compounds. We now have a strange situation in the United States where the standard for inorganic lead exposure at work (0.05 mg/m^3) is even lower than the standard for the organo-lead compounds. This is a ridiculous situation when one considers that in the metabolism of organo-lead compounds in the body, inorganic lead is actually a detoxification product.

Question: It seems to me that the regulating authorities either do not accept the evidence that you have presented or you have not got the message across to them. Is there in fact a lobby to reduce the legal maximum by a considerable amount?

Grandjean: Much of the evidence that I have presented has not yet been published. Thus, we have not reached the political level yet but I hope that this meeting may help us in reaching the right decision.

REFERENCES

Ahlbergh, J., Ramel, C., Wachtmeister, C.A., 1972, Organolead compounds shown to be genetically active, Ambio; 1:29-31.

Aldridge, W.N., Street, B.W., Skilleter, D.N., 1977, Oxidative phosphorylation, Halide-dependent and halide-independent effects of triorganotin and triorganolead on mitochondrial functions, Biochem, J.;168:353-364.

Chau, Y.K. and Wong, P.T.S., (1982), Organic lead in the aquatic environment. In Grandjean, P., (ed.) Biological Effects of Organolead Compounds, Boca Raton, Florida: CRC Press (in press).

Cremer, J.E., Specific toxic effects on the nervous system, 1981, In:S.S. Brown, D.S. Davies, eds.: Organ-Directed Toxicity. Oxford: Pergamon, p.213-217.

Davis, R.K., Horton, A.W., Larson, E.E., Stemmer, K.L. 1963. Inhalation of tetramethyllead. Arch environ Health, 6:473-479.

Grandjean, P., Nielsen, T., 1979, Organolead compounds: Environmental health aspects. Res Rev, 72:97-148.

Haring, M., 1980, Mortality and industrial hygiene study of workers exposed to tetraethyl lead, In:C.S. Muir, G. Wagner, eds: Directory of on-going research in cancer epidemiology 1980. Lyon: International Agency for Research on Cancer, p.428.

Harman, A.W., Frewin, D.B., Priestly B.G., 1981 Induction of microsomal drug metabolism in man and in the rat by exposure to petroleum. Br J Ind Med; 38:91-97.

Heard, M.J., Wells, A.C., Newton, D., Chamberlain, A.C., 1979, Human uptake and metabolism of tetra ethyl and tetra methyl lead vapour labelled with ^{203}Pb. In:R. Perry, ed:International Conference, Management & Control of Heavy Metals in the Environment. Edinburgh: CEP Consultants, p.103-108.

Hunter, D., 1975, The diseases of occupations. 5th ed. London: English Universities,p.291.

Huntzicker, J.J., Friedlander, S.K., Davidson C.I., 1975, Material balance for automobile-emitted lead in Los Angeles basin. Environ Sci Technol, 9:448-457.

Kehoe, R.A., Thamann, F., 1931, The behaviour of lead in the animal organism, II. tetraethyl lead. Amer J Hyg, 13:478-498.

Kennedy, G.L., Arnold, D.W., Calandra, J.C., 1975 Teratogenic evaluation of lead compounds in mice and rats. Food Cosm Toxicol, 13:629-632.

Laveskog, A., 1971, A method for determination of tetramethyl lead (TLM) and tetraethyllead (TEL) in air. In:H.M. Englund, W.T. Beery, eds: Proceedings of the 2nd International Clean Air Congress, p.549-557.

National Cancer Institute, 1978, Bioassay of 1,2-dichloroethane for possible carcinogenicity. Bethesda, Md.:National Cancer Institute, (Carcinogenesis, Technical Report Series No 55) (DHEW publication No (NIH) 78-1361).

National Cancer Institute, 1982, Carcinogenesis biossay of 1,2-dibromoethane in F344 rats and B6C3F$_1$ mice (inhalation study). Bethesda Md.: National Cancer Institute, (National Toxicology Program, Technical Report Series No 210) (NIH publication No 82-1766).

Nickerson, S.P., 1954, Tetraethyl lead: A product of American research. J Cehm Ed, 31:560-571.

Nielsen, T., Egsgaard, H., Larsen, E., 1981 Determination of tetramethyllead and tetraethyllead in the atmosphere by a two-step enrichment method and gas chromatographic-mass spectrometric isotope dilution analysis. Anal Chim Acta; 124:1-13.

Nielsen, T., Jensen, K.A., Grandjean, P., 1978. Organic lead in normal human brains. Nature; 274:602-603.

Razsudov, V.N., 1976. Toxicology of tetraethyllead (in Russian). Ministry of Public Health, Faculty of International Health of Medical Perf. Institute, 24pp.

Robinson, T.R., 1974. 20-year mortality of tetraethyl lead workers. J Occup Med; 16:601-605.

Robinson, T.R., 1976. the health of long service tetraethyl lead workers. J Occup Med; 18:31-40.

Roderer, G., Schnepf, E., 1977. Tetraethyl lead and triethyl lead inhibit cytokinesis of the chrysophycean flagellate poterioochromonas. Naturwissensch;64:588-589.

Seawright, A.A., Brown, A.W., Aldridge, W.N., Verschoyle, R.D., Street, B.W., 1980. Neuropathological changes caused by trialkyllead compounds in the rat. In:B. Holmstedt, R. Lauwerys, M. Mercier, M. Roberfroid, eds: Mechanisms of toxicity and hazard evaluation. Amsterdam:Elsevier, p.71-74.

Shapiro, H., Frey, F.W., 1968. The organic compounds of lead. New York: Interscience.

Tiravanti, G., Boari, G., 1979. Potential pollution of a marine
    environment by lead alkyls: The Cavtat Incident. Environ Sci
    Technol; 13:849-854.

EXPERIMENTAL STUDIES OF LEAD NEUROTOXICITY:
IMPLICATIONS FOR MECHANISMS, DOSE-RESPONSE,
AND REVERSIBILITY

Ellen K. Silbergeld, Ph.D.

Environmental Defense Fund
Washington DC
USA

INTRODUCTION

The study of low level lead poisoning has been characterized by an
unusually fruitful interconnection of clinical and experimental
research during the past ten years. Recent clinical studies, as
discussed in other papers of this volume, have substantiated new
appreciation of the adverse effects of lower levels of lead exposure
in children. In addition, experimental studies can provide
important information no available clinically. This paper summarizes
this research as it relates to the resolution of two issues: (1)
mechanisms of action of lead as a neurotoxin, and (2) the nature of
any apparent thresholds to lead in terms of dose-effects at the
neuronal level. Conclusions based on experimental research, in this
as in any area, must be tempered with reservations as to inter-
species comparability arising from differences in dose and chronicity
of exposure, and limitations on measurements of outcome,
particularly the expressions of neurobehavioral competence
measurable in rodents. With reference to models of lead toxicity,
these issues have been discussed at length elsewhere (Silbergeld
and Goldberg, 1979).

The discussion will be restricted to the neurotoxicity of lead. In
the child, the brain is probably one of the most sensitive targets of
lead. Also, adverse effects of lead on brain function are of the
greatest clinical concern, and it is in the area of neurological
toxicity, that the questions of mechanisms, threshold and
reversibility are most urgent. I will not attempt to provide a
complete summary of the evidence on review, the neurological
toxicity of lead in animals, since several reviews have been
published recently (Silbergeld, 1982a; Bornschein, et al, 1980;
Jason and Kellogg, 1980). After description of the primary animal
model for lead poisoning in children, four aspects of neurotoxicity
are reviewed: electrophysiology, behavior, anatomy and chemistry.
From the results of these studies, hypotheses on mechanisms are
presented, and implications for resolving questions of threshold for
neurotoxic effect and the potential reversibility of lead effects are
discussed.

ANIMAL MODELS

The animal model for the study of lead toxicity in children is based on the original work of Pentschew and Garro (1966), which utilizes neonatal rodents exposed indirectly, soon after parturition, by administering lead in food or water to their dams. It has been demonstrated that this method delivers significant doses of lead via maternal milk (Bornschein, et al, 1975). Although the model obviously does not replicate human exposure (since contamination of human milk or formula is usually a minor source of lead intake by infants), it preserves two essential aspects of lead exposure in children: the oral route of intake, and the timing of exposure during critical periods of brain growth. Studies on the comparability of brain growth patterns between rodents and humans support use of the preweaning period in the rat and mouse as analogous to the first two years of brain development in humans (Dobbing, 1972). It should be noted that these rodent models have been used almost exclusively for the study of postnatal lead exposure; the effects of prenatal exposure, currently of great clinical concern, have not been evaluated in animals. The relevance of those few studies that have been undertaken (Brady et al, 1975) is not known.

Several limitations on the rodent model have become apparent with its use. First, in several respects, rodents show differential sensitivity to lead, as compared with humans. For example, the rat appears more susceptible to cerebellar hemorrhage it may be uniquely sensitive to lead as a hepatic carcinogen; and the response of heme-dependent hepatic drug metabolizing enzyme systems to lead may also differ in rodents (Silbergeld and Goldberg, 1980). Second, both internal and external doses used in rodent studies appear high, in comparison with measurements of blood lead levels in exposed children and with the estimated exposure of children. Discrepancy in dose has provided some challenge to extrapolations from animals to humans, and questions on the reality of low level lead neurotoxicity, as demonstrated in animals (Michaelson, 1980).

In experimental toxicology, it is difficult to define equivalence of exposure. The relatively short life spans of experimental animals alter the relationship between dose and duration assumed for humans. This is further complicated in lead studies, because the relationship between these factors is not simple, i.e., in any species, long exposure to lead at a low dose is not equivalent to short exposure at high dose (Browder, et al, 1973). Moreover, comparing animals to humans solely on the basis of external dose may be misleading since there are significant species differences in absorption and retention of lead. A more appropriate defination of equivalence may be based on effect, which would encompass differences in absorption and dose and focus on equivalence of measurable outcome. Under this definition, the differences required in external dose to produce similar functional changes (or biochemical alterations) can form a basis for evaluating the comparability of particular studies to humans. Operationally, many experimental studies have been assumed to be of low level poisoning primarily on the grounds that no signs of overt toxicity, such as significant loss of body weight or anemia, were observed at the doses used. In general, this is not a very thoughtful approach, although changes in body weight appear to be a sensitive index of exposure in rodents.

EXPERIMENTAL MEASUREMENTS OF NEUROTOXICITY

The measurements of neurotoxic effect utilized in animal studies are not all comparable to those possible in children. Obviously, species differences and the ethics of clinical medicine prelude the use of similar techniques in both populations. Of all measures, electrophysiology and neurobehavioral methods are those most likely to be applicable to animals and humans, while neurochemical and neuroanatomic methods are, with rare exceptions, used only in experimental animals.

Electrophysiological studies, which in some cases might be feasible to apply clinically, have not been undertaken extensively in humans. Some recent reports have found striking differences in power output and pattern of cortical electrical activity in lead-exposed children as compared to controls (Thatcher, et al, 1982; Burchfield, et al, 1980). In rodents, more precisely defined electrophysiological as visual evoked response and hippocampal function (Fox, 1982) have been examined. The results suggest that stimulus dependent measures, such as evoked response, may be very sensitive indicators of adverse neurological effects, observable at very low doses. Two clinical studies confirm this (Otto, 1982; Thatcher, et al, 1982).

Electrophysiological measurements have been used in evaluating peripheral neurotoxicity in both adults and children exposed to lead. In sufficiently large populations, the results indicate that lead tends to slow ulnar and peroneal nerve conduction velocities at relatively low levels of exposure (Feldman, et al, 1977; Landrigan, et al, 1975). Comparable studies in rodents have not been performed.

Behavioral measurements have been extensively applied in animal studies of lead toxicity. In terms of behavior, lead is probably the most fully investigated neurotoxin and its study has advanced the field of neurobehavioral toxicology. Two types of behavior have been examined in animals: spontaneous behavior, and learned or scheduled behavior. As a preface to their discussion, it is important to be cautious in claiming homology between behavioral effects in animals and the clinical presentation of lead toxicity. The nature of behavioral dysfunction observed in lead-exposed animals has in some instances been compared to hyperkinetic behavior, aspects of which have been described in children with low level lead poisoning (David, et al, 1972; Needleman, et al, 1979). Also lead poisoning has been proposed as one etiological factor in minimal brain dysfunction/hyperkinesis/attention deficit disorders

(Schain, 1980). Nevertheless, the most appropriate definition of
the clinical entity "hyperkinesis" remains in dispute. As a result,
increased motoric activity may be less crucial to the syndrome than
distractibility and shortened attention span, behaviors which are
difficult to measure in rodents. Increases in spontaneous motor
activity have been frequently reported in lead exposed rodents
(Jason and Kellogg, 1980). However, it is apparent that this
phenomenon and its detection are largely dependent upon the age of
measurement as well as on the techniques used to measure activity
(Reiter, et al, 1975; Silbergeld and Goldberg, 1973). As shown in
figure 1,* in mice exposed to lead continuously from birth, a persistent hyperactivity is produced, which, while reduced with age,
still remains higher at all days measured than the activity of
age-matched controls.

The evaluation of studies of the effects of lead on learned or
scheduled behaviors is complex. Many different methods have been
applied, and different aspects of acquisition, performance, and
memory have been analyzed. An overview suggests that the results
are fairly consistent in demonstrating that lead-exposed animals
show reduced performance, with particular problems in three areas:
(1) the regulation of rate-dependent responses, (2) the suppression
of active behavior in a passive-response situation, such as shock
avoidance, and (3) the extinction or reversal of responses after
termination of eliciting stimulus conditions. Also, scheduled or
selective behaviors that require relatively fine visual distinctions
are performed less well by lead exposed primates, rodents, and
sheep (Bushnell, et al, 1977; Carson et al, 1974). This may
suggest specific effects of lead on components of the visual system
function, as distinct from visually-cued learning processes (Fox,
1982).

Learning, as measured operantly, involves the integrated function
of many parameters, including motor function, visual or auditory
activity. If food rewards are used, it also requires the intact
functioning of complex systems involved in motivation, hunger and
satiety. Lead is known to affect aspects of all of these functions.
Lead is a peripheral neurotoxic agent in the motor system (Manalis
and Cooper 1973; Silbergeld, et al, 1974); lead may have particular
affinity for precortical elements of the visual system, such as the
optic nerve (Tennekoon et al, 1978) and retina (Fox, 1982) and
lead can alter consummatory behavior and hypothalamic function
(Morrison, et al, 1974; Mailman, et al, 1978).

Clearly, it is difficult to make direct comparisons between the
behavioral observations of lead-exposed rodents and the behaviors
described in children. The most commonly used instrument for
determining adverse neurobehavioral effects of lead in children has
been the intelligence test (Needleman, et al, 1979; Rutter, 1980);
no battery of analogous complexity is available for rodents. Studies
in primates are perhaps suggestive of similar disturbances in higher
cortical function, but these have been less frequently done in
experimental studies (Bushnell and Bowman, 1979).

*Figure 1 at end of chapter

Another type of neurobehavioral method used with some success in experimental studies has been the measurement of drug-elicited behaviors. In many studies, it has been reported that lead exposure results in attenuation of response to stimulant drugs acting through catecholamingergic systems, such as methylphenidate, the amphetamines, and apomorphine (Silbergeld, 1982b). Pharacological probes for obvious reasons, are not applicable to clinical studies except in rare cases; the most that can be said is that it is consistent with the possible etiologic role of lead in hyperkinesis. Since many hyperkenetic children respond distinctively to stimulent medication, this may be another possible reason for exploring lead as both a cause and a model of the clinical disorder.

Neurochemistry and neuropathology, two methods not generally amenable to extensive use in humans, have been very important in understanding the mechanisms of lead neurotoxicity. Alterations in neurochemistry (see Tables 1 and 2) may precede other neurotoxic effects and may be the basis for expressions of altered behavior, pharmacological response, and cell pathology (Hrdina, et al, 1980; Silbergeld, 1982a). Although most neurochemical studies require fresh brain tissue for analysis, it is possible to study aspects of neurotransmitter metabolism with noninvasive techniques applicable to human research. As shown in Table 3, the appearance of aminergic metabolites in urine. have been studied in children and adults. In the study of urinary homovanillic acid in lead-exposed children, studies in mice were conducted in parallel (Silbergeld and Chisolm, 1976). The results taken together suggested that the observed increases in urinary metabolies seen in children were not inconsistent with changes in brain neurochemistry (see also Wince, et al, 1980; Lucchi, et al, 1981). However, the multiple sources for urinary HVA make it impossible to ascribe the observed increases exclusively or even immainly to effects of lead on the CNS. It is not known if the changes reported in urinary 5-hydroxindoleacetic acid of lead-exposed workers (Dugandzic, et al, 1973) are reflective of effects of lead on serotonergic function in the CNS, although some studies in rabbits suggest that lead can alter brain uptake of the serotonin precursor tryptophan (Lorenzo and Gewirtz, 1977) and regional neurochemistry (Hrdina, et al, 1980). Other neurochemical studies have not been done, and it is difficult to obtain any relevant measures on other types of chemical neurotransmission without recourse to such techniques as cerebrospinal fluid collection. However, the report that lead exposure in rodents alters plasma concentrations of pituitary hormones (Petrusz, et al, 1979) would suggest similar studies in humans.

TABLE 1. CHANGES IN BRAIN NE, DA, 5-HT AND 5-HIAA LEVELS IN RATS CHRONICALLY EXPOSED TO LEAD FROM BIRTH

Brain Region	Experimental group*	Levels (% control) and direction of changes			
		NE	DA	5-HT	5-HIAA
Cortex	Hyperactive (8 wk)	75 0	–	89	85
	Normal (12 wk)	91 0	110	87	120 0
	Withdrawn (10 wk)	95 0	107	87	110 0
Midbrain	Hyperactive (8 wk)	116 0	83	102 0	94 0
	Normal (12 wk)	97 0	95 0	101 0	95 0
	Withdrawn (10 wk)	92 0	88	100 0	91 0
Striatum	Hyperactive (8 wk)	73 0	99 0	104 0	107 0 →
	Normal (12 wk)	100 0	103 0	67 0	84 →
	Withdrawn (10 wk)	92 0	90 0	77	84 →
Hypothalamus	Hyperactive (8 wk)	99 0	80 0	86 0	82 → →
	Normal (12 wk)	104 0	97 0	97	77 →
	Withdrawn (10 wk)	107 0	97 0	86	86 →

NE   = Noreprinephrine
DA   = Dopamine
5-HT = 5-Hydroxy tryptophan
5-HIAA = 5-Hydroxy Indol Acetic Acid

TABLE 2 EFFECTS OF CHRONIC LEAD EXPOSURE ON VARIOUS PARAMETERS
OF ACETYLCHOLINE METABOLISM

Parameter studied	Species	Tissue	Results
Acetylcholine Turnover rate in vivo	Rat	Cortex, hippocampus, midbrain, striatum	33 – 54% decrease
Spontaneous release	Mouse	Cortical minces	40% increase
Potassium-induced release	Mouse	Cortical minces	16 – 30% decrease
Preganglionic stimulation-induced release	Cat	Perfursed superior cervical ganglion	Decrease
Size of endplate potential (epp) and frequency of miniature epps	Frog	Isolated sciatic nerve-sartorius muscle preparation	Reduction in size of epp; increased frequency of mepps
Force and latency of muscle contraction following nerve stimulation	Rat; mouse	Phrenic nerve-hemidiaphragm preparation	Reduction on force increase in latency
Choline High affinity transport	Mouse	Forebrain Synaptosomes	50% decrease
	Mouse	Cortical minces	No change
Low affinity transport	Mouse	Forebrain synaptosomes	No change
	Mouse	Cortical minces	No change
Spontaneous release	Mouse	Cortical minces	No change
Potassium-induced release	Mouse	Cortical minces	34 – 57% decrease

Data from Hrdina et al, 1980.

TABLE 3 EFFECTS OF LEAD EXPOSURE IN HUMANS ON
URINARY EXCRETION OF BIOGENIC AMINE
METABOLITES

Parameter	Controls	(n)	Lead-Exposed	(n)
5-hydroxyindoleacetic acid* mg/l	2.36	(23)	12.84	(50)
homovanillic acid** mg/m²/day	4.54	(6)	27.54	(6)
vanillymandelic acid** mg/m²/day	2.55	(6)	14.07	(6)

* measured in adults exposed occupationally to lead, in whom levels of spontaneously excreted urinary lead were (mean) 213 µg/l, as compared to 19 µg/l in controls. Data are from Dugandzic, et al, 1973.

** measured in children exposed to lead, in whom blood lead levels were between 59 and 68 µg/100 ml whole blood, as compared to less than 30 µg/100 ml in controls. Data are from Silbergeld and Chisolm, 1976.

TABLE 4 THICKNESS OF HIPPOCAMPAL CORTEX FROM
CONTROL AND LEAD-TREATED RATS[a]

	Thickness (um) of indicated brain sites	
Group	Dentate Gyrus	Cortex
Control	80.0 ± 2.1^{b}	1756.8 ± 53.1
Lead	68.4 ± 3.0^{c}	1528.3 ± 66.6^{c}
Percentage of control	98.2	87.0

[a] Neonatal rats given lead acetate (7.5 mg/kg ip) for the first 10 days of life.

[b] Mean $\pm$ SE from at least four 30-day old rats.

[c] Significantly different from that of respective control ($p < 0.05$).

Data from Louis-Ferdinand et al, 1978.

The neuropathologic studies of lead toxicity in animals cannot be compared to those in humans, except in fatal cases of acute lead encephalopathy, where tissue has been examined at autopsy. In these cases, good correlations with experimental animals exist in terms of edema, hemorrhage, and types of neuronal damage (Pentschew and Garro, 1966; Clasen, et al, 1974). However, significant morphological change has not been found to occur in experimental animals at doses of lead below these associated weight loss (Tennekoon, et al, 1978; Averill and Needleman, 1980). As shown in Table 4, altered synaptogenesis and decreased thickness of subcortical layers have been reported (Louis-Ferdinand, et al, 1978). The peripheral neuropathology produced by lead involves Schwann cell-associated demyelination and readily comparable effects can be observed in humans and experimental animals exposed to lead (Lampert and Schochet, 1968). The morphologic evidence of demyelination is associated with relatively high doses of lead (Winderbank, et al, 1980) and is not likely to underlie the functional observations of peripheral neurotoxicity, such as slowed conduction velocity.

In summary, neurophysiological, behavioral, and chemical studies of lead-exposed rodents demonstrate significant toxic effects associated with exposure comparable to the lower levels of increased lead absorption in children. In clinical terms, adverse effects have been described in animals with blood lead levels less than 30 µg/100 ml. In vitro, neurochemical parameters show effects within minutes of exposure to submicromolar concentrations of lead. The functional significance of such neurochemical effects may be difficult to assess, although any neurochemical change suggests a continuous dose-response relationship which eventually results in detectable dysfunction. This hypothesis of continuity can be demonstrated on the basis of studies utilizing pharmacological probes. Even in rodents not showing measurable changes in activity after lead exposure, motoric response to amphetamine is reduced (Silbergeld and Goldberg, 1980). In rats exposed to low levels of lead, GABAergic neurotransmission is inhibited rapidly and sensitively (Silbergeld, et al, 1981). At these doses, none of the expected behavioral manifestations of inhibited GABAergic neurotransmission - excitability or convulsions - are spontaneously shown. However, under conditions where this pathway is further challenged, by pharmacological intervention or other stress such as electroshock, the limitations imposed by lead are revealed. Sensitivity to drugs which act on GABAergic pathways is significantly increased, and can be measured in terms of lowered doses required to produce signs of convulsant activity (Table 5).

MECHANISMS OF ACTION OF LEAD AS A NEUROTOXIN

Fundamental to the investigation of the mechanisms of lead neurotoxicity, is the assumption that, as far as is presently known, lead has no role in cellular physiology. As a consequence, understanding its toxicity does not involve determining a relationship between the minimum requirements of nutrition and the

TABLE 5 EFFECTS   OF   LEAD   ON   SENSITIVITY   TO
GABAERGIC DRUGS

dose of picrotoxin required to elicit

Treatment	convulsions	hindlimb extension
acute lead*	3.3 ± 0.4 mg/kg	3.4 ± 0.2[a]
controls	3.7 ± 0.2	4.1 ± 0.2
chronic lead**	0.6 ± 0.3[a]	1.6 ± 0.2[a]
controls	3.2 ± 0.5	4.7 ± 0.7

* acutely treated rats were injected intraperitoneally with lead acetate, 10 μmol/kg/day, for 3 days.

** chronically treated rates were exposed from day 1 to 30 of life indirectly to lead in their dams' drinking water (10 mg/ml).

[a] lead-exposed significantly different from controls, p <0.025. Data are from Silbergeld, et al, 1981.

toxic effects of excessive exposure. This distinction is necessary in investigating the toxicity of such metals as copper and manganese, which, depending upon dose, are essential trace elements or neurotoxins. In addition, the lack of biological essentiality must suggest that there is no threshold for the toxic effects of lead at specific cellular sites of action.

Lead is also an elemental neurotoxin. Its toxic actions appear to be associated with its elemental state, and are not dependent upon a specific valence state or the metabolic or other conjugation of lead to a complex molecule or salt. Compositional differences in lead molecules affect its rate of uptake and compartmental accumulation; for example, organolead compounds have increased penetration to the brain and enhanced effects on myelin (Konat, et al, 1979).

Since lead is an element and a divalent cation, its effects are likely to involve interference with the normal role of other trace elements and physiologically important cations. Neuronal function is highly regulated by movements of charged ions across cell membranes. The chemical theory of neurotransmission postulates that information is propagated through the nervous system on the basis of such movements, in response to changes in membrane potential and chemicals binding to specifically reactive sites on cell membranes (Cooper, Bloom and Roth, 1970). Cellular fluxes of calcium, sodium, potassium, and chloride occur under conditions of changed membrane permeability of conductance, during which channels highly specific to these ions are opened to their entrance. Membrane-associated enzymes regulate their movement and limit the membrane excitability changes produced by their fluxes. Movements of these ions also initiate the events involved in propagating information exchange from cell to cell, by their involvement in the mechanisms of release and synthesis of neurotransmitters, transport and inactivation processes, and phosphorylation/activation of enzymes. Three important aspects of neurotransmission are controlled by ion movements: excitability state of the releasing cell; release of neurotransmitters from that cell; and translation of neurotransmitters action in the target cell.

Lead is known to affect the release of several neurotransmitters, including acetylcholine, Morepinephrine, dopamine, and g-aminobutyric acid (GABA). These effects can be demonstrated in experimental animals after in vivo exposure on the basis of turnover measurements and determination of metabolite or transmitter levels (reviewed by Hrdina, et al, 1980). Brain tissue has also been prepared from animals exposed in vivo, and specific aspects of neurotransmitter metabolism measured in vitro. These studies have shown effects of lead on dopamine uptake and release, ace-tylocholine release and choline uptake, and on GABA uptake and release. The results of such studies are summarized in Table 5. Cholinergic effects - decreased transmitter release - have also been shown in neuromuscular preparations taken from lead-exposed rodents (Silbergeld, et al, 1974).

Release of these transmitters from nerve endings, in response to stimulation of the nerves is a calcium-dependent process known as exocytosis. In preparations of peripheral tissue, it has been shown that the inhibitory effects of lead were limited to stimulus-coupled or calcium-dependent release of acetylcholine. The actions of lead could also be mimicked functionally and electrophysiologically by reducing calcium concentrations surrounding nerve cell preparations, while increasing calcium concentrations could reverse or suppress the effects of lead (Silbergeld, 1982a). When calcium flux into nerve endings was measured, it was shown that lead reduced calcium uptake during stimulation of the nerve. The site of action of this effect of lead, to block calcium entry into peripheral nerve cells, is not known. The reversability of peripheral neurotoxic effects of lead, with additional calcium or with washout, suggests that lead is not taken up by the neuron or tightly bound to the external membrane. The failure of lead to alter the nature of presynaptic neural electrical activity, in response to stimulation indicates that the actions of lead are relatively restricted to calcium. Changes in potassium or sodium flux, would have been reflected in altered compound action potential. Intracellular electrophysiological methods capable of detecting the contribution of calcium compound to presynaptic currents have not been applied to the study of lead.

TABLE 6 EFFECTS OF LEAD AND CALCIUM ON HIGH AFFINITY UPTAKE OF TYROSINE BY SYNAPTOSOMES

Lead	Calcium	^{14}C-Tyrosine Uptake
0	0	100%
0.1 uM	0	102
10.0 uM	0	143
100.0 uM	0	220
0	2.5 mM	100%
0	2.0 mM	94
0	1.0 mM	132
0	0.5 mM	148

Data from Silbergeld, 1977

Another calcium sensitive process which appears to be affected by lead is the high affinity uptake system for the dopamine precursor tyrosine. In vitor, both increased lead and decreased calcium concentrations act similarly to increase the uptake of tyrosine by rat brain synaptosomes (Table 6). In vivo, enhanced tyrosine uptake was also described in tissue prepared from lead-exposed mice (Silbergeld and Goldberg, 1975) although this was not found for a later study of rats (Wince, et al, 1980). Other important roles of calcium in nervous system function, such as calmodulin, have not been investigated for effects of lead. As shown in Table 7, the action of lead in vivo and in vitro to inhibit adenylyl cyclase activity (Nathanson and Bloom, 1976; Wince, et al, 1980) may involve calcium, but this has not been specifically studied.

It may be concluded, on the basis of these studies, that lead acts mechanically to antagonize calcium. However, blockade of release by lead is observed directly only at peripheral cholinergic synapses. In the CNS, lead in vitro does not block release of aceytcholine, dopamine, or GABA. In the CNS, lead does not interfere with cellular uptake of calcium; in contrast, the exposure of synaptosomes and isolated brain capillaries to lead in vitro increases uptake of ^{45}Ca (figure 2).* Thus the evidence is against the hypothesis that the neurotoxic effects of lead generally involve competition with calcium, although this mechanism may be the basis for some specific effects of lead, such as at peripheral cholinergic synapses.

*Figure 2 at end of chapter

TABLE 7 DOPAMINE STIMULATION OF ADENYLATE CYCLASE ACTIVITY IN HOMOGENATES OF 25- TO 35-DAY-OLD RAT PUP NEOSTRIATUM AFTER CHRONIC LEAD CARBONATE EXPOSURE

	Control			Lead	
Dopamine	Adenylate Cyclase activity[a]	% of basal	Dopamine	Adenylate Cyclase activity[a]	% of basal
0 (basal)	72.60 ± 1.69	100	0 (basal)	70.32 ± 1.95	100
10^{-6} M	74.28 ± 4.33	102	10^{-6} M	71.40 ± 4.67	101
10^{-5} M	87.00 ± 3.27^{b}	119	10^{-5} M	83.16 ± 6.02^{b}	118
10^{-4} M	106.88 ± 3.00^{b}	147	10^{-4} M	$94.20 \pm 3.47^{b,c}$	133
10^{-3} M	109.02 ± 5.22^{b}	150	10^{-3} M	$92.08 \pm 3.36^{b,c}$	130

[a] Pico-moles of cAMP per 50 µl/2.5 min; mean ± S.E.M. of five experiments in duplicate.

[b] $p < .05$ with respect to basal activity.

[c] $p < .05$ with respect to pair-fed control animals.

Data from Wince et al 1980.

Sodium is also importantly involved in neurotransmission. Sodium movements carry the major inward positive current to depolarize membranes. Rapid changes in its influx initiate nerve cell firing. Also, the nonenzymatic process by which neuronal communication si terminated in most cases -- the reuptake of released transmitters by the releasing cell -- is highly sodium-dependent. Effects of lead on sodium conductance have not been studied; effects of lead on several sodium-dependent high affinity uptake systems have been reported (Silbergeld and Goldberg, 1975; Bondy, et al, 1979). The uptake of sodium itself has not been studied at the neuronal level.

TABLE 8 EFFECTS OF LEAD IN VITRO ON CALCIUM UPTAKE BY SUBCELLULAR COMPARTMENTS OF SYNAPTOSOMES

Compartment	^{45}Ca bound [lead] = 0	(ng-atoms/mg protein/4 min)		
		1 µM	10 µM	100µM
vesicles	29.6	33.6	27.6	17.1[a]
mitochondria	7.2	11.3[a]	8.1	3.2[a]
membranes	4.3	8.6	2.6	4.9
microsomes	0.2	0.4[a]	0.4[a]	-

[a]significantly different from [lead] = 0, p<0.05.

Data are from Silbergeld and Adler, 1978.

Sodium also affects regulation of calcium and potassium in neurons by at least two actions, one at the membrane level and one intracellularly at the level of mitochondria. The efflux of calcium from neurons is strongly linked to sodium, through an exchange process driven by the membrane-bound enzyme Na, K-ATPase. Inhibition of this enzyme increases the concentration of calcium within nerve endings (Goddard and Robinson, 1976). Lead in vitro significantly inhibits the activity of Na,K-ATPase, with an apparent IC50 of 30-40 µM (Siegel and Fogt, 1977). Calcium concentrations within neurons are also influenced by uptake and release by intracellular organelles, of which vesicles, microsomes, membranes, and mitochondria have been proposed to be important elements. As shown in Table 8, lead at relatively low concentrations rapidly increases the retention of calcium by microsomes and mitochondria (Silbergeld and Adler, 1978). In mitochondria, this effect has been directly related to a sodium-calcium interaction. Sodium normally releases calcium from mitochondria; lead exposure at very low concentrations of mitochondria decreases this sodium stimulation of calcium efflux (Silberg and Adler, 1978).

Interactions between lead and sodium are likely to be intracellular, and thus depend upon lead gaining access to the cell to the mitrochondrion or the internal side of the ATPase molecule.   There is evidence that lead can enter nerve cells, after either in vivo or in vitro exposure (Holtzman, et al, 1980).   Figure 3[*] shows synaptosomes prepared by airdrying to minimize ion movements after in vitro exposure to 10 µM lead chloride.   Dense, intramitochondrial deposits are visible within the isolated nerve terminals; x-ray microanalysis shows that these cell deposits contain large amounts of lead, calcium, and phosphorus.   Their composition suggests that lead is bound to an ATP residue within the organelle.

IMPLICATIONS OF MECHANISTIC STUDIES

Experimental investigations of lead neurotoxicity indicate that the effects of lead are dependent upon changes in neurochemistry, which occur in vivo before consistent effects on behavior neuropathologic changes can be observed.   The types of changes which have been described include inhibition of transmitter release, as in the case of GABA and acetylcholine, and augmentation of release, as in the case of dopamine.   Mechanisms involving interactions of lead with calcium and sodium may explain some of these changes, but their diversity makes it unlikely that a single mechanism is sufficient to explain all the effects observed (Silbergeld, 1982a).   The neurochemical system most directly sensitive to lead appears to be dopamine in the CNS, although the production of acute in vitro effects appears in all cases to require higher concentrations than those found in brain affected animals exposed in vivo.   Presynaptic mechanisms - release and reuptake - appear to respond first to lead.   However, functional consequences may be better associated with consequent or delayed effects on postsynaptic parameters, such as increases in receptor density found in GABAergic pathways (Silbergeld, et al, 1981), alterations in dopamine receptor subtypes in certain brain regions (Lucchi, et al, 1980), and decreased responsiveness of cerebellar noradrenergic receptors (Taylor, et al, 1978).

Possibly because if its ionic mechanisms of action, neurochemical parameters are highly sensitive to lead.   The early biochemical changes associated with low levels of lead exposure are obviously connected to the full expression of greatly dysfunctional neurochemistry.   In those systems which have been examined pharmacologically, the dose-response relationship between lead and parameters of neurochemistry suggests a continuous, rather than step function correlation.   For example, the data on lead inhibition of adenylyl cyclase, acetylcholine release, and Na, K-ATPase are best fitted by smooth curves.   Extrapolations from these data may suggest a no-effect level in the nanomolar range, but this apparent lack of effect may represent the binding of lead to components not involved in the parameter being measured.   As a nonessential ion, its presence in any cellular compartment must be considered potentially toxic.   For example, while the nuclear sequestration of lead into inclusion bodies in the nuclei of kidney and liver cells is

*Figure 3 at end of Chapter.

considered to be protective, similar deposition in Schwann cells is apparently connected to the toxic sequelae of demyelination (Myers et al, 1980). The accumulation of lead, in the nanomolar range, in mitochondria may appear to protect adenylyl cyclase, a nonmito-chondrial enzyme, which shows response in the micromolar range. However, as discussed above, this "protection" of cyclase is not without effect on total cellular function, including neuro-transmission.

Animal experiments also permit investigation of an important question in clinical lead poisoning: the reversibility of lead neurotoxicity, in the presence or absence of therapeutic intervention. "Reversibility" encompasses a range of meanings, from the literal sense of reappearance of specific normal functions in place of altered ones, to more general concepts of compensation not necessarily involving the reversal or replacement of damaged elements. The relevant findings of experimental studies are several: first, effects of lead exposure on neurobehavioural function persist long after cessation of exposure. In fact, very limited exposure to lead in the neonatal period (as short as the first five days) is sufficient to produce later deficits in learning (Brown, 1975). These effects, and their persistence, may or may not depend on the actual presence of lead within the brain. Michaelson has shown that after cessation of early low level exposure, brain lead concentrations in rodents gradually decrease (although this may be reflective of decreases in blood lead concentrations).

Second, administration of chelating agents to rodents does little to remove lead from the brain, as shown in Table 9 (Goyer and Cherian, 1979). Since drugs such as EDTA and penicillamine do not readily cross the blood-brain barrier, if at all, it is not surprising that their administration does not quickly or extensively remove lead from the brain. Some decreases in brain lead concentration may be achieved by long-term equilibration of brain lead with other compartments, if these are lowered by chelating agents, but this is an indirect effect at the best.

TABLE 9 Soft Tissue Lead in Control and Lead Exposed Rats With Various Modes of Treatment (Mean ± S.E.M.)

	Group	Liver	Kidney	Brain
I	Control (6)	0.18 ± 0.06	0.49 ± 0.12	0.11 ± 0.0
II	Pb ± H$_2$0 (20)	5.53 ± 1.05	19.2 ± 6.2	1.70 ± 0.7
III	Pb ± Asc Ac (20)	3.02 ± 0.77	16.0 ± 9.3	1.33 ± 0.4
IV	Pb ± EDTA (12)	2.33 ± 0.69*	5.37 ± 2.17*	1.56 ± 1.2
V	Pb ± EDTA (10) + Asc Ac	2.70 ± 0.91*	11.5 ± 8.6	0.88 ± 0.1

* differs from Pb ± H$_2$O group (p < 0.05)

Data from Goyer and Cherian (1979)

TABLE 10 EFFECTS OF DIATHIOTHREITOL ON LEAD-INDUCED INCREASES IN SYNAPTOSOMAL CALCIUM UPTAKE

Treatment [lead]	(in order of addition) [dithiothreitol]	^{45}Ca uptake as percent of control
0	0	100
1 μM	0	124[a]
100 μM	0	229[a]
1 μM	5 mM	127[a,b]
100 μM	5 mM	190[a,c]
[dithiothreitol]	[lead]	
5 mM	1 μM	115[c,d]
5 mM	100 μM	123[a,c,d]

[a] Significantly different from control, p<0.01.
[b] Not significantly different from lead-treated in the absence of DTT.
[c] Significantly different from lead-treated in the absence of DTT, p<0.05.
[d] Significantly different from same treatment in opposite order of addition, p<0.005.

Data are from Silbergeld and Adler, 1978.

Experiments have been undertaken to determine if lead can be removed from brain cells in vitro. As shown in Table 10, a functional measure of lead neurotoxicity, its ability to increase synaptosomal calcium uptake, was unaffected by treatment of lead-exposed cells with a powerful sulfhydryl chelating agent, dithiothreitol. If dithiothreitol were present in the cell media before lead addition, then the effects of lead were bound before entering the cell. However, if lead was added only 2 minutes prior to dithiothreitol, then amounts of chelator several orders of magnitude greater than the added lead did not prevent the occurrence of lead effects. Electron microscopic examination of treated cells demonstrated that lead-containing deposits were still present in mitochondria, under these conditions of sequential addition, first lead, then dithiothreitol.

These experimental results strongly suggest that lead is an irreversible neurotoxin. While the growing nervous system may possess considerable reserve for functional compensation (involving plasticitity, regeneration, and redundancy of neural pathways) specific processes affected by lead are unlikely to be reversed, since intracellular lead in not removable. Also, the sensitivity of the period of maximal brain growth during the first two years of childhood tends to magnify over the longterm the severity of

consequences of any toxin encountered during that period
(Dobbing, 1982). Strategies of molecular compensation or
prophylaxis, which have been suggested for such ions as zinc and
calcium, will not change the course of lead neurotoxicity. The
neurochemical studies confirm that lead at very low dose is a potent
neurotoxin in several neuronal systems. Neurochemical effects may
preceed observable effects on electrophysiology, morphology, or
whole animal behaviour in terms of dose; nevertheless, these
biochemical effects are not separate from the functional effects
observable at higher levels. The nature of the dose-effect
relationships argues as well as our knowledge of mechanism against
any threshold for neurotoxic effect at the neuronal level.

DISCUSSION

David:

You mentioned the effects of lead on haem synthesis. Would you comment more specifically on its effects on ALAD (Amino-laevulinic acid dehydratase) and on the build-up of ALA (Amino-laevulinic acid)?

Silbergeld:

Yes. The porphyrias constitute a set of diseases that are not caused by lead but which are biochemically similar to the effects of lead intoxication. Some cases of porphyria are genetically determined; others are acquired after exposure to chemicals in the environment. Lead at very low dose, possibly without a threshold at the cellular level, affects the biosynthesis of haem in all cells that make this substance. This results in the build up of at least two haem precursors (amino-laevulinic acid, or ALA, and porphobilinogen or PGB) within the cells and within the plasma. ALA levels can rise very high, both in porphyria and in lead poisoning. Levels close to the millimolar range have been reported, so that it may not be necessary to demonstrate very great potency for ALA in order to suggest a role for this precursor in lead neurotocicity. ALA differs in structure from the neurotransmitter GABA by one carbon, and there has been interest in whether or not ALA is itself neuroactive. Several groups of investigators (Silbergeld and Lamon, 1980) have reported that ALA can interact with synaptic receptors for GABA, thus affecting the normal function of GABAergic pathways. It is not clear to what extent lead exposure affects haem synthesis in the brain, but Moore's group (Moore and Meredith, 1977) has shown that ALA can cross the blood-brain barrier. Therefore its documented overproduction in liver and kidney as a consequence of lead poisoning may influence neurotransmission. Disruptions in GABAergic function are associated with states of behavioural excitability, including seizures. The symptoms described by Needleman and David (see chapters 12 and 15) in children with low level lead exposure are also consistent with cerebral excitability. The question is whether this neurotoxic effect is reversible. The lead-induced inhibition of haem synthesis, which causes great elevations in ALA, is highly reversible. This happens rather rapidly after lead is removed from the erythropoietic tissue in bone marrow, or spleen, in humans or rats. Neurotoxic sequelae that might result from elevated ALA are therefore also potentially reversible. Because of the rapidity of the onset of the biochemical effects of lead on the GABA system and on seizure sensitivity, as well as reversibility of these effects, I would suggest that the elevated ALA levels, whilst not strictly a neurochemical effect, indeed constitute a neurotoxic effect of lead.

Davies:

Has any work been done to prevent the increased calcium influx resulting from lead toxicity?

Silbergeld:

In vitro, yes, but not in vivo. A key question was whether this increased amount of calcium within neurones was because lead was "punching" holes in nerve membranes that allowed excessive quantities of all ions to enter, or whether there was some effect specific to calcium. We do not have a complete answer, but it appears that inorganic lead at these levels is not punching holes in membranes. Other ions do not gain access in excess. Rather there seems to be a quite specific lead-calcium effect on neurones. However, it is not an effect on the calcium conductance channels. There is no change in those currents as far as we know, but the effect appears to be mediated through normal physiological processes. Agents such as ruthenium red, which block neuronal uptake of calcium by interfering with mitochondria, also interfere with this lead-induced excess of calcium transport.

Annest: If lead is so toxic to animals, why are there
                   not protective immune mechanisms to reject
                   lead from the body?

Silbergeld: In some senses perhaps there are some. For
                   example, the compartmentation process, the
                   sequestration of lead in bone, may be an
                   attempt by the body to keep lead away from
                   the brain. In other tissues, the intranuclear
                   inclusion bodies, in the kidney for example,
                   may well constitute a protective mechanism to
                   keep lead away from sensitive processes
                   mediated by mitochondria. Nevertheless, those
                   inclusion bodies may not always be benign.
                   there are recent data (Myers et al, 1980)
                   suggesting that the inclusion bodies which
                   occur in the Schwann cells of peripheral
                   neurones are precursors of demyelination.

Question: Could you comment generally on the problem of
                   a threshold dose response for lead in relation
                   to animal experiments?

Silbergeld: Many neurochemical studies concern disrupted
                   cells so that, whatever process is studied,
                   there is maximisation of lead's contact with
                   that process. Under these conditions there is
                   no detectable threshold. I think that whatever
                   thresholds may exist in vivo result from
                   barriers to lead access, something very
                   different from what we usually mean by
                   thresholds.

Rutter: It seems to me that animal studies are
                   extremely informative in pointing to possible
                   mechanisms; undoubtedly, this is their main
                   value. However, the findings raise the
                   question of how to extrapolate the particular
                   levels of experimental lead exposure to human
                   beings. In part, this is a matter of species
                   differences in response, but also, I presume,
                   it is a question of how far on can assume that
                   blood lead levels in different species mean the
                   same thing. Could you say how far you think
                   the animal studies help in the determination of
                   the level of lead exposure at which there are
                   effects in humans?

Silbergeld: There is a basic problem with respect to the
                   effects of lead on the brain in that the signs
                   and symtoms probably have very little to do
                   with the primary toxic effect. The
                   relationship between blood lead and brain lead

is species dependant, but it does appear to take a higher blood lead in a rat to produce a level of brain lead equivalent to that in clinical studies of humans. The assessment of comparability of effects is much more difficult. What one can do is take the spectrum of lead-induced neurotoxic effects in rats, from the first biochemical change up to gross pathology and cerebral haemorrhage, and superimpose that on the kinds of scales that Chisholm and others (Chisholm, 1971) have published for a similar range of effects on humans. Cross correlations could then be drawn. In terms of specific outcome measures in animals, obviously our tools for studying behaviour are very crude. It is unlikely that, with a neurotoxin which has its main effect on behaviour, we could detect it as sensitiveley in animals as in humans. However, some of the more refined tests used in animal studies, such as the fine discrimination between object sizes, are much more sensitive than measures of increased activity. Taken together, the evidence suggests that, in terms of the available measures, lead is an extremely powerful neurotoxin in comparison with the range of known psycho-active agents.

Grandjean: The half life of lead in the brain is relevant with respect to reversibility, but very little is known on that topic. However, pertinent findings are provided by Barry's (Barry and Mossman, 1970) study of the tissues of a former metal worker who died about ten years after the cessation of lead exposure. The important observation was that, although the lead levels in several soft tissues were normal, those in the bone, the aorta and the brain were some 5 to 10 times the normal level. As this was 10 years after exposure to lead ceased, it is clear that reversibility must be considered in terms of something happening over a very long period.

Silbergeld: With the brain, the only adequate approach is prevention of exposure. Obviously the term "reversibility" has several layers of meaning. There is a reversibility of function by which the brain can compensate for a tremendous amount of damage. Also there can be resprouting of neurones. I do not mean to suggest that there is total irreversibility.

Nevertheless, at the mechanistic level, because of the great resistance of lead to removal, the only adequate way to deal with the problem is to prevent lead gaining access in the first place.

Bevan: Would Dr. Barry like to comment?

Barry: Yes, the individual we studied had spent something like 40 years of his working life in a lead factory before dying from a coronary at the age of 65. There were very high levels of lead in bone, particularly in the dense bone, and we calculated a body lead burden of around 1600 milligrams, which is about ten times the normal level. Lead levels in the soft tissues were less elevated but that in the brain – about – 4 ppm – was much higher than that found in other samples, even for people working in the lead industry. I should perhaps mention though that his family said that he did not seem at all ill until he has his coronary.

Question: You mentioned that HVA (Homovanillic acid) in children did not appear to increase in urinary excretion until you had blood lead levels of 35 μgm/dl or more. What are the implications for thresholds?

Silbergeld: HVA is subject to many transformations before one can relate it in any way to CNS precursors. If one looks at concentrations of dopamine metabolites within the brain, effects occur at very, very low levels (Lucci et al, 1981; Wince et al, 1980). If one takes out synaptosomes to study direct effects of lead on catecholamines, again there is no observable threshold (Bondy et al, 1979). Between the brain in vitro and the child in vivo I think there are considerable thresholds, but these do not relate to mechanistic thresholds but to phenomena such as barriers to lead access.

REFERENCES

Averill, D.R., and Needlman, H.L. 1980. Neonatal lead exposure retards cortical synaptogenis in the rat. In Needleman, H.L., ed., Health Effects of Lead at Low Dose, Raven Press, New York. pp. 201-202.

Barry, P.S.I., Mossman, D.B., 1970. Lead concentration in human tissues. Brit. J. Industr. Med., 27: 339-351.

Bondy, S., Anderson, C.L., Harrington, M.E. and Prasad, K.N. 1979. The effects of organic and inorganic lead and mercury on neurotransmitter high-affinity transport and release mechanisms. Envir. Res. 19:102-111.

Bornschein, R.L., Michaelson, I.A., and Fox, D. 1975. Lead exposure in lactating rodents: a dose response determination of lead in maternal blood and milk and neonatal blood and brain. Pharmacol. 17:212.

Bornschein, R.L., Pearson, D., and Reiter, L. 1980. Behavioural effects of moderate lead exposure in children and animal models. CRC Critical Revicus in Toxicology 8:43-152.

Brady, K., Herrera, Y., Zenick, H. 1975. Influence of parental lead exposure on subsequent learning ability of offspring. Pharmacol Biochem Behav. 3:561-566.

Browder, A.A., Joselow, M.M., Louria, D.C., 1973. The problem of lead poisoning. Medicine. 52:121-139.

Brown, D.R., 1975, Neonatal lead exposure in the rat: decreased learning as a function of age and blood lead concentrations. Toxicol Appl Pharmacol. 32:628-637.

Burchfield, J., Duffy, F., Bartels, P.H., and Needleman, H.L. 1980. In Needleman, H.L., ed., Low Level Lead Exposure. Raven Press, New York. pp. 75-90.

Bushnell, P.J., and Bowman, R.E. 1979. Reversal learning deficit in young monkeys exposed to lead. Pharmcol. Biochem. Behav. 10:733-742.

Bushnell, P.J., Bowman, R.E., Allen, J.R., Marlan, R.J. 1977. Scoptopic vision deficits in young monkeys exposed to lead. Science. 197:333-335.

Carson, T.L., Van Geloer, G.A., Karas, G.C., Buck, W.B. 1974. Slowed learning in lambs prenatally exposed to lead Arch. Env. Hlth. 29:154-156.

Chisholm, J.J., 1971. Lead Poisoning, Scientific American, 224:15-23.

Clasen, R.A., Hartmann, J.F., Starr, A.J., Coogan, P.S., Pandolfi, S., Laing,I., Becker, R., and Hass, G.M. 1974. Electron microscopic and chemical studies of the vascular changes and edema of lead encephalopathy. Amer. J. Pathol. 74:215-233.

Cooper, J.R., Bloom, F.E., and Roth, R.H., 1970. The Biochemical Basis of Neuropharmacology. Oxford Union Press, New York.

David, O., Clarke, J., and Voeller, K. 1972. Lead and hyperactivity. Lancet II. pp. 900-903.

Dobbing, J., 1972. Vunerable periods of brain development in CIBA Foundation. Lipids, Malnutrition, and the Developing Brain. Elsevier, Amsterdam. pp. 9-20.

Dugandzic, M., Stankovic, B., Milovanovic, Lj., Koricanac, Z. 1973. Urinary excretion of 5-hydroxyindole acetic acid in lead exposed persons. Arh. Hig. Rada Toxsikol. 24:37-44.

Feldman, R.G., Hayes, M.K., Younes, R., Aldrich, F.D., 1977. Lead neuropathy in adults and children. Arch. Neurol. 34:481-488.

Fox, D.A. 1982. Effects of lead on usual function. Neurobehav. Toxicol. Teratol. In press.

Goddard, G.A., and Robinson, J.D. 1976. Uptake and release of calcium by rat brain synaptosomes. Brain Res. 110:331-350.

Goyer, R.A., and Cherian, M.G. 1979. Ascorbic acid and EDTA treatment of lead toxicity in rats. Life Sci. 24:433-438.

Holtzman, D., Herman, M.M., H.S.U., J.S., and Montell, P., 1980. The palliogenesis of lead encephalopathy. Virchons Arch. A. Pathol. Anat. Histol. 387:147-164.

Hrdina, P., Hanin, I., and Dubas, T.C., 1980. Neurochemical correlates of lead toxicity. In Singhal, R., and Thomas, J., eds., Lead Toxicity. Urban and Schwarzenburg, Baltimore. pp. 273-300.

Jason, K.M., and Kellogg, C.K. 1980. Behavioural neurotoxicity of lead. In Singhal, R., and Thomas, J.A. eds., Lead Toxicity. Urban and Schwartzenberg, Baltimore. pp. 241-272.

Konat, G., Offner, H., and Clausen, J., 1979. The effect of triethyllead on total and myelin protein synthesis in rat forebrain slices. J. Neurochem. 32:187-190.

Lampert, P.W., and Schochet, S.S. 1968. Demyclination and remyelination in lead neuropathy: electron microscopic studies. J. Neuropath Exp. Neurol. 27:527-545.

Landrigan, P.J., et al. 1975. Neuropsychologic disfunction in children with chronic low-level lead absorbtions. N.E.J. Med. 292:123-129.

Lorenzo, A.V., and Gewirts, M. 1977. Inhibition of 14C tryptophan transport into brain of lead exposed neonatal rabbits. Brain Research. 132:386-392.

Louis-Ferdinand, R.T., Brown, D.R., Fiddler, S.F., Daughtrey, W.C., and Klein, A.W. 1978. Morphometric and enzymatic effects of neonatal lead exposure in the rat brain. Toxicol. Appl. Pharmacol. 43:351-360.

Lucchi, L., Memo, M., Airaghi, M.L., Sapno, P.F., and Trabucchi, M. 1981. Chronic lead treatment induces in rat a specific and differential effect on dopamine receptors in different brain areas. Brain Res. 213:397-404.

Mailman, R.B., Krigman, M.R., Mueller, R.A., Mushak, P., Breese, G.R. 1978. Lead exposure during infancy permanently increases lithium - induced polydipsia. Science. 201:637-9.

Manalis, R.S., Cooper, G.P. 1973. Presynaptic and postsynaptic effects of lead at the frog neuromuscular junction. Nature. 243:354-356.

Michaelson, I.A. 1980. An appraisal of rodent studies on the behavioral toxicity of lead. In R. Singhaland, J.A. Thomas, eds., Urban and Schwarzenberg, Baltimore. pp. 301-365.

Moore, M., Meredith, P.A., 1977. The association of delta-aminolevulinic acid with the neurological and behavioral effects of lead exposure. In Trace Substances in Environmental Health, Vol. 10: 363-371, Ed. Hemphill, D., University of Missouri Press, Columbia, Missouri.

Morrison, J., Olton, D.S., Silbergeld, E.K., and Goldberg, A.M. 1974. Alterations in consuming behavior of mice produced by dietary exposure to inorganic lead. Dev. Psychobiol. 8:389-396.

Myers, R.R., Powell, H.C., Shapiro, H.M., Costello, M.L., and Lampert, P.W. 1980. Changes in endoneurial fluid pressure, permeability, and peripheral nerve ultrastructure in experimental lead neuropathy. Ann. Neurol. 8:392-401.

Nathanson, J., and Bloom, F.E. 1975. Lead-induced inhibition of brain adenyl cyclase. Nature. 255:419-420.

Needleman, H.L., Gunnoe, C., Leviton, A., Reed, R., Peresie, H., Maher, C., Barrett, P. 1979. Defects in psychological and classroom performance of children with elevated lead levels. N.E.J. Med. 300:689-695.

Otto, D., Benigus, V., Muller, R., Barton, C., Seiple, K., Prah, J., Schoroeders, S. Effects of low to moderate lead exposure on slow cortical potentials in young children. Toxicol. Teratol. In press.

Pentschew, A., and Garrow, F., 1966. Lead encephalo-myelopathy of the suckling rat and its implications for the porthrinopathic nervous diseases. Act. Neuropathol. 6:266-278.

Petrusz, P., Weaver, C.M., Grant, L.D., Mushak, P., and Krigman, M.R. 1979. Lead poisoning and reproductions: effects on pituitary and serum gonadotropins in neonatal rats. Environ. Res. 19:383-391.

Reiter, L.W., Anderson, G.E., Laskey, J.W., and Cahill, D.F. 1975. Developmental and behavioral changes in the rat during chronic exposure to lead. Envir. Health Persp. 12:119-124.

Rutter, M. 1980. Raised lead levels and impaired cognitive/behavioral function. Develop. Med. Child. Neurol. Supp. 42:1-36.

Schain, R.J. 1980. Medical and neurological differential diagnosis. In H.E. Rie, and S.D. Rie, eds. Handbook of Minimal Brain Dysfunctions. John Wiley, New York. pp. 338-406.

Siegel, G.J., and Fogt, S.K. 1977. Inhibition by lead ions of electrophorus electroplax (Na+K)-adenosine triphosphatase and K+-p-nitrophenylphosphatase. J. Biol. Chem. 252:5201-5205.

Silbergeld, E.K., 1977. Interactions of lead and calcium on the synaptosome uptake of dopamine and choline. Life. Sci. 20:309-318.

Silbergeld, E.K., 1982a. Neurochemical and ionic mechanisms of lead neurotoxicity. In K.N. Prosad, and A. Vernadakis, eds., Mechanisms of Actions of Neurotoxic Substances. Raven Press, New York. pp. 1-25.

Silbergeld, E.K., 1982b. Experimental and environmental neurotoxins: correlation of behavioral and biochemical effects. In A. Levy and M.S. Spiegelstein, eds., Behavioral Models and the Analysis of Drug Action. Elsevier, Amsterdam. pp. 1-25.

Silbergeld, E.K., Adler, H.S. 1982. Subcellular mechanisms of lead neurotoxicity. Brain Res. 148:451-467.

Silbergeld, E.K., and Chisolm, J.J. 1976. Lead poisoning: altered urinary catecholamine metabolies as indicators of intoxication in mice and children. Science. 192:153-155.

Silbergeld, E.K., Fales, J.T. and Goldberg, A.M. 1974. Lead: evidence for a prejunctional effect on neuromuscular function. Nature. 247:49-50.

Silbergeld, E.K. and Goldberg, A.M. 1973. A lead induced behavior disorder. Life. Sci. 13:1275-1283.

Silbergeld, E.K., Goldberg, A.M. 1975. Pharmacological and neurochemical investigations of lead-induced hyperactivity. Neuropharmacol. 14:431-444.

Silbergeld, E.K., and Goldberg, A.M., 1980. Problems in experimental studies of lead poisoning. In R. Singhal and J.A. Thomas, eds., Lead Toxicity. Urban and Schwarzenbeg, Baltimore. pp. 19-42.

Silbergeld, E.K. and Hskura, 1980. Neurochemical investigations of low level lead exposure. In Needleman, H.L. Low level lead exposure. The clinical implications of current research. Raven Press, New York. pp. 135-157.

Silbergeld, E.K., Lamon, J.M. 1980. The role of altered haem synthesis in the neurotoxicity of lead, J. Occup. Med., 25:680-684.

Silbergeld, E.K., Lamon, J.M., Bradley, D., Hruska, R.E., Pitman, K., Hess. R.A., and Frykholm, B.C. 1981. Heavy metal neurotoxicity: porphyrinopathic mechanisms. In Heavy Metals in the Environment, EEC-EPA-WHO, Amsterdam. pp. 561-564.

Taylor, D., Nathanson, J., Hoffer, B., Olson, L., and Sieger, A. 1978. Lead blockade of norepenephine-induced inhibition of cerebellar purkinje neurons. J. Pharmacol Exp. Ther. 206:371-381.

Thatcher, R.W., Lester, M.L. McAlaster, R., and Horst, R., 1982. Effects of low levels of cadmium and lead on cognitive functioning in children. Arch. Environ. Health. In press.

Tennekoon, G., Aitchison, C.S., Frangia, J., Price, D.L., and Goldberg, A.M. 1978. Chronic lead intoxication: effects on developing optic nerve. Ann. Neurol. 5:558-564.

Winderbank, A., McCall, J.T., Hunder, H.E., and Dyck, P.J. 1980. The endoneurical content of lead related to the onset and severity of segmental demyelation. J. Neuropathol. Exp. Neurol. 39:692-699.

Wince, L.C., Donovan, C.A., and Azzaro, A.J. 1980. Alterations in the biochemical properties of central dopamine synapses following chronic postnatal $PbCO_3$ exposure. J. Pharmacol. Exp. Ther. 214: 642-650.

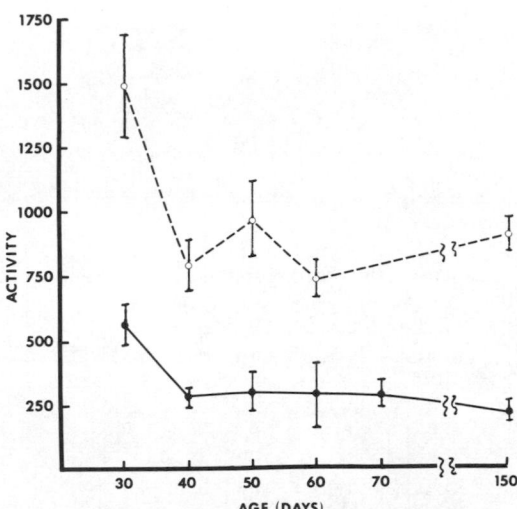

FIGURE 1. Effects of lead on motor activity in mice indirectly exposed to lead in drinking water (5 mg/ml) of their dams (open circles, dashed lines) as compared to that in age-matched controls (closed circles, solid lines). Activity was measured in cages using proximity counters; numbers on ordinate are counts/hr, for the second hour of testing, from day 30 to 150 after birth. Details are in Silbergeld and Goldberg, 1973.

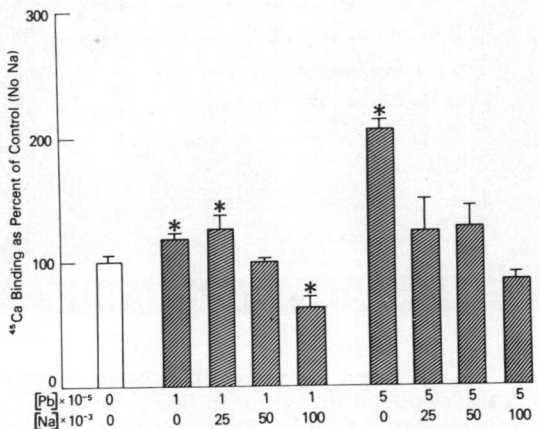

FIGURE 2. Effects of lead, in vitro, on uptake of ^{45}Ca by nerve terminals prepared from rat brain. Lead in concentrations greater that 0.1 μM increases ^{45}Ca uptake; this effect can be reversed by increasing sodium concentrations, as shown. Details are in Silbergeld and Adler, 1978.

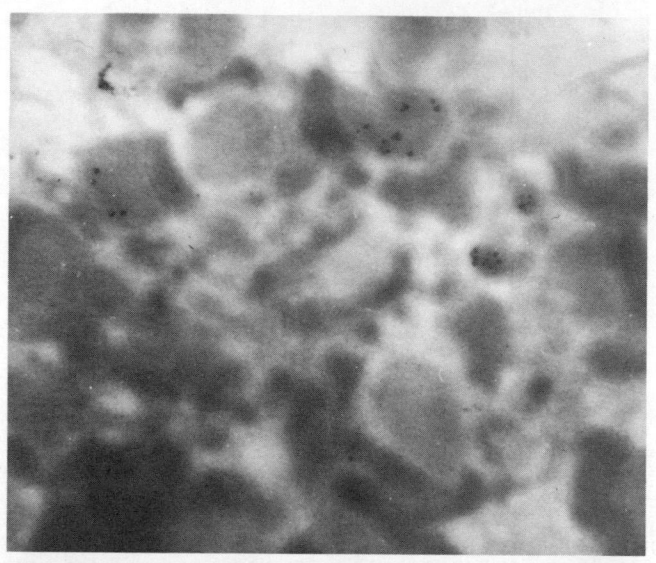

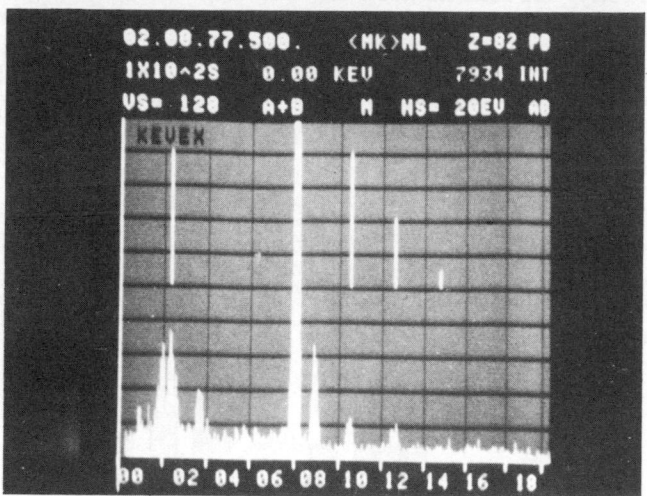

FIGURE 3. Top: Air-dried synaptosomes prepared from cortex of rats exposed in vivo to lead by the methods in Fig. 1. Note dense gradules in certain intracellular areas (magnification 50,000x, STEM micrograph). Bottom: X-ray spectrum of a dense granule, counted for 100 sec at 100 KeV (probe diameter 1000 Å). Vertical bars indicate position of peaks characteristic of lead; calcium, sodium, phosphorus, and copper (from specimen grid) are also detectable. Unpublished data of Silbergeld and Costa.

Lead Versus Health
Edited by M. Rutter and R. Russell Jones
© 1983 John Wiley & Sons Ltd.

EFFECTS OF LEAD ON REPRODUCTION: REVIEW OF
EXPERIMENTAL STUDIES

Ellen, K. Silbergeld, Ph. D.

Environmental Defense Fund,
Washington, DC

INTRODUCTION

Lead has an ancient history as a reproductive toxin. However, examination of the effects of lead on reproduction has mostly focused on post implantation aspects of reproductive function, with the mother and the fetus the subjects of study (Rom, 1976). In a more complete definition, reproductive toxicology includes the offspring and both parents. Reproductive toxins may exert their effects either directly on the developing fetus, after gestation hegins, or indirectly on paternal or maternal physiology before and during the processes of reproduction.

TABLE 1. Parameters of Reproductive Function: Effects of Lead

gonadal development

sexual behavior

potency/libido

pituitary releasing factors/gonadal hormones

target organ responsiveness

intact menstrual cycling

spermatogenesis

sperm viability/number

fertilization

implantation

embryonic/fetal development

placental integrity

parturition

lactation

postnatal development

maternal/paternal behavior

This chapter briefly reviews the experimental literature regarding
the effects of lead on several important physiological parameters of
reproduction (see Table 1). These parameters extend from the
sexual maturation of the parents, through conception and gestation
of the offspring, to such postnatal events as lactation, parenting
behavior and early development. As with all animal data, the
limitations of extrapolation across species to the implications for
human health must be acknowledged. In the area of reproduction,
thesμre are especially notable difficulties in comparing nonprimate
mammalian species to humans; for example, appropriate models for
many aspects of teratogenesis are not yet determined. It is also
important to emphasise that the definition and evaluation of toxic
effects on reproduction must include outcome measures more
sensitive than infertility or perinatal mortality. Such a restricted
view of reproductive toxicity is analogous to lethality tests for
general toxicology. Although reproduction may occur, in that
ostensibly viable offspring are produced, reproductive toxins acting
through such factors as hormones or sperm number may
significantly reduce the probabilities and the quality of reproductive
success. Appreciation of sublethal effects of prenatal exposure to
toxins is very recent (see for example, Schwarz & Yaffey, 1982).
Full evaluation of the importance of such effects of the offspring
require considerable sophistication of behavioral and biochemical
analysis. In addition, time may be required for the expression of
relatively subtle defects to appear, as the repertoire of cognitive
and behavioral tasks required of the offspring increases in
complexity.

Lead can affect reproduction in two ways: directly, by accumulation
in the reproductive organs of parents and in the tissues of the
developing fetus; and indirectly, through its ability to compromise
physiological functions involved in reproduction. In both parents,
lead exposure increases concentrations of lead in several organs of
importance in reproduction: median eminence of the hypothalamus,
pituitary, gonads, and seminal fluid (Thomas and Brogan, 1982;
Gunn and Gould, 1970). Additionally, lead exposure of the fetus
can occur through the plancenta and, after parturition, through the
mother's milk. Lead is known to cross the placental barrier, and
maternal: fetal blood lead concentrations are highly correlated
(Clark, 1977). In a study of 474 mother/infant pairs, Lauwerys et
al (1978) found a regression equation of fetal blood Pb = 0.90 +
0.73 x maternal blood Pb. In experimental animals, lead can be
shown to be secreted in milk in relation to exposure (and to
maternal blood lead). After a single intravenous dose of lead,
lactating rabbits secrete lead with a delay in peak concentrations,
which, while temporally lagging behind the peak blood lead levels,
persists longer and actually reaches a higher peak concentration
compared to the blood compartment (Lorenzo; et al, 1977).

Nonspecific toxic effects of lead may also compromise reproduction
indirectly. For example, the behavioral toxicity of lead, which
alters social interactions and reactivity (Chapter 10), may adversely
affect sexual receptivity and the complex behavioral patterns

involved in mating.   In this area, parallels between rodent and
human sexual behaviors may, however, be difficult to discern.
Another example of a toxic effect on lead that may indirectly
influence reproductive function is the inhibition of hepatic heme
synthesis.   Decreased biosynthesis of heme associated with lead
exposure reduces hepatic content of heme-containing cytochromes,
such as P-450, which are involved in drug and steroid hormone
metabolism (Alvares, 1979).   Interactions between steriod hormone
metabolism and the heritable conditions of porphyria are well known
(Welland, et al, 1964); lead, as an instance of chemically induced
porphyria, may be expected also to result in altered sex hormone
metabolism.

REPRODUCTIVE EFFECTS OF LEAD

1. Pregestational Effects   Exposure of animals to lead early in their
development appears to produce long-lasting effects which
compromise reproduction in later life.   Kimmel et al (1980) found a
significant delay in vaginal opening in female rats exposed to lead
from before their parents were bred through nine months after
parturition (mean blood lead levels in these animals ranged from 20
to 50 μg/100 ml).   Similarly, offspring of rats exposed during
gestation and lactation – that is, the F1 generation which were
never directly exposed – showed decreases in several measures of
reproductive success when these rats were bred at maturity (Stowe
and Goyer, 1971).   As shown in Table 2, some of these factors
were affected even when only one parent had been lead-exposed,
although more severe effects were found in reproduction by
offspring both of whose parents were lead-exposed.   The finding of
compromised reproduction in mating pairs where only the male was
exposed to lead points to long lasting gametotoxic effects of this
toxin mediated through alterations in sperm.

TABLE 2.   Effects of Lead Exposure on Reproduction in F1
Generation[a]

treatment of parents female - male	pups/litter	pup birthweight grams	survival rate at weaning
C - C	11.9 ± 0.4[b]	6.74 ± 0.15	89.8 ± 3.2
C - Pb	10.10 ± 0.5	5.92 ± 0.13*	73.7 ± 7.2
Pb - C	8.78 ± 0.3*	5.44 ± 0.13*	52.6 ± 7.2
Pb - Pb	7.75 ± 0.5*	4.80 ± 0.19*	30.0 ± 8.2

[a]Data from Stowe and Goyer, 1971.
[b]mean ± standard error of the mean; between 16 and 36 litters were
observed.
*significantly different from C-C group, p at least < 0.05.

Examinations of anatomic and biochemical pathology in lead-exposed animals has also been reported. Stowe and Goyer (1971), while not examining pathology in the male Fl parent, reported depressed stimulation of follicular development in females. In female mice exposed before mating to food containing 0.1% lead acetate, subsequent mating procedure significantly retarded embryos and lead containing dense granules were found in mitochondria of embryonic cells. (Maisin, et al, 1978). In mice exposed to lead 60 days after birth, testicular development was delayed, as well as sexual maturation in both sexes (measured as fertility) (Maker, et al, 1975).

2. Mutagenetic Effects   An important mechanism of reproductive toxicity is through mutagenic events at the level of the genome in germ cells (Bloom, 1981). Soluable salts of lead, including the organometals tetraethyl lead and tetramethlyl lead, are positive in a number of reliable in vitro assays for mutagenic activity. These include Chinese hamster cell cultures (Bauchinger and Schmid, 1972), human leucocytes (Beek and Obe, 1974), mouse kidney cells (Choie and Richter, 1974), Syrian hamster cells (DiPaolo, et al, 1978), the bacterial rec-assay (Kada, et al, 1980), and HeLa cells (Skreb, et al, 1981).

Clinically, mutagenic effects of lead have been studied in both males and females. In a report on women occupationally exposed to lead in the battery industry, significant increases in chromatid and chromosomal aberrations were found in lymphocytes cultured for 3 days. In this population, blood lead concentrations ranged from 24 to 59, with a mean of 42 ± 9.6 µg/100 ml (Forni, et al, 1980). Clinical studies in exposed men have also reported increased abnormalities in somatic cell chromosomes at levels of exposure associated with blood lead concentrations below 40 µg/100 ml (reviewed by Thomas and Brogan, 1982).

Several experimental studies have examined seminal cytology in mice exposed to relatively high doses of lead for several months. Sperm shape is a reliable assay for genetic mutations in mice; specific locus mutations have been associated with morphological abnormalities. Increased numbers of abnormally appearing sperm have been observed in mice exposed throughout development or semichronically only during adulthood (Varma, 1975; Eyden, et al, 1978).

Effects of sperm morphology appear to precede overt decreases in fertility. Mice exposed to 1% lead acetate diets had increased incidence of abnormal sperm, but no decreases in sperm number, motility, or ability to establish pregnancies. However, at 2% lead acetate exposure via drinking water, the fertility rate of exposed males also dropped by 50% (Eyden, et al, 1978).

Acute exposure also appears to cause mutations in sperm. Adult mice were exposed to lead acetate for five days by intraperitonel injection; sperm collected thirty days after the last injection were observed to have increased frequency of abnormal shape (Bruce and Heddle, 1979). Using a similar protocol, Wyrobeck and Bruce (1978), calculated a dose of 80 mg/kg (acute) required to produce in adult mice a doubling of the background level of sperm abnormalities. Relevant to the study of Stowe and Goyer (1971), discussed above, these researchers found that an increased incidence of sperm abnormalities was also seen in male progeny of males exposed acutely prior to mating. The possibility of transmission suggests a mutational event. However, abnormal shape may not be associated with changes in chromosomal or DNA content and the implications of sperm abnormalities for the viability or genetic status of the progeny is unclear. Further, with these exceptions, chromosomal studies in clinical lead toxicity have not been done on germ cells. It should also be noted that the studies described above refer to effects of inorganic salts of lead. More potent mutagenic activity has been recently reported for the organometals trimethyllead and tetraethyllead, as reviewed by Grandjean (Chapter 9).

TABLE 3. Effects of Lead Treatment on Pituitary FSH Content in Rats[a]

Treatment	Males	Females	Blood lead[b]
Control	21.4 ± 8.4[c]	56.7 ± 15.7	7.8 ± 2.1[d]
25 mg/kg	45.8 ± 23.0	N.S.	203.2 ± 53.4
100 mg/kg	37.8 ± 7.9	N.S.	1013.8 ± 218.0
200 mg/kg	N.S.	40.8 ± 3.6	1055.6 ± 645.7

[a]Data from Petrusz, et al (1979); results are for statistically significant differences, Pb-treated as compared to control, $p < 0.01$ "N.S." indicates no significant difference compared to controls.

[b]Blood lead data are pooled for males and females, assayed at day 15.

[c]μg/gland, mean ± standard deviation, assayed at day 20.

[d]μg/100 ml whole blood, mean ± standard deviation.

3. Hormonal Effects Effects of early lead exposure can also be observed on pituitary-gonadal hormone metabolism. In rats exposed from birth to lead, serum prolactin levels were higher in lead-treated males (Govoni, et al, 1978). As shown in Table 3, exposure of rats to lead for 20 days produced significant elevations

in pituitary FSH content of males and, at the highest dose, a
decrease in pituitary FSH in females.   The persistent estrus
reported in lead-exposed female rats (Grant, et al, 1980) may also
reflect effects on hormonal function.   The documented effects of
lead on hypothalamically mediated behaviors (such as polydipsia)
suggest that the neural axis of reproductive function may be
particularly sensitive to lead (Mailman, et al, 1978).   Further
studies on the effects of lead on pituitary/hypothalmic function have
not been done, although this area would seem opportune in light of
the growing body of information on the neurochemical effects of lead
on subcortial and limbic system dopamine pathways (Govoni, et al,
1980) as well as the relatively selective localization of lead in the
median eminence of the hypothalmus (Stumpf et al, 1980).

4. Gestational Effects   The effects of lead exposure in causing
impaired reproduction, after mating, as reported clinically and
experimentally in many studies, may be examined in terms of timing
of exposure.   For this purpose, post-breeding events are divided
into fertilization, implantation, gestational development, placental
integrity, and parturition.

The effects of lead specifically on the ability of sperm to fertalize
ova have not been examined, although some of the reports reviewed
above might suggest an impairment of such mechanisms.
Post-fertilization events have been examined by exposing rodents
soon after mating to lead acutely.   Exposure once on day 3 or
continuously from day 1 (timed from appearance of vaginal plug)
reduced pregnancy success.   Two studies using different
approaches indicate that the implantation phase of the fertilized
blastocyst may be specifically affected by lead.   In mice exposed
after fertilization but before implantation to 0.5% lead diets, no
successful pregnancies were established; this failure could be
significantly reduced by treatment of females with progesterone and
estradiol (Jacquet, 1978; Wide, 1980).

TABLE 4.   EFFECTS OF LEAD IN VITRO ON BLASTOCYST
DEVELOPMENT[a]

(lead)	percent blastocysts attached	percent without growth
0	91	91
5	84	61
10	80	39
20	25	0

[a]Data from Wide, 1978.

Wide (1978) also found that the interference of lead with implantation was probably not due to lead-induced defects in the blastocyst. (Table 4) Blastocysts exposed in vitro to lead at concentrations below 10 µM can directly decrease the ability of blastocysts to attach and develop. At 20 µM, no outgrowth was observed in the 25% of blastocysts which successfully attached. The viability of these embryos was also adversely affected (Wide, 1978). It is of interest to note that lead exposure affected not only processes of attachment but also of outgrowth (Table 4).

The possibility that these effects may represent some interference by lead with hormonal mechanisms involved in early stages of gestation is suggested by Jacquet (1978). Serum levels of estradiol were found to be normal on day 5 of pregnancy, but exposed females did not show the expected rise in progesterone after the fifth day (Jacquet, 1978; Wide, 1980). thus, the effect of lead on implantation may be caused by deficiencies in maternal gonadal hormone levels, or in reponsiveness of uterine tissue to hormones. There have been no studies on cytosolic estrogen or progesterone receptors in lead-exposed animals; one study of androgen receptors in mouse prostrate reported in vitro inhibition by lead (Thomas and Brogan, 1982).

5. Teratogenic Effects   Several studies demonstrate that post-implantation lead exposure during pregnancy adversely affects gestational development. Many of these effects may be due to effects mediated through the mother, by such mechanisms as interference in placental blood flow and transfer of amino acids to the fetus (Gerber, et al, 1978) or teratogenic effects of the fetus (Carpenter and Ferm, 1977; Jacquet and Gerber, 1979; Hilderbrand, et al, 1973). Teratogenicity of lead has also been demonstrated in the chick embryo assay, when lead was administered once on the four days after fertilization. (Gilain, 1973). The LD_{50} at day 4 was found to be 30 µg/embryo; at day 10, the LD_{50} was 1 mg/embryo (DeGennaro, 1978). Incresed frequency of congenital malformations was observed at doses as low as 5 µg/embryo. Interestingly, in mice, hamsters and chicks, a focus of malformations was the spinal cord (Carpenter and Ferm, 1977; DeGennaro, 1978; Gilani, 1973; Jacquet and Gerber, 1979.) These effects were observed with exposure to lead during the first half of pregnancy. Effects of exposure to lead late in pregnancy have not been described, although some of the clinical reports suggest that high levels of exposed may precipitate labour.

Another aspect of teratogenic effects of lead may be subsumed under behavioral teratology. Prenatal exposure to lead is hypothesized to affect neurological development, in large part on the basis that the younger the organism the more sensitive the CNS is to toxins like lead. Very few experimental studies have cleanly separated exposures between pre and postnatal periods; this requires crossfostering, since mothers leaded during pregnancy secrete lead into their milk from body stores long after external dosing ceases. One such study reported significant deficits in learning in offspring of rats of which either the male or female parent was exposed to lead before breeding (Brady, et al, 1975).

6. Postnatal Effects   Postnatal events in reproduction primarily focus on the progeny, rather than the parents. No measures of such factors as lactation or postpartum uterine physiology, or recovery of fecundity after pregnancy have been examined. Lead-exposed mothers appear to nature their offspring appropriately, at least in behavioral terms (Zenick, et al, 1979), although Mahaffey and Michaelson (1980) have suggested that lead exposure during lactation may affect the composition and nutritional value of milk. Mortality in the early neonatal period is increased, as demonstrated by Stowe and Goyer (1971), in examinations of the percentage of offspring surviving till weaning. Studies on rodents exposed through mothers' milk after parturition to lead also indicate that neonatal mortality is increased by lead exposure (Silbergeld and Goldberg, unpublished observations), but in these cases, exposure was initiated after parturition and thus cannot be separated from early developmental toxicity.

SUMMARY

Experimental data exist to indicate that lead, at relatively low levels, is a reproductive toxin. The effects of lead are likely to depend upon dose and timing of exposure. The assertion that lead exposure is associated with spontaneous abortion and still birth are probably only relevant to high levels of exposure during gestation. Animal experiments, at levels of exposure below overt toxicity, have not shown such effects (Kimmel, et al, 1980; Thomas and Brogan, 1982). At high levels, lead is toxic to the organs of reproduction in the adult and is lethal or teratogenic to the developing foetus. At lower levels of exposure, several parameters of reproduction are affected which may or may not significantly reduce fertility. These include: mutational effects on ovaries and sperm, reduced numbers of sperm, alterations of hormonal chemistry (basally and during important stages of reproduction), decreases in placental function; and compromised growth and development of the foetus, including neurobehavioral development. Little is known of the mechanisms of action associated with these effects, but their complexity and multiplicity suggests that several toxic actions, and several target systems, are likely to be sensitive to lead. Information on mechanisms of action would be of particular value in determining the relevance of many of the experimental findings to clinical lead toxicity, at various levels of exposure. Nevertheless, several conclusions may be drawn from the experimental studies, which are likely to be of relevance to human reproductive function: (1) lead at relatively low doses is a reproductive toxin in both male and female parents; (2) the reproductive toxicity of lead can be produced both after chronic exposure during early development, and after acute exposure of adults; (3) many of the effects of lead, particularly on early stages of reproduction, appear to result from actions on physiological functions in the parents rather than a consequence of a special sensitivity of the zygote/blastocyst/

embryo; (4) lead, both organonetal and inorganic compounds, is mutagenic in both somatic and germ cells; and (5) some reproductive effects of lead are transmissable and can affect the reproductive capacity of the offspring of the exposed generation, as shown for the male offspring of exposed males.

It is of concern to contrast the relative lack of corroborative clinical data on lead as a reproductive toxin, in comparison to other areas of lead toxicity, such as neurotoxicity. This may be due in part to the problems encountered in conducting clinical studies of reproductive toxicology in general (see Bloom, 1981). Information on other than the more drastic outcomes, fetal death or infertility, is not reliably collected, and clinical reproductive toxicology is still in its own developmental stages. In the case of lead, the experimental literature suggests areas of further research which are likely to be productive and important in fully assessing the toxicological impact of human lead exposure.

ACKNOWLEDGEMENTS

The author wishes to thank Dr. John A. Thomas and Dr. Philippe Grandjean for making available copies of papers in manuscript; and Dr. Max Costa for useful discussions on the mutagenic activity of lead. Thanks also to Judy Songco for typing this manuscript.

REFERENCES

Alvares, A.P., (1979): Lead and polychlorinated biphenyls: effects on heme and drug metabolism. Drug Metab. Rev. 10: 91-106.
Bauchinger, M., and Schmid, E., (1972): Chromosome analysis in Chinese hamster cell cultures after treatment with lead acetate (Ger.). Mutat. Res. 14: 95-100.
Beek, B., and Obe, G., (1974): Effect of lead acetate on human leukocyte chromosomes in vitro. Experientia 30: 1006-1007.
Bloom, A.D., (1981): Guidelines for the investigation of reproductive and mutagenic chemicals in the environment, New York, March of Dimes.
Brady, K., Herrera, Y., and Zenick, H., (1975): Influence of parental lead exposure on subsequent learning ability of offspring. Pharmacol. Biochem. Behav. 3: 561-565.
Bruce, W.R., and Heddle, J.A., (1979): the Mutagenic Activity of 61 Agents as determined by the Micronucleus, Salmonella, and Sperm Abnormality Assays. Can. J. Genet. Cytol. 21: 319-334.
Carpenter, S.J., and Ferm, V.H. (1977): Embryopathic Effects of Lead in the Hamster A Morphological Analysis. Lab. Invest. 37: 369-385.
Choie, D.D., and Richter, G.W., (1974): Cell proliferation in mouse kidney induced by lead. I. Synthesis of deoxyribonucleic acid. Lab Invest. 30:647-651.
Clark, A.R.L., (1977): Placental transfer of lead and its effects on the newborn. Postgrad. Med. J. 53:67-678.

De Gennaro, L.D., (1978): The Effects of Lead Nitrate on the Central Nervous System of the Chick Embryo. I. Observations of Light and Electron Microscopy. Growth 42: 141-155.

DiPaolo, J.A., Nelson, R.L., and Casto, B.C., (1978): In vitro neoplastic transformation of Syrian hamster cells by lead acetate and its relevance to environmental carcinogenesis. Br. J. Cancer 38: 452-455.

Eyden, B.P., Maisin, J.R., and Mattelin, G. (1978): Long-term Effects of Dietary Lead Acetate on Survival, Body Weight and Seminal Cytology in Mice. Bull. Environ. Contam. & Toxicol. 19: 266-272.

Forni, A., Sciame, A., Bertazzi, P.A., and Alessio, L., (1980): Chromosome and Biochemical Studies in Women Occupationally Exposed to Lead. Arch. Environ. Health 35: 139-145.

Gerber, G., Maes, J., and Deroo, J., (1978): Effect of Dietary Lead on placental Blood Flow and on Fetal Uptake of a-Amino Isobutyrate. Arch. Toxicol. 41: 125-131.

Gilani, S.H., (1973): Congential Anomalies in Lead Poisoning. Am. J. Obstet. Gynecol. 41 265-269.

Govoni, S., Memo, M., Lucchi, L., Spano, P.F., and Trabucchi, M., (1980): Brain Neurotransmitter Systems and Chronic Lead Intoxication. Pharmacol. Res. Commun, 5: 447-460.

Govoni, S., Montefusco, O., Spano, P.F., and Trabucchi, M., (1978): Neurochemical Correlates of Chronic Lead Treatment in Rat Striatum and Limbic Areas. Abst., 78th Int. Cong. Pharmacol. p. 765.

Grant, L.D., Kimmel, C.A., West, G.L., Martinez-Vargas, C.M., and Howard, J.L. (1980): Chronic Low-Level Toxicity in the Rat. II. Effects on Postnatal Physical and Behavioral Development. Toxicol. Appl. Pharmacol. 56: 42-58.

Gunn, S.A., and Gould, T.C., (1970): Cadium and other mineral elements. In Johnson, A.D., Gomes, W.R., and Vandemark, N.L. (eds) The Testis, vol. III, New York, Academic Press, p. 411.

Hilderbrand, D.C., Der, R., Griffin, W.T., and Fahim, M.S., (1973): Effect of Lead Acetate on Reproduction. Am. J. Obstet. Gynecol. 115: 1058-1065.

Jacquet, P., (1978): Influence de la progestérone et de l'estradiol exogenés sur le processus de l'implantation embryonnaire, chez la souris femelle intoxiquée par le plomb. C.R. Soc. Biol. 172 1037-1040.

Jacquet, P., and Gerber, G.B., (1979): Teratogenic Effects of Lead in the Mouse. Biomed. 30: 223-229.

Kada, T., Hirano, K. and Shirasu, Y. (1980): Screening of environmental chemical mutagens by the rec-assay system with Bacillus subtilis. Chem. Mutagens, 6 (in press).

Kimmel, C.A., Grant, L.D., Sloan, C.S., and Gladen, B.C., (1980): Chronic Low-level Lead Toxicity in the Rat. Toxicol. Appl. Pharmacol. 56: 28-41.

Lauwerys, R., Buchet, J.P., Roels, H., and Hubermont, G., (1978): Placental Transfer of Lead, Mercury, Cadmium, and Carbon Monoxide in Women. Environ. Res. 15: 278-289.

Lorenzo, A.V., Gewirtz, M., Maher, C., and Davidowski, L.I.

(1977): The Equilibration of Lead Between Blood and Milk of Lactating Rabbits. Life Sci., 21: 1679-1684.

Mahaffey, K., and Michaelson, I.A., (1980): Interactions between lead and nutrition. In Needleman, H.L. (ed) Low Level Lead Exposure, Raven Press, New York, pp. 159-200.

Mailman, R.B., Krigman, M.R., Mueller, R.A., Mushak, P., Breese, G.R., (1978): Lead exposure during infancy permanently increases lithium - induced polydipsia. Science 201: 637-9.

Maisin, J.R., Lambiet-Collier, M., and De Saint-Georges, L., (1978): Toxicité du plomb pour les embryons de la Souris. C.R. Soc. Biol. 172: 1041-1043.

Maker, H.S., Lehrer, G.M., and Silides, D.J., (1975): The Effect of Lead on Mouse Brain Development. Environ. Res. 10: 76-91.

Petrusz, P., Weaver, C.M., Grant, L.D., Mushak, P., and Krigman, M.R., (1979): Lead Poisoning and Reproduction: Effects on Pituitary and Serum Gonadotropins in Neonatal Rats. Environ. Res. 19: 383-391.

Rom, W.N., (1976): Effects of Lead on the Female and Reproduction: A Review. M. Sinai J. Med., Vol. 43, No. 5, 542-552

Schwarz, R.H., and Yaffe, S.J., (eds.) (1982): Drug and Chemical Risks to the Fetus and the Newborn. Alan Liss, New York.

Skreb, Y., Habazin-Novak, V., and Hors, N., (1981): The rate of DNA synthesis in hela cells during combined long-term and acute exposures to lead. Toxicology 19: 1-10.

Stowe, H.D., and Goyer, R.A., (1971): The Reproductive Ability and Progeny of F1 Lead-Toxic Rats. Fertil. Steril. 22: 755-760.

Stumpf, W.E., Sar, M., and Grant, L.D., (1980): Autoradiographic Localization of (210)Pb and its Decay Products in Rat Forebrain. Neurotoxicol. 1: 593-606.

Thomas, J.A., and Brogan, W.C., (1982): Some Actions of Lead on the Sperm and Upon the Male Reproductive System. Amer. J. Indust. Med., In press.

Varma, B., (1975): Embryonic Death in Mouse due to Lead Exposure Experientia 31: 1312-1313.

Welland, F.H., Hellman, E.S., Collins, A., Hunter, G.W., and Tschudy, D.P., (1964): Factors Affecting the Excretion of Porphyrin Precursors by Patients with Acute Intermittent Porphyria. II. The Effect of Ethinyl Estradiol. Metab. 13: 251-258.

Wide, M., (1978): Effect of Inorganic Lead on the Mouse Blacstocyst In Vitro. Teratol. 17 165-170.

Wide, M., (1980): Interference of Lead with Implantation in the Mouse: Effect of Exogenous Oestradiol and Progesterone. Teratol. 21: 187-191.

Wyrobek, A.J., and Bruce, W.R., (1978): The induction of sperm-shape abnormalities in mice and humans. Chemical Mutagens. 5: 257-285.

Zenick, H., Pecorraro, F., Price, D., Saez, K., and Ward, J., (1979): Maternal Behavior During Chronic Lead Exposure and Measures of Offspring Development. Neurobehav. Toxicol. 1: 65-71.

PART 4
Neuropsychological Effects of Lead

Lead Versus Health
Edited by M. Rutter and R. Russell Jones
© 1983 John Wiley & Sons Ltd.

LOW LEVEL LEAD EXPOSURE AND NEUROPSYCHOLOGICAL
PERFORMANCE

Herbert L. Needleman

University of Pittsburgh
Western Psychiatric Institute and Clinic
Children's Hospital of Pittsburgh
Pittsburgh
USA

Corde was beginning to think that with pure scientists,
when they turned their eyes from their own disciplines,
there were occasionally storms of convulsive clear
consciousness; they suffered attacks of confusing lucidity.

Saul Bellow: "The Dean's December" p139

Here science itself, which was designed for deeper
realization, experienced a singular failure. The genius of
these evils (lead exposure) was their ability to create
zones of incomprehension. It was because they were so
fully apparent that you couldn't see them.

Ibid, p140

In these sentences, Albert Corde, Dean of a Chicago university, is
speaking of lead's millenial pollution of our planet and its possible
role in contemporary social disorder. Bellow tells us here of the
brilliant light that scientific consciousness can throw on our world,
and of the parallel-perhaps fused-potential to mask reality.

There are still questions to be asked about lead in this decade, and
I shall mention two. The first is: "Is there a threshold for lead's
effects?" This question has been illuminated by science, and I
shall comment primarily on the work of my own group in this
terrain. In attending to this question, one confronts a formidable
set of causal questions. Many things, after all, affect the
development of the growing child's brain, and many of these factors
interact with the effects of lead. It is essential to separate out
these effects to the maximum extent possible in naturalistic studies.
Statistical control of these variables has become possible through
the use of multivariate techniques, but these techniques, powerful
as they are, require proper experimental design and verdical causal
modelling if they are to function optimally.

The second question is: "Why does this problem continue to vex us
200 years after Benjamin Franklin noted lead's effects on tinkers,
painters, and printers; 80 years after J.L. Gibson's discovery of

childhood lead poisoning in Australia; 40 years after Randolph
Byers showed that behaviour disorder in children was a common
consequence of lead exposure; and 20 years after Clair Patterson's
pioneering first paper on the subject of global pollution with lead?"
(Needleman and Landrigan, 1981). Multivariate techniques and
causal models have little to contribute in response to this question;
its answer lies in a transscientific domain. Any fit response
engages our understanding of economics-money is made from the
distribution of lead; of politics-money can influence decision
making; and ethics - a parody of the scientific method has on
occasion been employed to blur our vision and to retard attempts to
act on the problem.

While scientific enterprises must be prepared to be exposed to stern
testing and critical analysis, scientists should at the same time be
making discriminations between essential rigor and scepticism, and
the erection of zones of incomprehension. There are times when
the data speak clearly.

THE THRESHOLD QUESTION

If one molecule of lead enters a cell, it will bind to a ligand. This
binding is itself a change of state or effect. What then is meant by
an adverse health effect? In the absence of a commonly accepted
defination of "health", this question assumes metaphysical
proportions. At the same time, the answer has immediately
practical consequences, since alterations in blood chemistry (i.e.
d-ALAD activity and FEP concentrations) are altered at blood lead
levels borne by large segments of the population (Hernberg, 1973,
Piomelli et al, 1982). Are these alterations to be considered health
effects by regulatory agencies when they take decisions on the
setting of standards? Some critics on the U.S. Environmental
Protection Agency's partial reliance on FEP levels to determine a
"safe" blood lead level, have claimed that FEP and d-ALAD changes
were merely biochemical changes, and of themselves, without health
consequence. This issue will not be debated any further in this
paper. However, I shall take as axiomatic the belief that any
impairment in the neurobehavioural adaptation of a child, of
whatever magnitude, is to be considered an adverse health effect.

In the 1960's screening studies in large American cities found that
as much as 10 per cent of the population of children had blood lead
levels over 40 µg/dl. The level of blood lead defined as hazardous
at that time was 60 µg/dl. This slender margin caused a number of
pediatricians to wonder whether some of these children were
intoxicated, but not recognized as such. Randolph Byers (Byers
and Lord, 1943) had asked whether many of the cases of school
failure or behaviour disorder were not due to undiagnosed
plumbism.

A directed response to Byers' question required a means by which
to look back into a child's history of lead exposure. Because blood
lead levels indicate recent exposure, they may missclassify a child

who was exposed years before the level was obtained. Lead goes to
bone and stays there, but one cannot do bone biopsies on
ostensibly healthy children. It occured to me that a universal,
spontaneous and painless biopsy was available for the investigator:
the decidous tooth. With Irving Shapiro of the University of
Pennsylvania, I showed that dental lead levels were elevated in lead
poisoned children, in children from the "lead belt", and in children
from good housing stock who lived near a major lead processor
(Needleman et al, 1974).

We now possessed a marker for past lead exposure which gave us
confidence that we could classify children with accuracy. Alan
Levitton and I then set out to design a study which attempted to
deal in direct fashion with problems in design which had troubled
other investigations (Needleman et al, 1979). The most common
problems in design were: 1) inadequate classification of past
exposure. Almost all studies had used blood lead levels in older
children. Blood lead declines once exposure ceases, and children
could therefore be missclassified readily. 2) inadequate control of
other variables which affect development. The growing child's
development is influenced by manifold factors, genetic,
psychosocial, and physical, some of which may be correlated with
lead exposure and thus could confound its effects. Measurement
and then control of covariates, by subject selection of biostatistical
analysis, are necessary to make valid inferences about lead's
effects. 3) insensitive measures of neuropsychologic outcome. To
find subtle changes, sensitive, appropriate measures of performance
are required. Group tests, or screening tests are not adequate in
this regard. 4) selection bias. Subjects who participate in a study
may differ in some systematic way from those who are excluded, or
who refuse to be tested. Because these differences may be
correlated with the outcome of interest, an ignoring of this issue
may bias the results.

AN EPIDEMIOLOGIC STUDY OF DENTINE LEAD LEVELS AND NEUROPSYCHOLOGIC FUNCTION

In an attempt to address the above issues, we collected shed
decidous teeth from 70 per cent of the 3329 children attending
ordinary (non-remedial) first and second grade classes in two white
working class towns near Boston, Massachusetts (Needleman et al,
1979). We compared children who participated with those excluded,
and found that they did not differ on either teachers' ratings of
classroom behaviour or on distribution of dentine lead levels. The
sample was thus shown to be an unbiased representation of children
in those towns. Children with dentine lead levels, which were in
the highest 90th percentile or lowest 10th percentile for lead were
invited for neuropsychologic evaluation if they met the following
criteria: 1) they had no history of lead intoxication. 2) English
was the primary language of the home. 3) they were born at term.
4) they had no history of noteworthy head injury.

The mother accompanied the child to the laboratory and filled out a lengthy questionnaire which scaled 39 non-lead covariates of potential influence on development. These were compared by univariate t-tests, and those that differed at p=0.1 or less were entered into the biostatistical analysis and thus controlled. (Table 1). In addition to family size, mother's age at subjects birth, mother's education, and father's socio-economic status, parental IQ was entered into the analysis of covariance (ANCOVA).

TABLE 1. COMPARISON OF NON-LEAD VARIABLES IN HIGH AND LOW LEAD GROUPS

Variable	Low Dentine Lead	High Dentine Lead	P Value
General			
% Male	49.5	55.9	NS
% White	97.0	98.3	NS
% Father Head of Household	77.2	67.8	NS
% Positive Pica	10.9	28.8	0.008
Physical Variables			
Age (mo)	87.2 ± 7.7	90.7 ± 8.4	0.009
Height (cm)	126.6 ± 6.3	126.4 ± 6.3	NS
Weight (kg)	25.8 ± 4.9	26.5 ± 4.6	NS
Head Circumference	51.8 ± 1.6	51.7 ± 1.5	NS
Past Medical History			
Birth Weight (gm)	3400.0 ± 448.6	3346.0 ± 514.0	NS
No. of hospital admissions	0.47 ± 1.2	0.42 ± 1.6	NS
Parental Variables			
No. of Pregnancies	3.3 ± 1.8	3.8 ± 2.3	0.10
Mother's age at subjects birth (yr)	26.2 ± 5.5	24.5 ± 5.8	0.07
Mother's social class	4.1 ± 0.8	4.2 ± 0.8	NS
Mother's education (grade)	11.9 ± 2.0	11.4 ± 1.7	0.08
Father's social class	3.8 ± 1.0	4.1 ± 0.8	0.02
Parent IQ	111.8 ± 14.0	108.7 ± 14.5	NS

Sixteen of 39 non-lead variables are summarized here. For brevity, 23 variables are not shown. None of these differed at P(0.1 between groups.

High and low lead subjects (N=58 and 100 respectively) were then evaluated with a number of tests which probed psychometric intelligence, speech and language processing, visual motor function, attention, concrete operational intelligence, and motor coordination. The results are summarized in Tables 2 & 3, which shows only those outcomes that differed at the level of $p < 0.05$.

TABLE 2. COMPARISON OF OUTCOMES ON THE WECHSLER INTELLIGENCE SCALE OF CHILDREN (REVISED) BETWEEN HIGH AND LOW LEAD SUBJECTS (ANALYSIS OF COVARIANCE)

	Low Lead (Mean)	High Lead (Mean)	P Value
Full Scale	106.6	102.1	0.03
Verbal IQ	103.9	99.3	0.03
Information	10.5	9.4	0.04
Vocabulary	11.0	10.0	0.05
Digit Span	10.6	9.3	0.02
Arithmetic	10.4	10.1	0.49
Comprehension	11.0	10.2	0.08
Similarities	10.8	10.3	0.36
Performance IQ	108.7	104.9	0.08
Picture Completion	12.2	11.3	0.03
Picture Arrangement	11.3	10.8	0.38
Block Design	11.0	10.3	0.15
Object Assembly	10.9	10.6	0.54
Coding	11.0	10.9	0.90
Mazes	10.6	10.1	0.37

Herbert L. Needleman, M.D.

TABLE 3. COMPARISON OF AUDITORY PROCESSING SCORES AND REACTION TIME UNDER VARYING DELAY BETWEEN HIGH AND LOW LEAD SUBJECTS

Test	Low Lead (Mean)	High Lead (Mean)	P Value
Seashore Rhythm Test			
Subtest A	8.2	7.1	0.002
Subtest B	7.5	6.8	0.03
Subtest C	6.0	5.4	0.07
Sum	21.6	19.4	0.002
Token Test			
Block 1	2.9	2.8	0.37
Block 2	3.7	3.7	0.90
Block 3	4.1	4.0	0.42
Block 4	14.1	13.1	0.05
Sum	24.8	23.6	0.09
Sentence Repetition Test	12.6	11.3	0.04
Reaction Time Under Varying Intervals of Delay			
Block 1 (3 sec)	0.35 ± 0.08	0.37 ± 0.09	0.32
Block 2 (12 sec)	0.41 ± 0.09	0.47 ± 0.12	0.001
Block 3 (12 sec)	0.41 ± 0.09	0.48 ± 0.11	0.001
Block 4 (3 sec)	0.38 ± 0.10	0.41 ± 0.12	0.01

High lead children showed significant impairment on the WISC-R, especially on the Verbal and Full scale IQ measures, and on almost all of the verbal subtests. Impaired function associated with lead exposure was also found on the Seashore Rhythm Test, a test of auditory memory and discrimination, on the Token test which evaluates verbal comprehension, and the Sentence Test which is a measure of memory for language. Reaction Time Under Varying intervals of Delay, a measure of the subjects' ability to maintain an additional set, was also sensitive to the lead burden of the subjects.

Teachers were given an eleven item, forced-choice questionnaire which evaluated general classroom behaviour, with particular focus on attention. (Table 4).

TABLE 4. TEACHER'S BEHAVIOURAL RATING SCALE

1. Is this child easily distracted during his/her work?
2. Can he/she persist with a task for a reasonable amount of time?
3. Can this child work independently and complete assigned tasks with minimal assistance?
4. Is his/her approach to tasks disorganized (constantly misplacing pencils, books, etc)?
5. Do you consider this child hyperactive?
6. Is he/she over-excitable and impulsive?
7. Is he/she easily frustrated by difficulties?
8. Is he/she a daydreamer?
9. Can he/she follow simple directions?
10. Can he/she follow a sequence of directions?
11. In general, is this child functioning as well in the classroom as other children his/her own age?

The teachers' ratings for high and low lead subjects are shown in Table 5. The item scores were transformed so that a good outcome was given a score of =1, and a bad outcome a score of =0. This enabled us to compile summed scores for the teachers' ratings, and analyze the scores by ANACOVA, thus controlling for the five covariates.

TABLE 5. COMPARISON OF HIGH AND LOW LEAD SUBJECTS ON TEACHERS' BEHAVIOURAL RATING SCALE. THE PERCENT OF STUDENTS IN EACH GROUP RECEIVING A NEGATIVE RATING IS SHOWN.

Item	Low Lead (%)	High Lead (%)	P Value
Distractable	14	36	0.003
Not persistent	9	21	0.05
Dependent	10	23	0.05
Disorganized	10	20	0.14
Hyperactive	6	16	0.08
Impulsive	9	25	0.01
Easily frustrated	11	25	0.04
Daydreamer	15	34	0.01
Does not follow			
Simple directions	4	14	0.05
Sequence of directions	12	34	0.003
Low overall functioning	8	26	0.003
Sum Score (Mean)	9.5	8.2	0.02*

* Analysis of covariance

In addition, teachers' ratings were available for 2146 subjects for whom we had a dentine lead level on file. The subjects were classified according to increasing dentine lead levels in six classes arranged to give a symmetrical distribution around the mean, and the proportion of negative reports for each group was calculated. (Fig 1). A strong dose-response relationship for each item is seen.

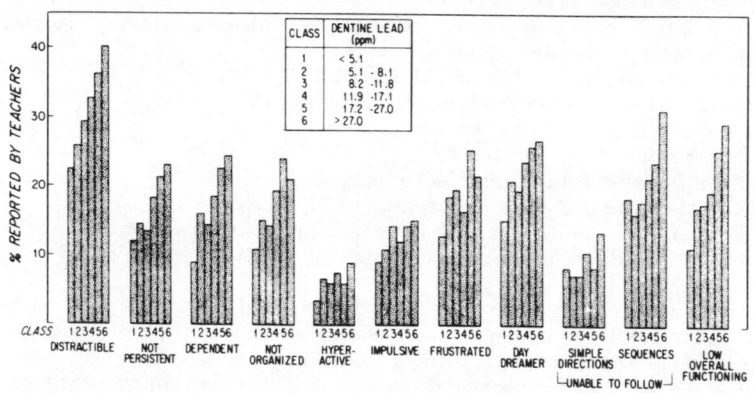

DISCUSSION

These data show a significant difference between high and low lead subjects on a number of outcomes, including verbal and full scale IQ, attention (reaction time under varying intervals of delay), auditory and language processing, and behaviour in class as evaluated by teachers (who were kept blind to the childrens' lead burden). These differences persisted after partialling out the contribution of those psychosocial variables that differentiated between high and low lead subjects.

These findings were accompanied by parallel changes in brain electrophysiology. Burchfiel et al (1980) studied a subset of these children using quantative electroencephalography, and showed

lead-related changes in mid-line EEG leads (decreased amounts of alpha frequencies and increased delta). This finding has been recently supported by the work of Otto and colleagues, using evoked potentials (1981). The psychometric changes measured here appear to be associated with consequent alterations in the real life classroom behaviour of the children measured four years later by observers blind to the children's lead levels. Bellinger et al (1981) measured on and off-task behaviour of a sample of these subjects, and found on that high lead children, during quiet academic work, spent more time staring at their classmates, or the observer, or out the window than low lead controls. The data based on 144 7-second observation periods for each of the 41 children in the sample (see Table 6).

TABLE 6. PERCENTAGE OF INTERVALS IN WHICH CLASSROOM BEHAVIOURS OBSERVED

| | Category | Dentine Lead Level | | | |
		Elevated (n=13)	Middle (n=13)	Low (n=15)	
1.	On-task	81.1 ± 16.4*	92.8 ± 8.7	88.8 ± 15.0	++
2.	Out-of-seat: unrelated to task	0.8 ± 1.4	0.7 ± 1.7	0.3 ± 0.7	**
3.	Glances at peer	9.3 ± 7.4	6.0 ± 2.8	6.5 ± 2.4	
4.	Glances at group	6.8 ± 12.8	4.6 ± 4.5	4.1 ± 5.3	**
5.	Glances at observer	10.1 ± 4.0	7.4 ± 6.1	5.6 ± 3.3	**+
6.	Glances at desk: unrelated to task	5.5 ± 8.0	1.7 ± 2.0	3.9 ± 8.5	
7.	Glances away	4.2 ± 3.1	2.4 ± 2.3	2.2 ± 1.9	**++
8.	Peer interaction	12.0 ± 8.1	8.0 ± 8.1	7.9 ± 8.4	**

*   mean ± standard deviation
** scores dose-related to lead grouping
+ $p < .05$
++ $p < .10$

probability that the elevated lead children would display the least appropriate behaviour in all 8 categories: .0002 (expansion of binomial)

probability that scores would be dose-related with respect to lead grouping on 5 of the 8 categories: .0046 (expansion of Binomial)

(From Bellinger et al. 1981)

An estimate of the amount of impaired classroom performance attribute to lead exposure may be obtained through the used simple formula applied to the estimates of low overall functioning provided by the teachers in the highest and lowest exposure groups in Table 5 (Cowan and Leviton 1980). It was found that 69% of the low overall classroom performance in the children with high lead can be attributed to their lead exposure.

$$\text{Attributable risk} = \frac{Ie - Io}{Ie}$$

where Ie = Incidence of trait in the exposed group and Io = incidence of the trait in the unexposed group

$$AR = \frac{.26 - .08}{.26}$$

$$= 69\%$$

George Provenzano (1980), using data from this study and health care costs measured in 1979, estimated that the cost for remedial education provided for US children reached $951 million in 1979. These data should be considered conservative estimates given the incidence of elevated blood lead levels estimated by the National Centre for Health Statistics (Annest, this volume) and the inflation of health care and education dollars since the publication of his paper.

More recently, Yule and colleagues (1981) have shown IQ and reading deficits in children with blood lead levels > 13 µg/dl when compared to controls below 13µg/dl. In this study, Yule controlled for age, sex and socioeconomic status. In the present volume, the same investigators (chapter 14) evaluated classroom behaviour by the same teacher rating scale used by my group. Their findings correspond strikingly to ours. The attributable risk for low overall classroom performance in their subjects is 0.63. This similarity, in children of a different culture, scaled by teachers in a different school system, suggests that the effect of lead on classroom behaviour is remarkably robust.

A number of questions and criticisms have been raised about the data and interferences presented here. One criticism has been that while the difference between groups is statistically significant, the difference is small, and of questionable biological import. Figure 2 plots the actual cumulative frequency distribution of verbal IQ scores in high and low lead subjects, and shows that a difference between groups of this magnitude is associated with an almost four-fold difference in the number of children with severe deficits,

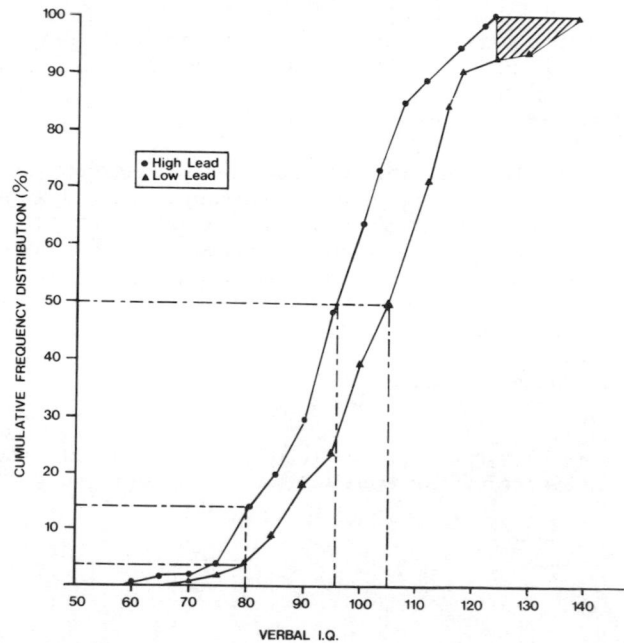

that is IQ scores below 80. In addition, 5 per cent of the low lead children reached the superior range of over 125, while none of the high lead subjects did so. Perhaps one of the costs of low level lead exposure is its effects at the upper end of the distribution, where one child in twenty is prevented from achieving superior function - surely an important phenomenon.

It has been argued that the differential distribution of pica between high and low lead subjects confounds the effect of lead. It is true that children with psychological deficit may display more pica, and may as a result have higher blood and tooth lead levels. We therefore controlled for the effect of pica, using the elegant technique of James Schlesselman, and found that pica did not affect the relative risk of low IQ (Needleman et al, 1982).

One critic has suggested that since we measured a large number of outcomes, and a certain number could be expected to achieve a difference at $p<0.05$ on the basis of chance, the differences reported here are due to chance. Of 66 outcomes evaluated, 15, or roughly 1 in 4 were significant. On the basis of chance, if the outcomes were uncorrelated, one would expect 1 in 20 to differ. The most persuasive response to the question of multiple comparisons lies in whether the findings are replicable. The replication of studies, even if they report p values below the sacrosant 0.05 level, increase the likelihood that the differences observed are not due to chance. The findings of Yule (Chapter 14) and Winneke (Chapter 13) reported in this volume are the strongest response to this criticism.

Is the relationship between lead and neurosychologic deficit causal in nature? In the real world, multivariate space has infinite dimensions. Epidemiologic investigations by their nature cannot hope to achieve complete control of all variables, and cannot prove causality. Indeed, as David Hume has shown, causality is a construct not accessible empirical proof. What has been demonstrated here is a dose-dependent association between lead and neuropsychologic function which persists after control for a large number of relevant covariates, and which has now been supported by careful studies by independent investigators.

Not mentioned in this paper, but of direct relevance to the causal question, is the enormous literature of experimental animal studies in which systematic administration of lead to rodents and subhuman primates produces neurochemical, anatomical, and behavioural deficits (see chapter 10).

CONCLUSIONS

Lead at low dose is seen to be associated with a spectrum of behavioural alterations in these areas: psychometric intelligence, auditory and language processing, reaction time under varying intervals of delay, quantitative electroencephalography, and classroom behaviour as rated by teachers and outside observers.

The findings with respect of IQ and teachers' ratings have been replicated by independent investigators in different cultures.

The question of whether low level lead exposure is associated with significant brain alterations no longer needs - or deserves - prolonged and debilitating debate. Action on lead, clearly warranted, long delayed, and easily obtained, could be the first in a series of steps to protect the legacy we owe to our children - a world in which the physical and social arrangements we provide permit their brains and futures to achieve their full reach.

DISCUSSION

Rutter: What are the problems of using tooth lead as a marker of lead exposure?

Needleman: Unlike blood, teeth are not homogenous. As a consequence, different types of teeth may differ somewhat in their level of lead and, more importantly, different sections of the same tooth may give different values. This means that a single sample of tooth might result in misclassification because of some localized concentration of lead. It was for this reason that we excluded all cases in which the results of the analysis seemed unreliable or in which the results of two analyses were discrepant. For those subjects included I have great confidence that our separation of high lead and low lead groups was both reliable and valid.

Grandjean: The NHANES data (see chapter 3) showed that children from low income groups had a blood lead level that was twice as high as that for the high income group. If that finding applies to the Boston area, could you have over-corrected by allowing for socio-economic factors when you analysed your results according to lead levels? In other words, if the low social class children truly had higher lead levels (as they did in the NHANES data) could you have inadvertently removed a genuine lead effect by your introduction of controls for socio-economic factors?

Needleman: That is an important point. Of course, in ordinary circumstances, multivariate analyses should provide the appropriate degree of correction. But this may be influenced by the causal connections between the independent variables. Let us suppose that the lead exposure of the parents correlates with that of their children (a not unreasonable assumption), and also that the parental lead exposure has affected their IQ and social status. In that situation, lead may exert an indirect effect on the child through its impact on the parents, as well as through direct actions on the child's brain. If so, it is possible that statistical controls for parental IQ and social status may over-control to some extent, and hence underestimate the effect of lead.

Rutter:

It might be helpful if you indicated how much the social class correction changed your findings. What was the IQ difference between your high dentine lead and low dentine lead before this correction was made?

Needleman:

The initial between-group difference was about 2 IQ points more than that found after the correction. The fact that the lead effect was or roughly the same order before social variables were entered into the analysis makes it most unlikely that over-correction had occurred. But, by the same token, it also suggests that if it had been possible to add still more social variables into the analysis probably this too would have made very little difference to the broad pattern of findings.

Delves:

We have been involved in a study looking at 2,000 children using whole tooth lead rather than dentine lead. We found vales very similar to Winneke's - about 4 ppm. However, for children who gave two teeth there was some discordance between them. For example, 15-20% of the children sampled had differences of 3 ppm between the two teeth. This constitutes rather a large difference in relation to a mean value of 4ppm. Such discrepancies provide the possibility of substantial errors in classification, particularly in the middle of the range. What level of variation did you find in you dentine leads, and what implications might possible misclassification have for your findings and conclusions?

Needleman:

We did not encounter such large differences as those you report. Nevertheless, we shared your concern regarding errors of misclassification and it was for this reason that we took two important steps to avoid that error. Firstly, we employed very strict criteria for concordance between samples and discarded all subjects for whom these criteria could not be met. Secondly, for most analyses we focused on the more extreme high lead and low lead groups, omitting the middle group in which errors of classification were likely to be greatest. We felt that the best approach in an epidemiological study was to confine analyses to samples in which the measures of crucial variables (in this case dentine lead) were thoughly reliable. However, we also sought to check on the consequences of this rigorous approach through an examination of the psychological outcome measures of the discarded group. The findings showed that they were intermediate between the high and the low lead groups; accordingly, it seems likely that the discrepant tooth lead analyses reflected exposures in the middle range.

Rutter:

In that connection, it is important to differentiate between the effects of random error and of systematic error. Systematic error refers to the tendency to systematically overestimate measures in one group and to underestimate them in another group. Such errors, which may arise through biased sampling or through wishful thinking in making measures with knowledge of which child is in which group, are very likely to lead to seriously misleading positive findings. That is to say, systematic errors are liable to cause biases leading to a finding of an apparent difference between groups, when in reality no such difference exists. Random error, in sharp contrast, tends to have the opposite effect of reducing differences between groups so that, in truth, the real difference is greater than it appears. Random error is most likely to be caused by weak measurement – a problem in many branches of science. In your study it does not seem likely that there was systematic error, but as in all research, there is bound to have been some random error – although great care was taken to keep error to a minimum. In so far as there was any random error, it is likely to have led to an underestimate rather than an overestimate of the effect of lead on psychological functioning.

Needleman:

I think that is probably correct.

Pocock: You said there was an age difference between
                  the high and low lead groups, which you
                  described as an artefact. I wonder if you
                  could elaborate on that?

Needleman: Yes, I wanted my technicians to get some
                  experience with normal children, so I
                  arranged, without their knowledge, for the
                  first group of children to be low lead children.

Pocock: Dosen't that introduce the possibility of bias?

Needleman: While it does constitute a minor departure from
                  an ideal design, it is not easy to see how it
                  could have led to any bias. After all, the
                  technicians were unaware of which group they
                  were testing and, of course, they were kept
                  blind to the neuropsychological findings.

Pocock: You seem to have moved rather directly to a
                  causal interpretation of your results. But, is
                  it not possible that the cause and effect
                  relationship might work in the opposite
                  direction? In other words, perhaps children
                  of lower IQ or those with disturbed behaviour,
                  may be more liable to pick up lead through
                  putting dusty hands in their mouth or through
                  eating paint or some other toxic material.

Needleman: I agree that that constitutes a serious design
                  issue of particular importance in my study
                  because there was indeed a marked difference
                  between the rate of pica in the high lead
                  group (29%) and that in the low lead group
                  (11%). Certainly, that suggests that some of
                  the high lead children were especially subject
                  to excessive lead exposure by virtue of
                  putting things in their mouth. However, that
                  does not in itself invalidate the causal
                  argument. The matter may be systematically
                  examined by repeating the statistical
                  comparison of the high lead and low lead
                  groups after stratification according to the
                  presence or absence of pica. In effect, this
                  means that the IQ levels in the two groups
                  were being compared separately in the children
                  without pica and then again in those with pica
                  (with these two comparisons being then
                  statistically recombined in order to give an
                  overall measure of comparison between the two
                  groups). This procedure was undertaken
                  using Schlesselman's alogorithm; the results
                  indicated that still, high lead dentine levels

were associated with a similarly increased risk for an IQ below 80 (Needelman et al, 1982).

Rutter:

Could you comment on the possible confounding effect of pica with respect to the association you found between high lead levels and inattentive behaviour?

Needleman:

We tackled that problem by determining both the strength of the association between pica and behaviour (as assessed by a summation of scores on the teacher's questionnaire), and that between behaviour and dentine lead levels. (Needleman et al. 1982).   The children with pica did not differ from those without pica on their behaviour ratings (t = 0.93; NS) but the high lead group did differ significantly in behaviour scores (t = 3.18; p<0.001) from the low lead group.   The clear implication is that the presence of pica does not account for the association between high lead levels and inattentive behaviour.   These two sets of analyses provide important support for the argument that the high lead levels caused the children to show disturbed behaviour and impaired intelligence, rather than the other way round.

Murgraff:

Would it be a crucial addition to the sum of knowledge on this matter if children presenting behavioural and psychological symptoms or with low IQ were routinely examined for lead levels, and are there any contraindictions for such routine checking?

Needleman:

Blood lead levels have been measured routinely in many parts of the USA and this has proved to be a very productive means of lead screening.   The prevalence of high lead levels dropped dramatically after a few years, partly because of public awareness and partly because some children were picked up very early before their lead levels rose to a point where there was a risk of severe encephalopathy.   Some screening tests are very cheap and cost effective.   The FEP (free eythrocyte protoporphyrin), for example, costs less than 50 cents a test.   Until we get lead out of the environment, such screening procedures have an important role.

Question:

What is the cost of dentine tests and would you consider it advisable to include them as a routine part of the school entrance examination at age 5½ to 6 years?

Needleman: The measurement of dentine lead has serious drawbacks for routine screening purposes. First of all, it is necessary to wait for the tooth to fall out. Secondly, it is rather an expensive procedure. The tooth has to be sliced, then dried to a standard weight, and finally it has to be digested in acid. The FEP, in contrast, is cheap, easy to undertake, and can be done on all children. It is based on just a simple finger prick and the result is immediately available at the time. Dentine lead analysis constitutes a useful epidemiological tool, but it is not yet suitable for screening purposes.

Question: Have you looked at the school environment as a possible explanation for the different lead burdens in the children in your study? Also, what was the sex ratio of the groups you examined? Dr. David indicated that 90% of the individuals he examined were male. I wondered if you noticed a preponderance of males in your high lead group as well?

Needleman: No, we did not look at lead in schools, as the study was concerned with the effects of high lead, rather than with the sources of lead in the environment. In answer to your second question, the sex ratio was approximately equal. Epidemiologcial studies show that lead levels tend to be slightly higher in boys than in girls (see chapter 3) but the difference is not particularly large in the age group with which we were concerned. Dr. David's design was quite different in that his sample was initially defined in terms of the children having been referred for hyperactivity, rather than for high lead levels. Hyperactivity is well known to be very much more frequent in boys than girls and it is for that reason (as well as the fact that his was a clinical rather than epidemiological study) that his sample showed such a marked ,ale preponderance.

Hartley: In your study you looked at a large number of outcomes, including many not reported in your paper. Inevitably, when a large number of comparisons are made, some will be statistically significant by chance alone. Did you make appropriate corrections for that possibility?

Needleman: We did make an estimate of the reduced P values for multiple comparisons; there is a footnote in the New England Journal of Medicine article (written in consultation with their statistical consultant) that deals with that point. However, there are also other ways of approaching the problem. One way is to examine the direction of the statistically significant inter-group differences. If they were due solely to chance (i.e. if there were no true lead effect), then 50% of the tests should favour the high lead group. As it was, 65 out of 66 favoured the low lead group. Obviously, the likelyhood of that happening by chance is astronomically small.

Russel Jones: When the minister responsible for the decision about lead was interviewed last week on BBC radio, he said that what was needed was medical evidence which was robust enough to withstand scientific scrutiny. What questions do you think that future studies will answer that have not been answered by your own work?

Needleman: I do not know. But I do think we have enough information to act responsibly now, especially when the animal data are taken into consideration. Many of the problems associated with the epidemiological studies (such as dose-response, controlling for socio-economic class, etc.) are answered by the animal studies. Similarly, many of the problems with the animal studies, such as applicability ti the human situation, are answered by the epidemiological enquiries. I think that the case against lead is more solid than for any other neurotoxin, and if we are not prepared to act on that, then I question whether we are prepared to act on any toxin. It has been suggested in Developmental Medicine and Child Neurology, and in the British Medical Journal, that attention to lead distracts attention from other factors that influence intellectual development. That is nonsense. If society is not prepared to do anything about lead, I am pessimistic that it will do anything about poverty, or hunger, or racial antagonism. In fact, lead provides a pathway to the solution of other important problems in the social domain.

Rutter: In the subgroup you studied using the
                     computerized EEG's, were the EEG findings
                     related either to your IQ measure, or
                     behavioural measure; if they were, that would
                     constitute a most useful way of examining the
                     possibility that the neurophysiological
                     dysfunction (as reflected in the EEG) served
                     as a meditating variable.

Needleman: I cannot answer your question directly, but
                     Burchfiel did a linear discrimination function
                     analysis using psychological measures. Without
                     the EEG there was some separation of the high
                     lead and low lead groups but the addition of
                     EEG data pulled the groups apart quite
                     dramatically (Burchfiel et al, 1980).

Question: With respect to your comment on the need for
                     society to take much more vigorous steps to
                     remove lead from the environment, I would
                     have thought that during the last ten to
                     fifteen years a great deal had been done
                     already. A recent EEC study of blood leads
                     showed a mean value across the countries of
                     roughly 13 µg/dl.

Needleman: Of course, that is good news, but I do not
                     think it is a source for complacency. Dr.
                     Yule has shown that around a mean level of 13
                     µg/dl there is still a 7 point IQ difference
                     between children with higher and lower lead
                     levels. We should not be content to rest at a
                     level of 13 µg/dl; the evidence suggests that
                     it is not low enough.

REFERENCES

Bellinger, D., Needleman, H.L., Hargrave, J., Nichols, M. (1981).
    Elevated dentine lead levels and school success. Paper
    presented at the Biennial Meeting of the Society for Research in
    Child Development, Boston, Mass.
Burchfiel, J., Duffy, F.H., Bartels, P. and Needleman, H.L.
    (1980). The combined discriminating power of quantitive
    electroencephalographic and neuropsychologic measures in
    evaluating CNS checks of lead at low levels, in Needleman, H.
    (ed.) Low Level Lead Exposure : The Clinical Implications of
    Current Research. New York : Raven Press. pp 75-89.
Byers, R., and Lord, E., (1943) Late effects of lead poisoning on
    mental development. Am J Dis Child. 66:471:494.
Cowan, L., and Leviton, A., (1980) Epidemiologic considerations in
    the study of the sequellae of low lead exposure in Low Level

Lead Exposure: The Clinical Implications of Current Research
(ed H.L. Needleman) pp91-120 Raven Press, New York.

Hernberg, S., (1973). Biological effects of low lead doses in
International Symposium Environmental Health Aspects of Lead
(eds D. Barth, P. Recht, R Engel, J. Smeets) pp617-629, CEC,
Luxembourg.

Needleman, H.L., Davidson, I., Sewell, E., Shapiro, I.M. (1974)
Subclinical lead exposure in Philadelphia school children:
Identification by dentine lead analysis. N Engl J Med
290:245-248.

Needleman H.L., Gunnoe, C., Leviton, A., Reed, R., Peresie, H.,
Maher, C., Barrett, P., (1979). Deficits in psychologic and
classroom performance of children with elevated dentine lead
levels. N Engl J Med 300:689-695.

Needleman, H.L. and Landrigan, P. (1981) The health effects of
low level exposure to lead. Ann Rev Pub Health. 2:277-298.

Needleman, H.L., Leviton, A., and Bellinger, D. (1982).
Lead-associated intellectual deficit. N Engl J Med 306:367.

Otto, D.A., Benignus, V.A., Muller, K.E., and Barton, C.N.
(1981). Effects of age and lead burden on CNS function in
young children. I. Slow cortical potentials. EEG and Clin
Neurophysiol 52:229-239.

Piomelli, S., Seaman, C., Zulow, D., Curran, A. and Davidow, B.
(1982). The threshold for lead damage to heme synthesis in
urban children. Proc Nat Acad Sci 79:335-339.

Provenzano G., (1980) Social costs of excessive lead exposure
during childhood in Low Level Lead Exposure: The Clinical
Implications of Current Research (ed H.L. Needleman) pp299-316
Raven Press, New York.

Yule, W., Lansdown, R., Millar, I.B., and Urbanowicz, M. (1981)
The relationship between blood lead concentrations, intelligence
and attainment in a school population: A pilot study. Dev Med
Child Neurol. 23:567-576.

Lead Versus Health
Edited by M. Rutter and R. Russell Jones
© 1983 John Wiley & Sons Ltd.

NEUROBEHAVIOURAL   AND   NEUROPSYCHOLOGICAL
EFFECTS OF LEAD

Gerhard Winneke, Ph.D.

Head, Psychophysiology Section
Medical Institute of Environmental Hygiene
University of Dusseldorf
Gurlittstrasse 53
D-4000 Dusseldorf, F.R.G.

During recent years our group has investigated the neurobehavioural effects of lead, using both experimental animal-models and epidemiological studies of lead-exposed children, in order to determine the effects of low-level lead exposure on the developing brain. This chapter summarizes the main findings from both approaches and compares some results from animal-experimentation with observations made in children, in order to discuss the cause-effect issue.

Two double-blind neuropsychological investigations of lead-exposed children were conducted in 1977/78 and in 1980/81, both of which relied on tooth lead-concentrations (PbT) as indices of longterm past cumulative lead-intake. Lead-concentrations in whole incisor-teeth were measured by means of atomic absorption spectrophotometry (AAS), according to the procedures described in detail elsewhere (Ewers et al., 1979, 1982). Basically, the teeth are dissolved in a mixture of nitric acid and perchloric acid diluted with ammonium citrate-solution. Lead is extracted from the aqueous solution using the ADPC/MIBK-system and determined by AAS. Over the entire range of concentrations the reproducibility of analyses was 6% on the average, and the detection-limit was found to be 0.15 $\mu g/g$; the correlation-coefficient for the comparison of 1st and 2nd incisor-teeth was 0.86 (Ewers et al., 1982).

Our first study was undertaken in Duisburg (Hrdina, 1978; Winneke, 1979; Winneke et al., 1982c) - a city of about 500,000 inhabitants, located in the "Ruhrgebiet", and characterized by heavy industry and high air pollution. Its industrial structure is made up of coke oven-plants, coal power-plants, and a number of metal processing factories, some of which are non-ferrous smelters. Airborne lead-concentrations (annual averages) were between 1.5 and about 2 $\mu g/m^3$ in 1976 and 1977 (Brockhaus et al., 1978).

Shed baby-teeth were collected in a press-supported campaign in 1976. Our of 1238 children who between them had delivered 3127 teeth, we used only the 458 children aged between 7 and 10 years who had delivered at least two incisor-teeth and who were representative of the total child population. The distribution of tooth-lead-concentrations was log-normal. The geometric mean was

4.6 µg/g with individual values ranging from 1.4 to 12.7 µg/g.
From this basic sample those with tooth-leads ⟨3 µg/g (control
group) or ⟩7 µg/g (lead group) were provisionally selected for
participation in the neuropsychological examinations. Of those
invited, 77% (controls) and 61% (lead group) agreed to participate.
From this pool, matched pairs were formed by assigning a
"best-fitting" control-partner to every child from the lead-group
using age, sex, and father's occupational status as matching
criteria. 26 pairs of children were finally selected. The average
PbT of the controls was 2.4, that of the lead-group 9.2 µg/g.

Psychometric and simple neurological tests were selected to cover as
broad a range of neurobehavioural characteristics as possible. In
addition to cognitive performance, visual-motor integration, gross
motor coordination and general test-behaviour of the children were
assessed. Also information was sought on risk factors during birth
as well as during pregnancy and early postnatal life.

General intelligence was measured by means of the German version
of the WISC (Hardesty and Priester, 1956). Visual "Gestalt"-
perception, known to be easily disturbed in cases of brain-
dysfunction, was assessed by 3 tests: The Benton-test (Benton,
1974), the German version of the Bender-Gestalt-Test (Schlange et
al., 1972), as well as the "Diagnostics for cerebral damage"
(Weidlich, 1972). Gross body coordination was assessed by means
of the "body coordination-test for children" (Schilling and Kiphard,
1974), yielding age standardized motor-quotients as indices of
normal or retarded motor-development. In addition, the test
behaviour of the children were rated by means of rating-scales
adapted from the CONNERS-scales (Conners, 1969).

The neuropsychological examinations were carried out by three
advanced psychology students who were kept unaware of the tooth
lead findings and of any other background measures on the
children. Children were assigned at random to each examiner as
pairs, in order to rule out any possibility of differential treatment
of control- and lead-children. Finally, the child's mother was
asked about possible risk-factors during pregnancy, birth and the
first year of life, as well as about the child's later general
development.

The main results from this study are given in Table 1.

We obtained an IQ deficit of 5 to 7 points for the high lead group,
which in this sample size was of only borderline significance
($p < 0.1$). We also obtained a significant ($p < 0.05$) increase of 2.4
points in the error-score for the high lead group using the
"Gottinger Form-reproduktionstest" (Gottinger Form Reproduction-
Test), the German version of the Bender Gestalt-test which is often
used for the clinical diagnosis of "brain-damage". Furthermore,
significantly fewer children ($p < 0.05$) from the high-lead group
were able to solve the reproduction problems posed by the
"Diagnostikum fur Cerebralschadigung (DCS)" (Diagnostics-for-

Cerebral-Damage-Test), which also is a clinical test used to confirm tentative diagnoses of "brain damage" by testing perceptual motor integration.   The other inter group differences were statistically non-significant.

TABLE 1. Summary of main results from our pilot study run in 52 school age children living in the city of Duisburg (FRG). Significance levels refer to paired t-tests

| Pilot-Study (Duisburg): Main Findings | | | | |
Area	Test-Scores	"Low-Pb"	"High-Pb"	Level of Significance (one-tailed)
Intelligence (WISC)	Verbal-IQ	122±18.9	117±16.6	n.s.
	Performance-IQ	130±14.8	124±17.1	p < 0.1
	Fullscale-IQ	130±17.1	123±17.6	p < 0.1
Visual-Motor Integration	GFT-errors	17.2±6.0	19.6±4.8	p < 0.05
	DCS-Score	6.9±2.7	7.2±2.9	n.s.
	BENTON-Score	10.4±3.5	10.2±3.2	n.s.
Gross Motor-Coordination	KTK-MQ total	97±19	95±15	n.s.

These results supported the hypothesis of a correlation between increased lead-exposure during childhood and disturbances of neuropsychological development.   However, they were not unequivocal and pronounced enough to prove a relationship between the lead burden and the observed neuropsychological deficit.

For this reason we decided to run a second study in Stolberg (Winneke et al., 1982b) - a small, highly industrialized city near Aachen of about 60,000 inhabitants with a century-old history of metal-mining and processing. The principal source of lead-pollution is a large primary lead-smelter. Airborne lead-concentrations, given as one year-averages, ranged from 1.3 to 7.6 $\mu g/m^3$ in 1973, and were reduced by various preventive measures to 0.4 - 2 $\mu g/m^3$ in 1980. In the same period, lead-depositions in the vicinity of the primary lead-smelter were reduced from as high as 10 to about 2 $mg/m^2/day$. The parents of all children born between July 1, 1968 and June 30, 1973 (N = 3669) were requested to submit shed baby-teeth, emphasizing incisor-teeth. We finally analyzed the shed teeth of 317 school-age children (311 incisors and 6 molars - having discarded various teeth and those with fillings).

Again the tooth-lead values were found to have a normal logarithmic distribution. The geometric mean was 6.0 µg/g (Ewers et al., 1982), and the extremes were substantially higher than those found in our Duisburg-study (Ewers et al., 1979). For example, in Duisburg only 2.2% of the tooth-lead-concentrations were higher than 10 µg/g, whereas in Stolberg 13.6% exceeded this value. For neuropsychological testing children with low, average and high values were selected from the total sample of 317 children in such a manner as to set up a more or less continuous range of tooth lead values extending from 1.5 to 38 µg/g. Thus, contrary to the Duisburg-study, we were able to exploit fully the information contained in the data by evaluating them by means of stepwise multiple regression analysis, considering the effects of several confounding variables.

In addition to tooth lead analyses, capillary blood leads were available for a subgroup of 83 children (who volunteered). The average blood lead level (geometric mean) for this subsample was 14.3 µg/dl; blood lead levels correlated 0.47 with tooth lead levels.

The mothers in Stolberg were extensively interviewed on the case histories of their children in order to obtain as much background information as possible. More than 50 possibly confounding variables were collected on the social environment, the family, and the case history of each child. Each one of them was tested to determine whether it correlated with the tooth lead level. Only three of the variables showed a significant correlation with the tooth lead values: duration of parturition according to the mother's recollections (p = 0.05), occupational status of the father (p = 0.02) or the mother (p = 0.01), and type of school attended by the child (p = 0.05). Neither parental education nor net income correlated with tooth lead level.

Those children attending schools that did not lead to higher education (secondary school or "Hauptschule") had significantly higher tooth lead values than those children attending other types of schools. In addition, children of parents belonging to the unskilled workers-category also had elevated tooth lead levels. Because of their high intercorrelations, the type of school attended by the child and the occupational status of the parents were grouped together as one category called "socio-hereditary background", for the purpose of testing the statistical significance of associations with neuropsychological dependent variables, using a stepwise multiple regression analysis, with tooth lead being entered as the last step.

The battery of performance-measures was somewhat different from the one used in the Duisberg study: the Benton-test and the body coordination-test (KTK) were omitted. Instead, the Vienna reaction device (Wiener Determinations test), a serial reaction-time task (Klebelsberg, 1960), a cancellation-test for the assessment of perceptual speed (Kleber and Kleber, 1974), as well as a simple tapping-test were added. In addition, standardized behaviour rating-scales for mothers and teachers were used to rate classroom and homework behaviour, respectively.

The main results of this study in 7 to 12 year old children from the city of Stolberg are given in Tables 2 (data before correction for confounding variables) and 3 (data after correction). For the sake of clarity the continuous tooth lead variable (see Winneke et al. 1982c) was broken down into subgroups of children with low ($<$ 4 ppm), moderate ($>$ 4-10 ppm) and high ($>$ 10 ppm) tooth lead concentrations.

TABLE 2. Results for main variables ($\bar{x} \pm s$) for groups of children with low, moderate and high tooth lead-concentrations (age-adjusted values, except for IQ), before correction for confounding variables (Stolberg-study).

Variables	"low" $<$ 4 ppm	"moderate" $>$ 4-10 ppm	"high" $<$ 10 ppm	level of significance[+]
	n = 36	n = 56	n = 23	
Verbal IQ	116.6±13.0	115.0±12.8	109.0±12.9	p $<$ 0.1
Performance IQ	115.3±13.8	114.1±14.3	114.7± 9.9	n.s.
Full Scale IQ	118.3±12.7	116.6±13.1	113.3±11.6	n.s.
GFT (errors)	21.2± 6.1	20.6± 5.1	23.9± 3.5	p $<$ 0.05
DCS-index	1.1± 1.9	1.1± 2.0	1.2± 1.5	n.s.
Wiener CR	101.7±30.3	108.1±36.4	108.2±30.6	n.s.
Wiener LR	48.7±19.8	43.2±24.8	44.1±18.1	n.s.
Wiener FR	3.7± 3.2	4.8± 3.0	5.0± 4.3	n.s.

[+] two-tailed probabilities from analysis of variance

High lead level children had a verbal IQ 7.6 IQ-points below that of the low level children before correction for confounding variables, with the moderate group being in between both extreme groups (Table 2); these differences were of borderline significance (F=2.62; p=0.08). For both performance and full scale IQs group differences were smaller and clearly not significant. After correcting for the effects of confounding variables (socio-hereditary background (SHB) and duration of parturition), the inferiority of the high level group was reduced to 4.6 IQ points (verbal IQ). Whereas SHB alone accounted for 10.1% of total variance (F=8.33; p=0.005), lead exposure contributed only an additional 0.5%

(F=0.91; p=0.41). Basically the same situation pertained to the performance IQ, although the social factor was much less influential here (F=1.55; p=0.22).

TABLE 3. Results for main variables ($\bar{x}$ ± SD) <u>after</u> correction for confounding variables (Stolbert-Study).

Variables	"low" < 4 ppm	"moderate" > 4-10 ppm	"high" < 10 ppm	level of significance[+)]
Verbal IQ	115.9±12.7	114.6±12.4	111.3±10.2	n.s.
Performance IQ	114.5±13.5	114.5±12.6	115.2± 9.4	n.s.
Full Scale IQ	117.3±12.6	116.5±11.8	115.0± 9.9	n.s.
GFT (errors)	21.0± 5.8	20.6± 4.8	23.8± 3.2	p < 0.05
DCS-index	1.1± 1.9	1.1± 1.9	1.3± 1.4	n.s.
Wiener CR	105.0±29.6	106.4±36.4	107.2±27.5	n.s.
Wiener LR	47.3±19.9	43.4±24.0	45.6±17.4	n.s.
Wiener FR	3.5± 3.2	5.1± 2.8	5.1± 3.8	n.s.

[+)] two-tailed probabilities from analysis of variance

On the "Gottingen-Form-Reproduktionstest (GFT)" for perceptual-motor integration there was a significant (p<0.01) positive correlation (r=0.22) between number of errors and tooth lead concentration. In terms of group-means before correction (Table 2) this corresponded to an age-adjusted error-increase from 21.1 (low lead) to 23.9 (high lead), a statistically significant difference on an analysis of variance (F=3.48; p=0.03). This effect remained after correction (Table 3), and still was significant on an analysis of covariance (F=3.27; p=0.04). Performance on the "Diagnosticum fur Cerebralschadigung (DCS)" was not affected.

Reaction-performance, as measured by hits (CR) and late reactions (LR) on the "Wiener Determinationsgerat" (Vienna Reaction-Device), did not correlate significantly with lead exposure; however, "false reactions (FR)" did show a significant correlation (r=0.18; p<0.05) before correction, and a nearly significant one (p<0.10) after correction. This is at least partial confirmation of similar findings reported by Needleman et al (1979) for attention-bound reactions. Due to the loss of information involved in breaking down the continuous tooth lead variable in three subgroups, this association is not borne out significantly in Tables 2 and 3.

Behaviour ratings, given by the testers, the mothers and the teachers, using almost identical 7-point rating scales, emphasised different aspects of attention, organisation and endurance displayed by the children during testing, when doing the homework, or in the classroom, respectively. Borderline to significant (one-tailed tests) associations were observed between four of the single item mother-ratings and tooth lead levels, after correction. These items were: (1) "Is easily distracted" ($F=1.72$; $p =0.07$); (2) "Is restless" ($F=2.08$; $p=0.04$); (3) "Doesn't know his homework" ($F=2.64$; $p=0.01$); and (4) "Keeps poking around and doesn't start with his homework" ($F=5.38$; $p=0.001$). The associations were much weaker for the teacher-ratings, which exhibited a much stronger relationship with the SHB variable than did those of the mothers.

CONCLUSIONS

From these two studies carried out in the cities of Duisberg and Stolberg the following conclusions may be drawn as to the effect of low level lead exposure on neuropsychological development:

1. Raised lead levels were associated with an increased error score on the "Gottinger Form-Reproduktionstest (GFT)" (The German version of the Bender Gestalt-Test); this reflects an impairment of perceptual-motor integration. This dysfunction may be considered as having been caused by lead, since it remained significant after having taken social background into account. In addition, this effect was clearly established in both independent studies. The small degree of the effect and the lack of corresponding deficit in functionally related tests, such as the DCS or some sub-tests of the WISC, run contrary to an interpretation in terms of organic brain damage. The error-increase in the GFT is much more readily explained by an inaccuracy of perception, based on disturbances of the attention-process. The general direction of this interpretation is supported by the behaviour-ratings of the mothers and, possibly, even by the finding of an increase of errors in the Wiener-Reaction-device.

2. The association between childhood lead-exposure and impairment of intellectual development, as measured by the verbal IQ, has been confirmed as a correlation, although probably this is not a cause-effect relationship. Our results rather suggest, that when sufficient differentiation is applied to the consideration of social background, IQ-deficits as well as elevated lead-exposure can both be considered as resulting from factors determined by the social environment. Many uncertainties still remain in this area of research. Using a cross-sectional approach, the evidence for lead being the causative factor for the observed intellectual effects can at best be considered suggestive.

Quite apart from the outcome of our Stolberg-study there are three main reasons which, in my opinion, cast doubt on the idea of an intelligence-deficit being causally related to childhood lead-exposure:

(1)   Although there were indications of dose-effect charac-
        teristics for verbal IQ within the Stolberg-study (tables
        2,3), the lack of correspondence between our studies must
        be mentioned. Tooth lead-concentrations were lower in the
        high level-group of the Duisburg-study ($\bar{x}$ = 9.2 µg/g)
        than in the high level-group of the Stolberg-study ($\bar{x}$ =
        15.7 µg/g) as defined in Table 2, but the lead-values of
        the low level-groups of both studies were very similar,
        namely 2.4 µg/g (Duisburg) versus 3.1 µg/g (Stolberg).
        Despite these differences of tooth lead-concentrations
        between the extreme-groups of both studies, the verbal
        IQ-differences (corrected values) were roughly the same
        for both studies. The same holds true when comparing
        Needleman's results with the outcome of our studies, if
        dentine lead can be compared with whole tooth-lead.

(2)   There is some lack of consistency with clinical experience
        as far as the differential vulnerability of the various
        IQ-measures is concerned. The verbal IQ has been shown
        to be influenced more profoundly by socio-economic factors
        than the performance IQ, which corresponds to our
        findings. Most recent studies, including our Stolberg-
        study, show closer associations between verbal IQ and
        markers of lead-exposure than between performance IQ and
        lead. Clinical experience indicates, however, that
        exogeneous factors, such as excessive alcohol intake or
        brain injury, if it inteferes with IQ at all, has its main
        impact on performance IQ, with verbal intelligence
        relatively unimpaired.

(3)   Neurobehavioural data from animal experiments run in our
        laboratory, again do not support the idea of lead being
        detrimental to "intellectual" development, either, although
        they clearly support the hypothesis that lead causes
        certain CNS-dysfunctions at low blood lead-levels - as
        explained below in more detail.

In an earlier study (Winneke et al., 1977) we demonstrated a task-dependent performance-deficit in visual discrimination-learning in rats at blood lead-levels around 30 µg/dl. These experiments were run in a Lashley jumping-stand and, through food-reward, the animals learned to discriminate between different visual patterns, namely vertical vs horizontal stripes or large vs small discs. Whereas there was no lead-related performance-deficit for the easy task (orientation), there was a pronounced lead-related performance-deficit for the difficult size-discrimination. A similar performance-deficit in visual discrimination-learning has recently been demonstrated by our group at even lower blood lead-values of near 20 µg/dl (Winneke et al., 1982a).

Performance-deficits in the learning tasks used in animal models may come about by a disruption of several underlying processes including disturbances of associative-processes, of sensory functions, of memory-storage or of emotional-motivational conditions.

Learning ability as such, namely the ability to form and to retain stimulus-response-associations, does not seem to be impaired by lead in our animals, because the easy discrimination was learned equally quickly by both groups. It is still uncertain if visual functions are disturbed by lead at low blood lead-levels; according to findings from our laboratory they are not. Amplitudes of visual evoked potentials recorded from freely moving animals did not exhibit a decrement until blood lead levels were clearly in excess of 30 µg/dl (Winneke, 1979).

Some behavioural findings in lead-exposed rats are consistent with the hypothesis that lead may increase emotional reactivity. Increased locomotor activity in the novel surrounding of the open field has, for example, been demonstrated at blood leads between 20 and 30 µg/dl (Winneke et al., 1977; Schlipkoter and Winneke, 1980). These effects are more compatible with an interpretation in terms of lead-induced behavioural reactivity than with hyperactivity. If this interpretation is essentially correct, even lead-induced improvement should occur in suitable learning tasks, such as active avoidance-learning. This has in fact been shown to be so (Winneke et al., 1982a): With increasing lead-dose (0, 80, 250 and 750 ppm in the diet) the animals needed progressively fewer trials to reach the criterion of successful avoidance-learning. This finding demonstrates that learning-performance in animals being exposed to lead from early developmental stages to adulthood may either be disrupted, as in the difficult visual discrimination task, or even improved, as in the active avoidance-paradigm, depending upon the specific task requirements. In other words, an explanation of Pb-induced performance inhibition in learning-tasks in terms of an impairment of cognitive processes, e.g. learning-capacity or/and memory functions, is not convincing if the different findings from different learning-tasks are taken together. Lead-induced increase of reactivity of response disinhibition (Overman, 1977) would, indeed, be expected to be disruptive in attention-demanding, difficult discrimination learning, but facilitating in active avoidance-learning.

Although these findings from controlled animal-studies cannot be extrapolated to children in any quantitative manner, they agree largely with the symptom pattern observed in our epidemiological studies in children with elevated tooth lead-levels, and, in addition, support the hypothesis that these symptoms may be caused by long term low-level lead-exposure.

DISCUSSION

Russell Jones: As I understand it, you are suggesting that the
                   behavioural and attentional deficits found in your
                   population were caused (in part) by lead,
                   whereas probably the variations in verbal IQ were
                   not due to lead. Is that not a difficult position
                   to maintain?

Winneke: No. In the first place, it is important to
                   emphasise that the causal inference necessarily
                   relies on the pattern of cross-sectional
                   associations found in circumstances in which many
                   of the variables overlap and in which many
                   variables apart from lead are known to affect
                   intelligence and behaviour. These other variables
                   have to be taken into account in the analyses.
                   The conclusion that the lead-behaviour or lead-
                   intelligence association is likely to reflect a
                   causative influence stems from the demonstration
                   that the association remains even after controlling
                   statistically for the effects of the other con-
                   founding variables. It was an empirical finding
                   (and not any theoretical assumption of mine) that
                   that was so for some of the associations with
                   lead, but yet not with others. Secondly, it is
                   well known that both social and physical factors
                   often have differential effects on different
                   psychological functions. Moreover, the
                   differential pattern associated with biological
                   impairment tends to be rather different from that
                   associated with psychosocial disadvantage. As a
                   consequence, both our findings and the
                   inferences based on them are consistent with the
                   available knowledge.

Needleman: Would you comment on the social scale that you
                   used in your analysis, and on its derivation?

Winneke: We used two measures. First, we utilized a
                   socio-economic index that is widely employed in
                   Germany. That is based on a cumulative score
                   that takes account of the net income, education
                   and occupational status of the father. That index
                   did not correlate with lead exposure. So, if we
                   had relied on the index alone we would have
                   concluded that the decrease in verbal IQ was
                   related to lead and not to the social factors. But
                   then we took an additional step and created a
                   further index, based on observed correlations
                   with tooth lead that also took into account the
                   mother's occupational status, and the type of
                   school attended by the child. This second

composite index did show a significant correlation with lead exposure. Moreover, when the composite index score was taken into account, the verbal IQ no longer showed a significant association with lead exposure.

Needleman: I appreciate that the inclusion of the mother's occupational status was appropriate in order to provide a better control for non-lead familial factors likely to influence intelligence and behaviour. But, it seems to me that the inclusion of the child's school may have created a bias through a confusion of independent and dependent variables. The point is that insofar as schools exercise selection over the pupils they admit they are likely to do so on the basis of their behaviour and intelligence. If this occurs there is the likelihood that lead-induced changes in behaviour and cognition will be misleadingly 'removed' because the social index takes account of, not only school influences (which are appropriately included), but also variations in the child's pre-admission behaviour and attainments that influenced school selection. As a result are you not in danger of confusing effect with cause?

Winneke: I would not rule out that possibility completely but I do not think that it is likely. It would be difficult to investigate in my study because the IQ differences between schools were very much larger than those usually observed with the effects of lead exposure.

Needleman: But, it is the very existence of those large school differences that raises the problem. Insofar as they were present at the time of school entry and insofar as they were not accounted for by your family variables, they could have been due in part to the effects of lead that were the subject of your investigation. If you cannot determine whether that was so, you may have concealed a real effect of lead by inadvertently 'over-controlling' for other variables. If you had stayed with conventional methods of assessing socio-economic status for inclusion in your analysis of variance a lead effect would have been apparent.

Winneke: That is so, but I do not believe in convention! The possibility you raise is a real and important one but, of course, there is a parallel danger of 'under-controlling' for family variables. The point of including the child's school in the index was two-fold: firstly, to take account of family variables more adequately (as these, too, are likely to influence choice of school); and, secondly, to provide coverage for non-family school influences on the children's behaviour and attainments. In addition, it must be pointed out that school-attendance is highly correlated with the occupational status of the parents. Moreover, only 8 out of 115 children attended secondary schools so that there was very little opportunity for school selection to be influenced by the children's own characteristics. In only 2 out of those 8 cases was there discordant classification between parental occupation rating and the school rating.*

Bryce-Smith: Did you analysis treat the socio-hereditary factors and the tooth lead as wholly independent alternatives for the effects on IQ and other outcome measures?

Winneke: Clearly the two are not independent in that the socially disadvantaged do not have the resources to move into the cleaner areas of cities or of the countryside; as a result they suffer greater exposure to lead. Accordingly, in any statistical analyses it is necessary to take into account the social class-lead association. Of course, the results differ slightly according to the method by which that is done. If use is made of a model in which the effects of lead are entered into the analyses before controlling for social factors, there is a slight - but only slight - increase in the variance accounted for by lead (from about 0.5% to 2%).

Question: Western Germany has decreased the amount of lead in petrol. Is there any correlation between the lead levels of the children and the comparatively lower amount of lead in the petrol in Germany?

---

*   Following the Symposium, the findings have been re-analysed omitting school measures from the confounding variables. On this re-analysis the findings are virtually the same as in the chapter in this volume; in no case has it altered the significance or non-significance of any differences.

Winneke:

I am not aware of any such study using tooth lead as a marker of lead exposure. The lead reduction from 0.40 grams per litre to 0.15 grams per litre was introduced in 1976. It has been shown that this was followed by a dramatic reduction in air lead concentrations - to approximately 50% of what they were before at different measuring stations. To the best of my knowledge, there has been only one study (in Frankfurt) which has related these changes to blood lead.   The results were not as dramatic as those seen in the NHANES study, in that the reduction in blood lead (between 1 and 2 micrograms) was only about 10% of the original. However, the subjects in that study were adults, and did not include the critical child population.

Needleman:

I am disappointed to hear you say that, because I think that you are making the same kind of mistake as people who say that a 4 point difference in mean IQ is small. The shift of 10% in the Frankfurt mean blood lead constitutes a very important difference. It would lower substantially the proportion of people with blood lead levels over 30.

Winneke:

Yes, but it is considerably less than that evident in the NHANES study. I agree that 10% is a remarkable reduction but still it is much smaller than obtained in the United States.

Russell Jones:

When you were interviewed on BBC radio recently you were asked whether you felt that the evidence so far justified a further reduction in the lead level of German petrol. You replied that the evidence was not strong enough to justify further legislative action at the moment. On the basis of the NHANES study from America, would you revise that opinion at all?

Winneke:

I said that the German study should be prolonged to determine whether a further reduction would be obtained over a 3 to 5 year time span. If the trends demonstrated in the NHANES study are correct, then certainly I would revise my opinion. If the reduction of lead in petrol in the USA truly caused a 50% decrease in blood lead, then clearly that constitutes an effective measure that should be introduced.

Russell Jones:

Is the Frankfurt study still continuing?

Winneke: I don't know but I hope that it is.

Turner: On a point of information I understand that the
                  Frankfurt study has been continued and that a
                  further series of blood leads have been obtained
                  for many of the people who were in the original
                  series. The results have not yet been published.

Ward: With respect to the Frankfurt study, the findings
                  from my New Zealand study during the 1970s may
                  be relevant.   Sheep that
                  grazed on grass adjacent to a busy motorway had
                  lead levels considerably above those from a rural
                  area. Once those sheep were removed from the
                  motorway their blood lead levels fell dramatically,
                  but still they did not approach those seen in
                  their rural counterparts. Even after six months
                  there was a threefold difference in blood lead
                  between the two groups of sheep, although
                  presumably their lead intakes were then similar.
                  These findings suggest that a new equilibrium
                  between lead intake and blood lead is achieved
                  only slowly. The recycling of skeletal lead
                  deposits may delay equilibrium for a considerable
                  time after exposure has been lowered. This
                  observation is relevant to the Frankfurt studies.

Winneke: I agree that this study should be prolonged in
                  order to assess the long term reduction of lead in
                  the whole ecosystem. For this a two-year period
                  is certainly too short.

Barlett: Why were your tooth lead levels so much lower
                  than those in Needleman's American study?

Winneke: I am not really qualified to comment on that.
                  There are quite a number of imponderables here.
                  For example, Dr. Needleman used dentine lead
                  and we used whole tooth lead. The American
                  values may be higher because the children's
                  exposure was aggravated by lead paint which we
                  do not have in Germany (Needleman's association
                  between pica and blood lead suggests that
                  possibility). Our data agree very well with Dr.
                  Delves' data so I do not feel that it reflects the
                  type of analysis so much as the degree of
                  exposure. In comparing our studies we are
                  probably talking about different points on the
                  dose/effect curve.

Grandjean: Children of unskilled workers had the highest
                  tooth lead levels did they not? That suggests a
                  possible pathway that is not related to lead in

	petrol; namely, occupational exposure of the father in this little town with a primary lead smelter. In my country the highest levels in children were found in the children of workers with occupational lead exposures.
Winneke:	You are correct. The children of fathers who are occupationally exposed to lead clearly suffer excessive exposure themselves; nevertheless, in the total sample of unskilled workers in our study, only three or four were occupationally exposed.
Russell Jones:	In your animal studies, you found a dose dependent relationship between blood lead and the number of trials to attain criteria on a learning task. The dosage rates administered in the diet were 80, 250 and 750 ppm for your rats and these were producing blood lead levels of about 10, 20 and 30 μg/dl. Could you say how applicable that sort of experimentation is to the human situation?
Winneke:	Great care is needed in making quantitative extrapolations from rats to humans. Nevertheless the animal studies are important for two different reasons. Firstly, experimental studies in animals can determine whether there are cause/effect relationships. Secondly, animal studies are important in showing the patterns of effects. Biochemical measures constitute one crucial way of comparing results between rats and humans. As far as delta-amino-laevulinic acid dehydratase is concerned, 20 μg/dl in the rat corresponds to approximately 40 μg/dl in the child. But this comparison should be treated very carefully since the enzyme system of the rat is very different from that of the child.
Russell Jones:	I gather that urinary ALA starts going up in human subjects when blood lead levels are around 20 μg/dl. What is the equivalent level in the rat at which urinary ALA starts to rise?
Winneke:	We have not measured ALA in rats. Perhaps Ellen Silbergeld can provide an answer?
Silbergeld:	We have measured ALA, or rather Dr. Donals Chew's laboratory has measured these parameters for us, and in rats with blood lead levels in the high 20s and 30s there is a significant increase in ALA concentrations. But I would stress that, unlike the studies with humans, we were able to control diet.

Russell Jones: In effect, so far as ALA is concerned, is there
                    then equivalence between the human and animal
                    studies for the level at which ALA starts to rise?

Silbergeld: I think that it is very dangerous to try to attach
                    direct equivalents in terms of blood lead. There
                    are too many discontinuities in the data. I want
                    to repeat again that all of us who have worked
                    with animals would suggest that it is much better
                    to look at a spectrum of effects.

Winneke: I would agree, with one exception. In order to
                    bridge the gap between lower animals and man,
                    primate studies are relevant. The preliminary
                    results of a rhesus study by a collaborator of
                    mine are very interesting in this respect.
                    Although this experiment is not yet fully
                    completed the existing results indicate that a
                    deficit of visual discrimination learning may be
                    associated with blood lead levels around 30 µg/dl
                    in the rhesus monkey.

Edwards: Dr. Winneke said that the enzymes of a rat are
                    very different from man. I was a little surprised
                    at this. Could you elaborate on the differences -
                    it always struck me that the mammals were extra-
                    ordinarily uniform in their enzyme systems.

Silbergeld: As you probably know, in humans it has been
                    shown that there is a feedback system for the
                    control of haemsynthesis which involved the
                    expression of ALAD activity. This system does
                    not appear to be as active in rats. Obviously the
                    enzymes are the same, in fact they are producing
                    the same products and their basic functional
                    purpose is the same, but still there are signifi-
                    cant differences between the two systems in the
                    ways in which they work.

REFERENCES

Benton, A.L. (1974), 'Der Benton-Test', Handbuch, Deutsche
    Bearbeitung von O.Spreen, Huber Verlag, Bern-Stuttgart-Wien,
    4. Aufl.
Brockhaus, A., Jermann, E., and Freier, I., (1978), 'Bestimmung
    der Blutbleikonzentration bei Schulkindern aus funf unter-
    schiedlich belasteten Wohngebieten der Bundesrepublik',
    Arbeitstagung d. Ges.f.Hygiene u. Mikrobiol. am 02.-03.10.1978
    Vortrag in Mainz.
Conners, C.K. (1969), 'A teacher rating scale for use in drug
    studies with children', Am. J. Psychiatry 126, 884-888.
Ewers, U., Brockhaus, A., Genter, E., Idel, H., und Schurmann,
    E.A., (1979), 'Untersuchungen uber den Zahnbleigehalt von

Schulkindern aus zwei unterschiedlich belasteten Gebieten in Nordwestdeutschland', Int. Arch. Occup. Environ. Health 44, 65-80.

Ewers, U., Brockhaus, A., Winneke, G., Freier, I., Jermann, E., and Kramer, U. (1982), 'Lead in deciduous teeth of children living in a non-ferrous smelter area of West-Germany', Int. Arch. Occup. Environ. Health, 50, 139-151.

Hridina, K.G. (1978), 'Neurophysiologische Untersuchungen an Kindern mit erhohtem Zahnbleigehalt', Med. Diss. (Dusseldorf).

Klebelsberg, D. (1960), 'Wiener Determinationsgerat', Diagnostica VI.

Kleber, E.W., und Kleber, G. (1974), 'Differentieller Leistungstest-KE', Hogrefe-Verlag, Gottingen.

Needleman, H.L., Gunnoe, C., Leviton, A., Reed, R., Peresie, H., Maher, C., and Barrett, P. (1979), 'Deficits in psychologic and classroom performance of children with elevated dentine lead levels', N. Eng. J. Med., 300, 689-695.

Overmann, S.R., (1977), 'Behavioral effects of asymtomatic lead exposure during neonatal development in rats', Toxicol. appl. Pharmacol., 41, 459-471.

Schilling, F., und Kiphard, E.J. (1974), 'Korperkoordinationstest fur Kinder', KTK. Beltz-Verlag, Weinheim.

Schlange, H., Stein, B., Boettcher, J., und Taneli, S. (1972), 'Gottinger Formreproduktionstest (G-F-T)', Handbuch, Hogrefe, Gottingen.

Schlipkoter, H.W., and Winneke, G., (1980), 'Behavioral studies on the effects of lead in the developing central nervous system of rats', in Commission of the European Community (ed) Environment and the quality of life, 2nd environment research programme, ECSC-EEC-EAEC, Brussels-Luxembourg, pp. 127-134.

Weidlich, S. (1972), 'Diagnostikum fur Cerebralschadigung (DCS)', Handbuch, Huber-Verlag, Bern-Stuttgart-Wien.

Winneke, G. (1979a), 'Modification of visual evoked potentials in rats after longterm blood-lead elevation', Activ Nerv. Sup, 21, 282-284.

Winneke, G. (1979b), 'Neuropsychological studies in children with elevated tooth-lead levels', Paper presented at the symposium, Toxic effects of Environmental lead, London.

Winneke, G., Brockhaus, A., and Baltissen, R. (1977), 'Neurobehavioral and systemic effects of longterm blood lead-elevation in rats', Arch. Toxicol., 37, 247-263.

Winneke, G., Lilienthal, H., and Werner, W. (1982a), 'Task dependent neurobehavioral effects of lead in rats', Arch. Toxicol., Suppl. 5, 84-93.

Winneke, G., Hrdina, K.G., and Brockhaus, A. (1982b), 'Neuropsychological studies in children with elevated tooth lead-concentrations', Part I, Pilot study Int. Arch. Occup. Environ. Health, (in press).

Winneke, G., Kramer, U., Brockhaus, A., Ewers, U., Kujanek, G., Lechner, H., and Jahnke, W. (1982a), 'Neuropsychological studies in children with elevated tooth lead-concentrations', Part II, Extended study, Int. Arch. Occup. Environ. Health, (in press).

BLOOD LEAD, INTELLIGENCE, ATTAINMENT AND
BEHAVIOUR IN SCHOOL CHILDREN: OVERVIEW OF A
PILOT STUDY

Richard Lansdown,[1] William Yule,[2]
Marie-Anne Urbanowicz,[2] and Ian B. Millar[3]

1. Department of Psychological Medicine, The Hospital
    for Sick Children, Great Ormond Street, London,
    W.C.1.

2. Department of Psychology, University of London,
    Institute of Psychiatry, de Crespigny Park, London,
    SE5 8AF.

3. District Community Physician, Greenwich Health
    District, London.

INTRODUCTION

Our research had its origins during the meetings of the DHSS
Working Party on Lead in the Environment - the Lawther Committee
(DHSS, 1980) - of which the first two authors were members. The
Committee was acutely aware of the paucity of studies examining the
effects of lead on children in the general population. It concluded
that there was, at the time, no convincing evidence of deleterious
effects on children at blood lead concentrations below 35 µg/100 ml.
However, the Committee's report made it clear that its conclusions
were based on a lack of evidence rather than on firm evidence to
the contrary.

During its deliberations, the results of the 1979 European Economic
Community (EEC) surveys on blood lead were published. The EEC
surveys fulfilled the directive on biological screening of the
population for lead (Directive 77/312/EEC). Adults in major urban
areas, persons specifically exposed to lead and those at special risk
were screened, data being available on 39 groups in the United
Kingdom. The "persons specifically exposed" were mainly children
of leadworkers or children who lived near a leadworks, but also a
small number of children living near very busy roads were
included.

Strictly speaking, none of these constituted a random sample from
the general population. However, even though they had been
selected as being at risk of elevated exposure to lead, in 7 of the
19 samples of children, all children had lead levels below 31 µg/100
ml. In only two samples did more than 3% of the children have
blood lead levels greater than 35 µg/100 ml. In other words,

all samples consisted of children with comparatively low blood lead levels.

The Boston survey of tooth lead levels (Needleman et al, 1979) as the most extensive and systematic study available, was given particular attention by the Lawther Committee. Like them, we were impressed by the dose-response relationships between tooth-lead levels and teachers' ratings of children's behaviour. These were found across the total sample and at low levels of lead exposure. In our own work, therefore, it was decided to apply Needleman et al's (1979) teacher rating scale to children in one of the EEC survey samples. For ease of access, we selected a group living in the London area near a lead works.

METHOD

Full details of the sample and of our methodology are available elsewhere (Yule, Lansdown, Millar and Urbanowicz, 1981; Yule, Urbanowicz, Lansdown and Millar, 1982) and will not be repeated here. Suffice it to say that we successfully traced and tested 85% of the sample in the 6 to 12 year old age range. As Table 1 shows, the sample largely comprised children of skilled manual workers. Classification of occupation was based on information on fathers' occupations as coded by the Registrar General (1966).

TABLE 1. Social-class composition of sample

SOCIAL CLASS	NO.	%
I	3	1.8
II	11	6.6
III Non-manual	17	10.2
III Manual	77	46.4
IV	19	11.4
V	2	1.2
Single parent	12	7.2
Unemployed	2	1.2
Not Known	23	13.9
TOTAL	166	

Blood samples had been taken by venepuncture and analysed in the Department of Chemical Pathology and Human Metabolism, University of Southampton, under the direction of Professor Clayton and Dr. Trevor Delves. As Table 2 shows, the blood lead concentrations formed a lognormal distribution, as expected for measures of natural phenomena in which there is a fixed lower and open-ended upper limit. The overall distribution of lead levels conformed with

that prescribed in the EEC directive. Only two children had levels
above 30 μg/100 ml. One of these had a level of 60 μg/100 ml,
which was found to be associated with the ingestion of paint. As
she had been chelated prior to the study, the results from this
little girl were omitted from the findings. Otherwise, as can be
seen in Table 2, the range of blood level concentrations was from 7
to 32 μg/100 ml, with an arithmetic mean of 13.52 μg/100 ml. Half
the sample had blood leads below 13 μg/100 ml.

TABLE 2. Distribution of blood lead levels
classified into quartiles

μg/100 ml	No.	%	GROUP	NO.	%
7	6	3.6			
8	6	3.6			
9	12	7.2			
10	10	6.0	1	34	20.4
11	22	13.3			
12	26	15.7	2	48	29.0
13	13	7.8			
14	11	6.6			
15	17	10.2			
16	8	4.8	3	49	29.4
17	11	6.6			
18	6	3.6			
19	8	4.8			
20	2	1.2			
21	1	0.6			
22	1	0.6			
24	2	1.2			
25	1	0.6			
26	2	1.2			
32	1	0.6	4	35	21.0

Mean Pb = 13.52 μg/100 ml (SD 4.13)

The tests (listed in Table 3) were selected to be similar to those
used in previous studies (Lansdown et al, 1974; Needleman et al,
1979). General intelligence was assessed on the Wechsler Intelligence   Scale   for   Children   (Revised)   (Wechsler,   1974);   and
educational attainment on well standarised tests of reading (Neale
1958), spelling (Vernon, 1977) and mathematics (Vernon and Miller,
1976).   The intelligence and reading tests were administered
individually; the spelling and mathematics tests were administered to
small   groups.   All   testing   was   undertaken   by   clinical   and
educational psychologists trained and experienced in the assessment
of children. The psychologists were kept unaware of the children's
blood lead levels.

TABLE 3. The test battery

Educational Attainment

Neale Reading - Comprehension Accuracy
Vernon Spelling
Vernon Mathematics

Intelligence

WISC-R - Verbal Scale IQ
Performance Scale IQ
Full Scale IQ

Behaviour Ratings

Needleman Questionnaire
Rutter B(2)
Conners Scale

Teachers were asked to complete three behaviour rating scales on each child. Firstly, there was the 11-item forced-choice scale used by Needleman et al (1979). Secondly, we used the 26-item Teacher Rating Scale B2 (Rutter and Yule, 1968). Thirdly, we used the 40-item Conners (1969) scale. The B2 scale is a screening instrument and high scores are known to be reasonable indicators of behavioural and emotional difficulties (Rutter, 1967; Rutter, Tizard and Whitmore, 1970; Rutter, Graham, Chadwick and Yule, 1976; Rutter, Cox, Tupling, Berger and Yule, 1975). This questionnaire, then, tapped more general areas of disturbance than those apparently measured by the Needleman et al (1979) scale. The Conners scale was included because it has been widely used in the study of hyperactivity, particularly in relation to treatment by drugs (Conners, 1969; Sandberg, Rutter and Taylor, 1978). With all these scales, we hoped to examine the claims that increasing lead levels were related to increasing levels of activity and other behavioural problems.

Testing and behavioural ratings were completed in the summer term of 1980, some 9 to 12 months after the blood samples had been taken.

RESULTS

a) Intellectual and Educational Attainment

As shown in Table 4, it is apparent that this sample was well within the normal range of educational attainment and intelligence. The children were reading at age level and there was no indication that the sample was in any way deviant.

TABLE 4. Means and standard deviations on criterion
(attainment) measures

Variable	No.	Mean	SD
Chronological age (mths)	166	102.44	21.70
Reading : Accuracy (mths)	164	102.88	23.68
Comprehension (mths)	164	101.87	24.79
Spelling (standard score)	162	94.24	14.81
Mathematics	161	94.38	13.29
WISC-R: Verbal IQ	166	96.75	14.24
Performance IQ	166	100.25	13.44
Full-scale IQ	166	98.21	13.44

The question of interest was whether, within this essentially normal
sample (both in terms of blood lead distributions and educational
attainments) there was any relationship between lead level and the
outcome measures. The matter may be tackled by means of several
different statistical techniques. Full details are contained in our
earlier paper (Yule et al, 1981). Here one set of analyses is
presented to illustrate the findings.

The children were divided into four quartiles according to their
blood lead levels. There are reservations about this procedure in
that the band width of the quartiles was roughly equivalent to the
standard error of estimate of the blood lead measure, namely 2 μg.
However, since other statistical techniques produced essentially
similar results, this objection has less force than it might otherwise
have had.

A central problem in the analysis and interpretation of the
associations between lead levels and psychological impairment
concerns the role of social factors. This was explicitly recognised
by Needleman et al (1979) in their Boston study (see also chapter
12), and the same issues arose with our data. As Annest and
Billick report (chapters 3 and 4), all studies have shown that
children of lower socio-economic status tend to have higher lead
levels than those from a more privileged background. The problem
stems from the fact that both social class and level leads are
associated with differences in psychological performance. In other
words, all three sets of variables are inter-linked. The question
then arises as to what mechanisms or casual processes underlie this
three-way pattern of associations. Various competing alternative
explanations have to be considered (chapter 1); multivariate
statistical analyses were originally developed for just that purpose -
to investigate associations when the possibly causal variables are
not independent of one another. It is important to emphasize that
attempts to unravel this complex set of interactions are not part of
a plot to deny the possibility of a causal relationship between lead

and adverse development, as some commentators have argued
(Jones, 1982; Rogers, 1982). Rather, they constitute essential
basic steps in which the findings are likely to have important social
policy implications. Unless we fully understand the extent, nature
and direction of these relationships, we will not be in a position to
take the most effective actions. For example, one issue is whether
there is an interaction between social factors and lead exposure
such that disadvantaged children are most likely to suffer
psychological impairment as a result of raised body lead burdens -
a question for which multivariate analyses were particularly
designed.

Table 5 shows that there was, indeed, a strong association between
social class and blood lead levels with higher levels in those from
lower socio-economic backgrounds. It was essential to control
statistically for this. This was done by means of analysis of
covariance to partial out the effect of social class (see Table 6).
This table illustrates the trend of the results and is not, in itself,
definitive. For example, also there were close relationships between
age and blood lead levels - younger children having high lead
levels. This was not taken into account in Table 6, but when age
was controlled statistically, essentially the same effects remained.

TABLE 5. Analysis of variance: lead x social class

Social Class	No.	Mean	SD	F	P
I + II	14	12.07	3.17	3.19	0.0153
III Non-manual	17	11.94	2.82		
III Manual	77	13.47	4.24		
IV + V	21	16.10	4.83		
Single parents	12	13.17	3.97		
TOTAL	141	13.51			

N.B. The results are presented here in terms of observed blood
lead values ($\mu g/dl$). Strictly speaking, the log values should be
used, and when the ANOVA is performed using Log Pb, F = 3.18,
p = 0.0155. Therefore the untransformed values are presented as
being more readily understandable.

Table 6 shows a number of important findings. Firstly, reading
and spelling scores were significantly lower in the children with
higher blood lead levels. Secondly mathematics scores did not vary
according to blood lead levels. Thirdly, the differences between
blood lead groups in IQ (particularly verbal IQ) remained statistically significant, even after social class was controlled. The
difference amounted to some 7 IQ points between the 'lowest' and
'highest' lead groupings.

TABLE 6

Summary Analyses of Covariance – Social Class Partialled Out.

Pb Group	Accuracy (adj. mean)	Comprehension (Adj. mean)	Spelling (Adj. mean)	Mathematics (Adj. mean)	Verbal IQ (Adj. mean)	Performance IQ (Adj. mean)	Full-scale IQ (Adj. mean)
1 Low	121.36	117.17	104.41	96.78	101.48	105.09	103.32
2	109.69	110.32	97.69	97.18	101.48	103.43	102.68
3	98.48	95.07	92.01	95.44	94.69	97.90	95.75
4 High	89.23	87.79	89.19	94.54	93.93	98.80	95.70
Social Class	NS	$p = 0.095$	$p = 0.060$	$p = 0.013$	$p = 0.009$	NS	$p = 0.029$
Pb	$p = 0.001$	$p = 0.001$	$p = 0.001$	NS	$p = 0.043$	$p = 0.102$	$p = 0.027$

Looked at another way, we found a correlation of -0.26 between
$\log_e$ Blood Leads and Full Scale IQ. This reduced to -0.21 after
the effects of age, sex and social class were all partialled out.
This correlation is statistically significant at the 0.05 level, but it
means that only $4\frac{1}{2}\%$ of the variance in intelligence scores is shared
with blood lead levels independent of these other factors. The
interpretation of these results is discussed below.

(b) Teachers' Ratings of Behaviour. The Lawther Committee
concluded that "... up to the present no study has satisfactorily
demonstrated a relationship between increasing body lead burden
and either educational attainment or hyperactivity. Measuring
subtle effects requires sophisticated techniques and these have not
so far been employed. There are far fewer data on all aspects of
behaviour and adjustment other than intelligence" (Department of
Health and Social Security, 1980). However, we had been
impressed with Needleman et al's (1979) findings of dose-response
relationships between tooth lead estimates and teachers' ratings of
behaviour. Those findings are shown graphically in chapter 12 (p
-).

It is psychometrically surprising that a non-standard, forced-choice
rating scale should appear to work so well. To date, there are no
published data on the derivation of the scale, its reliability or
validity (although the new data reported by Needleman in this
volume do attest to its reliability). Needleman et al (1979) found
that the proportion of negative teacher ratings increased parallel
with tooth lead levels on the following items: distractable, not
persistent, dependent, not organized, frustrated, day dreamer,
unable to follow sequence of directions, and low overall functioning.
No such linear relationships were obvious on the remaining three
items: hyperactive, impulsive, unable to follow simple directions.

These were challenging findings that needed to be checked in a
British sample. Since we wanted to know more about what the scale
might be measuring, we decided to use in addition the two other
rating scales described above.

Figure 1 and Table 7 show the findings on the Needleman et al
questionnaire in our London sample. The group was split into four
quartiles according to lead level - the numbers were too small to
divide into six groups as Needleman had done. Allowing for that
difference, it can be seen that the pattern of our results was very
similar to his. In 5 of the 11 items - Impulsive, Day Dreamer,
Does not follow Simple Directions, Does not Follow Sequence of
Directions and Low Overall Functioning - the associations between
blood lead level and behaviour rating were statistically significant
(see Table 7 for details). In a further 4 items - Distractable, Not
Persistent, Dependent and Disorganized - it seems that children
with blood lead levels of 12 µg/100 ml and below receive fewer
negative ratings than those above this median level. As in
Needleman's study, Hyperactivity was noted in very few children
and was not associated with blood lead level.

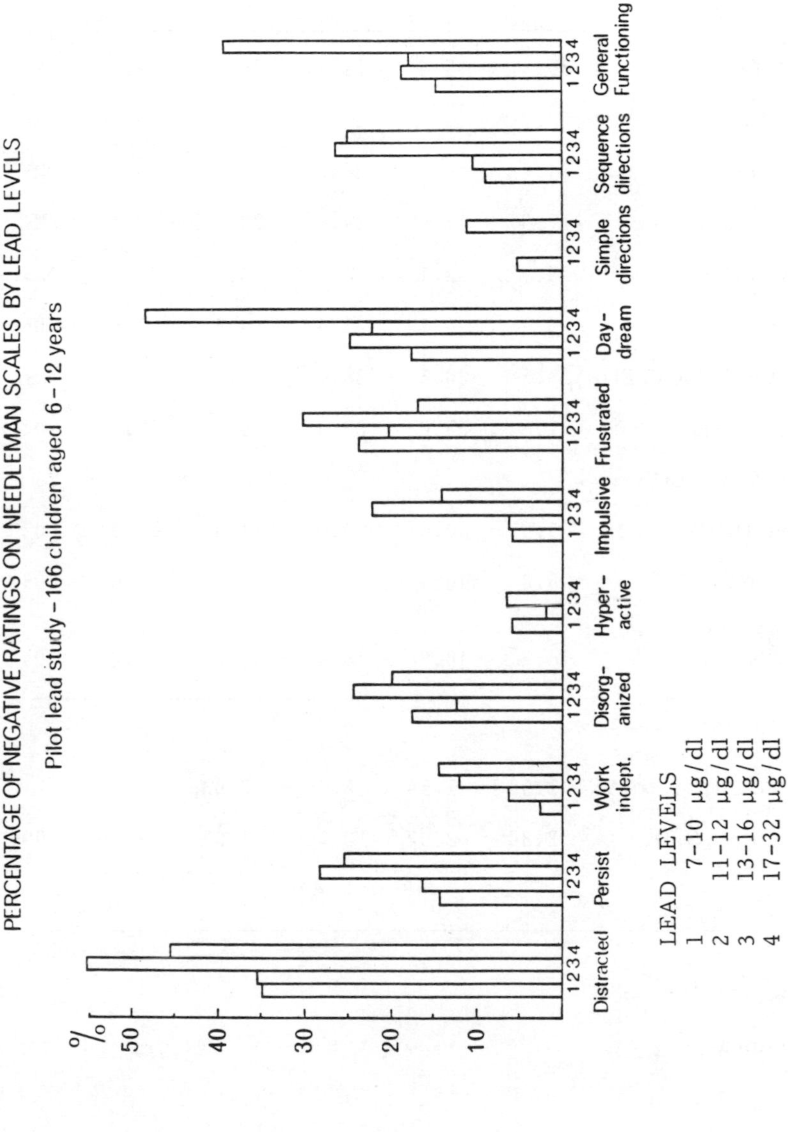

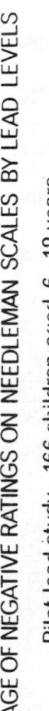

PERCENTAGE OF NEGATIVE RATINGS ON NEEDLEMAN SCALES BY LEAD LEVELS

Pilot lead study – 166 children aged 6–12 years

LEAD LEVELS
1   7–10 μg/dl
2   11–12 μg/dl
3   13–16 μg/dl
4   17–32 μg/dl

Fig. 1.   Percentage of negative ratings on Needleman scales by lead levels
Pilot lead study – 166 children aged 6–12 years.

TABLE 7.   % children receiving negative rating on Needleman
scales

ITEM	BLOOD LEAD LEVEL (μg/dl)					
	7-10	11-12	13-16	17-32	X^2	P
DISTRACTABLE	35.3	35.4	53.1	45.7	4.1	NS
NOT PERSISTENT	2.9	6.3	12.2	14.3	3.8	NS
DEPENDENT	14.7	16.7	28.6	25.7	3.4	NS
DISORGANISED	17.6	12.5	24.5	20.0	2.4	NS
HYPERACTIVE	5.9	2.1	6.1	0.0	3.0	NS
IMPULSIVE	5.9	6.3	22.4	14.3	7.5	.06
EASILY FRUSTRATED	23.5	20.8	36.6	17.1	2.4	NS
DAY DREAMER	17.6	25.0	22.4	48.6	10.2	.02[+]
DOES NOT FOLLOW -						
SIMPLE DIRECTION	5.9	0.0	0.0	11.4	10.3	.02[⌀]
SEQUENCE OF "	8.8	10.4	26.5	25.7	7.6	.05[+]
LOW OVERALL FUNCTIONING	14.7	18.8	18.4	40.0	8.2	.04[+]
					F	P
TOTAL SCORE : MEAN	1.53	1.54	2.45	2.63		
S.D.	2.34	2.02	2.70	3.01	2.15	.096
No.	34	48	49	35		

+ = linear

⌀ = non-linear

The total scores on the Needleman et al questionnaires differ across the four blood lead groupings at a level which is not statistically significant (F = 2.15, P = 0.096). There was, however, a trend for the total scores to increase with increasing lead levels with, again, the greatest difference occurring at the 12 µg/100 ml cut-off point.

Overall, it appears that the level of negative ratings in the Boston sample differed somewhat from this outer London sample. More London children were rated as distractible; fewer as persistent; fewer as hyperactive; more as easily frustrated. It is impossible yet to say whether this reflects differences in teacher usage, differences in ages of the two samples, or real differences in behaviour.

Before considering the validity of these findings further, it must be emphasized that, as in Needleman's study, these results were not controlled for social class.

Table 8 shows the results from the Rutter B(2) Teacher Rating Scale. When the children in the top 50% of the lead distribution were compared with the remainder, the higher PbB group were more often deviant on 20 of the 26 items. For only two items – "Squirming" and "Fights" – was this difference statistically significant at the 5% level; in 5 others the difference was significant at the 5 to 10% level – "Sucks Thumb", "Bites Nails", "Inert", "Disobedient" and "Truants". Truancy was more frequent in children with lower blood lead levels but the other behaviours were associated with higher lead levels. The increase in thumb sucking and nail biting in the higher lead group is of interest in so far as it indicates one behavioural mechanism whereby increased lead can get into the body. Overall, however, the associations with individual items were small. This probably indicates that only a small proportion of the variance of behavioural deviance and lead levels is shared and that larger sample numbers will be needed to understand more fully the nature of the association.

Recently a factor analysis of the B(2) scale (Schachar, Rutter and Smith, 1981) showed a separate "overactivity" factor, defined by summating scores on the following three items – "Restless", "Squirming" and "Can't settle". Children were operationally classified as "overactive" if their score was 3 or more on these items. Children with lead levels below 13 µg/100 ml had lower mean activity scores than did those with higher lead levels (see table 9).

TABLE 8. B-Scale (O 1,2) x PB (7 - 12 v 13 - 32),
        % "deviant" at 2 Blood Lead Levels

	Item	Blood Lead Level		X^2	P
		7 - 12 %	13 - 32 %		
1.	RESTLESS	26.8	33.3	0.55	NS
2.	TRUANTS	6.1	0	3.4	0.07
3.	SQUIRMY	13.4	32.1	7.21	0.007**
4.	DESTROYS	3.7	9.5	1.46	NS
5.	FIGHTS	6.1	20.2	6.04	0.014*
6.	NOT LIKED	11.0	16.7	0.70	NS
7.	WORRIED	30.5	35.7	0.30	NS
8.	SOLITARY	19.5	26.2	0.70	NS
9.	IRRITABLE	8.5	15.5	1.29	NS
10.	MISERABLE	17.1	16.7	0.02	NS
11.	TWITCHES	6.1	9.5	0.28	NS
12.	SUCKS THUMB	1.2	8.3	3.16	0.08
13.	BITES NAILS	3.7	11.9	2.85	0.09
14.	ABSENT	14.6	13.1	0.00	NS
15.	DISOBEDIENT	9.8	21.4	3.44	0.06
16.	CAN'T SETTLE	14.6	25.0	2.19	NS
17.	FEARFUL	28.0	35.7	0.80	NS
18.	FUSSY	17.1	15.5	0.00	NS
19.	LIES	8.5	16.7	1.80	NS
20.	STEALS	1.2	6.0	1.48	NS
21.	INERT	9.8	20.2	2.79	0.09
22.	ACHES	13.4	10.7	0.09	NS
23.	TEARS	11.0	4.8	1.44	NS
24.	STUTTERS	6.1	9.5	0.28	NS
25.	RESENTFUL	11.0	15.5	0.39	NS
26.	BULLIES	8.5	14.3	0.84	NS

P Values

 * = <0.05

** = <0.01

TABLE 9

B(2) overactivity scale and blood lead
levels

(a)   Analysis of Variance

PB Group	OVERACTIVITY SCORE			
	Mean	S.D.	F	P
7 - 11	0.68	1.32	2.15	0.096
11 - 12	0.58	0.94		
13 - 16	1.27	1.83		
17 - 32	0.91	1.38		

- - - - - - - - - - - -

(b)   Chi² analysis - Children categorised as "overactive" if
score on 3 items is 3 or over.

PB Group	OVERACTIVITY SCORE	
	0 - 2	3 - 6
7 - 11	32(94.1%)	2 (5.9%)
11 - 12	46(95.8%)	2 (4.2%)
13 - 16	39(79.6%)	10(20.4%)
17 - 32	29(82.9%)	6 (17.1%)

Chi² = 8.12, 3df, P = 0.04

(c)   Analysis using a 12 µgm/dl cut-off

PB Group	OVERACTIVITY SCORE		
0 - 2	3 - 6		
12 or less	78	4 (4.1%)	82
13 or more	68	16(19.0%)	84

166

The difference was not statistically significant when the data were
analysed by Analysis of Variance (P = 0.096). However, a
non-parametric chi-square analysis is more appropriately applied to
categorical data such as those 4.9% of children below the median
lead level compared with 19.0% above the median were classified as
"overactive". This difference was statistically significant (P =
0.04).

A similar picture emerged from the results of the Conner's Questionnaire - few individual items related significantly to blood lead levels, although there were many trends for greater behavioural deviance to be associated with higher lead levels. The scale has been shown by factor analysis to yield a number of sub-scales which have been replicated several times (Conners, 1969; Taylor and Sandberg, 1982; Thorley, 1982). Table 10 summarizes the results of five one-way analyses of variance in which the children have been divided at the median score into low and high blood lead groups. As can be seen, on every sub-scale the children with higher blood lead values were rated as more deviant; this reached statistical significance with Conduct Problems, Inattentive-Passive and Hyperactivity. These differences remained when chronological age was controlled by analysis of covariance.

TABLE 10. Lead level and Conner's factor
scores summaries of analyses
of variance and covariance

FACTOR	N	Mean	SD	F	P	Controlling for Age F	P
1. Conduct Problems							
7 - 12 µg/dl	82	0.04	0.26	4.21	0.04	4.02	0.05
13 - 32 µg/dl	84	0.15	0.40				
2. Inattentive-Passive							
7 - 12 µg/dl	82	0.41	0.56	5.16	0.02	5.68	0.02
13 - 32 µg/dl	84	0.62	0.64				
3. Tension-Anxiety							
7 - 12 µg/dl	82	0.38	0.34	0.18	0.67	0.52	0.47
13 - 32 µg/dl	84	0.41	0.46				
4. Hyperactivity							
7 - 12 µg/dl	82	0.27	0.41	4.50	0.04	5.88	0.02
13 - 32 µg/dl	84	0.44	0.61				
5. Total Score							
7 - 12 µg/dl	82	0.26	0.28	4.22	0.04	4.97	0.03
13 - 32 µg/dl	84	0.37	0.39				

Taylor and Sandberg (1982) subjected their London data on 6 to 9 year olds to factor analysis and derived a more complex factor-score loading on "hyperactivity". Applying this derived score to our 6 to 9 year olds only (see table 11) we again found that children above the median blood lead level were significantly more hyperactive than those below (p = 0.03).

TABLE 11. Taylor/Sandberg hyperactivity score

6 - 9 year olds only

BLOOD LEAD LEVEL	No	MEAN	S.D.	F	P
7 - 12 µg/dl	40	-2.68	2.60		
				4.69	0.03
13 - 32 µg/dl	65	-1.36	3.30		

↑ negative because our data had
uniformly lower mean scores on all
items.

Similarities Across the Behaviour Rating Scales. Findings on
individual items should be treated with caution for two reasons.
Firstly, the shorter the scale, the less reliable it is, and one
cannot get a shorter scale than a single item. Summated scores or
factor scores are always more reliable than individual items.
Secondly, with so many individual items being examined, some
differences are bound to arise by chance. Over all the three
teacher rating scales, 77 individual items were rated. By chance
alone, 4 can be expected to be "significant" at the 5% level of which
2 would be in the predicted direction. In fact, 7 items were found
to be significantly related to lead level. This might be regarded as
indicating only chance levels of associations but for two features:-
firstly, 4 of the 7 items were on the much shorter Needleman scale,
secondly, the results on the Needleman scale broadly replicate the
earlier study. Therefore, it is important to examine the present
data further to try to explain why the one scale should apparently
be sensitive to lead level and why activity ratings on the other two
scales should also relate to lead level.

Table 12 examines the relationship between adverse ratings on each
individual item on the Needleman scale with the overall scores on
the Rutter B(2) scale. As can be seen, there were significant
associations on 9 of the 11 items - the two exceptions being
"hyperactivity" and "does not follow single directions". This
indicates that, in general terms, the two scales were measuring
broadly similar child behaviours.

Our data allowed us to examine the concurrent validity of the
Needleman scale. Table 13 summarizes relationships with age, sex,
social class and WISC-R Full Scale IQ. Unlike the B(2) scale, the
Needleman items showed no age loading and only one sex difference,
on the item "Distractable" on which boys were more frequently
rated as distractable. The scale resembled the B(2) scale in
displaying only two significant associations with social class:
children from working class backgrounds were more likely to be
rated as distractable or lacking in persistence.

TABLE 12. Relationship between
Needleman items and B(2)
total score

% scoring negative ratings on needleman

ITEM	NON-DEVIANT 0 - 8 (N=135) %	DEVIANT 9+ (N=31) %	Chi²	P
DISTRACTABLE	32.6	87.1	28.4	.001
NOT PERSISTENT	5.2	25.8	10.7	.01
DEPENDENT	12.6	61.3	32.4	.001
DISORGANISED	13.3	41.9	11.8	.001
HYPERACTIVE	2.2	9.7	2.2	NS
IMPULSIVE	5.9	41.9	26.4	.001
EASILY FRUSTRATED	14.8	61.3	27.8	.001
DAY DREAMER	22.2	51.6	9.5	.01
DOES NOT FOLLOW -				
SIMPLE DIRECTIONS	2.2	9.7	2.2	NS
SEQUENCE OF				
DIRECTIONS	12.6	41.9	12.7	.001
LOW OVERALL				
FUNCTIONING	14.1	58.1	25.7	.001

With respect to Full Scale IQ, 9 of the 11 items showed significant
relationships with intelligence – the two exceptions being
"Hyperactive" and "Day Dreams". In all other cases, more deviant
ratings were given to children with lower IQs. Clearly, this
overlapping relationship between lead level, IQ and behaviour rating
must be examined more fully on a larger sample size than available
at present.

TABLE 13.   Concurrent validity of the
Needleman teacher rating scale

ITEM	SIGNIFICANCE (P) OF RELATIONSHIP (X^2) WITH			
	AGE	SEX	SOCIAL CLASS	FS IQ
DISTRACTABLE	NS	.04*	.01*	.006**
NOT PERSISTENT	NS	NS	.03*	.001***
DEPENDENT	NS	NS	.11	.001***
DISORGANISED	NS	NS	.23	.04*
HYPERACTIVE	NS	NS	.10	.36
IMPULSIVE	NS	NS	.22	.02*
EASILY FRUSTRATED	NS	NS	.37	.003**
DAY DREAMER	NS	NS	.19	.41
DOES NOT FOLLOW –				
SIMPLE DIRECTIONS	NS	NS	.84	.001***
SEQUENCE OF DIRECTIONS	NS	NS	.28	.001***
LOW OVERALL FUNCTIONING	NS	NS	.35	.001***

P Values

  * = <0.05

 ** = <0.01

*** = <0.001

From the similarities and differences in content between the three scales, it would appear that whilst the Needleman items broadly reflect the behaviours covered by the two other scales, also they are more specific in their apparent focus on an ability to focus attention in a relatively structured classroom learning situation.

DISCUSSION

Although we gathered many data on 166 children, our investigation constituted only a pilot study to examine the use of the Needleman teacher· questionnaire in relation to blood lead levels in a British sample.   From the outset, we were aware that we could get only one datum – father's occupation – as an index of social factors, a serious weakness indeed.   Furthermore, we relied on a single estimate of blood lead level taken some 9 to 12 months prior to psychological testing as our index of body lead burden.   Despite these obvious weaknesses what can be concluded from our results and how can the results lead on to better designed studies?

Intelligence and Educational Attainment. The results on the WISC-R
are broadly keeping with other recent studies (Needleman et al,
1979; Hrdina and Winneke, 1978; DHSS, 1980; Rutter 1980). There
was a tendency for the effect to be greater on verbal than on
non-verbal tasks. Not all previous studies have found such a
relationship and it is possible that any relationship between body
lead burden and intelligence is not linear across the range. This
study found a significant relationship within a predominantly
working class sample at blood lead levels much lower than
previously reported (Lansdown et al, 1974; Needleman et al, 1979).
Whether the effect is stronger within working class samples (as a
closer examination of our data suggests) or whether there is a
threshold effect at comparatively low lead levels, or more likely,
whether there is a complex interaction among all these variables
remains to be examined in larger studies.

We noted that less than 5% of the variance in intelligence was
shared with lead. To some readers, this may appear to be a trivial
amount. However, intelligence has long been recognized as being
multifactorially determined and to be able to identify even 5% of the
variance reliably would be an important advance. Had the
association been much stronger, then it would surely have been
found in many more previous studies. Some support for our
findings comes from Otto et al which reports a correlation of +0.20
between blood lead levels and developmental quotients in pre-school
children.

Another way of considering the potential importance of a 5 to 7
point difference in IQ between the lower and the higher lead groups
is to consider the effects in population terms. If, and it is a big
'if', lead is causally related to a lowering in IQ and if it has similar
effects at all IQ levels, then it can easily be demonstrated from the
properties of the normal curve of distribution of intelligence that a
5 point lowering in IQ would be associated with a doubling of the
numbers of children with IQs below 70. This effect has been
demonstrated empirically by Needleman, Leviton and Bellinger
(1982). In their Boston data, their high lead group contained 15%
of the children with a Verbal IQ below 80 compared with 5% in the
low lead group. No child in the elevated lead group scored a
Verbal IQ above 125 whereas 5% of the low lead group did so. In
other words, whilst any one individual child's IQ score may
fluctuate over time, nonetheless, the implications of a 5 point
difference between groups are very considerable.

On the three verbal measures of educational attainment, the higher
lead groups were again placed at a disadvantage. The effect
remained after partialling out age, sex and social class. Thus, it
could appear that the IQ effect is indeed being generalized with a
resulting interference with scholastic progress. However, the
scores on the mathematics tests did not follow the same pattern.

This was an unexpected finding. No one has previously reported
on academic attainment in such detail. There is no way from one

study to be certain that this is a real finding or a chance result peculiar to this set of data. However, the failure of the mathematics score to relate to lead is internally consistent with the lack of relationship with the Arithmetic sub-test on the WISC-R – an effect also to be found in Needleman et al's (1979) data. If it turns out to be true that lead levels differentially affect verbal/language scores as compared with mathematics scores, this could provide clues as to the seat of action of lead within the central nervous system – but that requires many further studies.

BEHAVIOUR

Our findings on behaviour broadly replicate the findings of Needleman et al (1979). On the same items, there are indications of a dose-response relationship between increasing lead levels and an increased likelihood that teachers' record deviant behaviour. Nevertheless, a number of differences between the studies must be noted. Firstly, Needleman's scale was, of course, used with American teachers and had not previously been used in Britain. However, it does appear that it is being used in a similar way. Secondly, the present study has smaller numbers and a wider age range of children. Thirdly, the estimate of body lead burden came from a single determination of blood lead level taken some nine months prior to the teachers ratings of behaviour. With these differences in mind, the similarity to Needleman's findings is all the more impressive.

The results on the factor scores derived from both the Rutter B(2) scale and the Conner's scale provide harder evidence for an association between increasing blood lead levels and increasing ratings of hyperactivity by teachers. It must be remembered that this is an association within an essentially normal sample of children. Previous studies of hyperactivity and lead levels (Baloh et al, 1975; David et al 1972, 1976, 1977) have been with very deviant groups of children.

More recently, David, Hoffman and Kagan (1979) report on the relationship between lead levels and Conner's score in a sample of 428 children attending an out patient clinic. The children were predominantly black from poor homes in an inner city. The data are presented in correlational form with correlations of 0.09 to 0.15 between lead levels at overactivity. Because of the large numbers, the correlations were statistically significant. Unfortunately, the data as reported do not allow us to compare the strength of the effects in the two studies.

Ernhart, Landa and Schell (1981) used the Conner's scale with 62 black children whose blood leads were assessed at two points in time separated by 5 years. They failed to find relationships with either lead level and any of the Conner's factor scores. Unfortunately, they do not report the scores obtained so its uncertain whether small differences failed to reach statistical significance because of their relatively small sample size.

Thus, we would claim that with our broad replication of Needleman et al(1979) findings, and their extension to the association between lead levels and activity levels measured on the Rutter and Conner's scales, we have provided harder evidence of an association between increasing lead levels and an interference with focussed attention and socially modulated activity. We emphasise that because of our small numbers, because the metric properties of the measures and because of our limited information on social factors, we have not, at this point, attempted to partial out the effects of social class or intelligence.

OUR FURTHER STUDIES

Each of the authors is engaged in a number of other studies concerned with lead. Each study has been designed to examine different problems, but, wherever possible, all studies have used similar methodologies and measures so that results can be compared across the studies.

Together with colleagues in the Institute of Child Health in London and the University of Southampton, Lansdown has undertaken a study of some 450 children. The main index of body lead burden was tooth lead, but in addition blood lead was estimated on some children. In this study, a large semi-structured interview was developed to investigate in detail a wide range of social factors and other potentially confounding variables. The study is financed by the British Government's Department of the Environment.

All four authors have recently completed the data collection on a second London sample. In addition to the measures detailed in this paper, we used the social interview developed by the Institute of Child Health group. Further, we assessed the intelligence of both parents and had parents complete parental versions of the behaviour scales. Finally, the estimation of blood lead levels was repeated after the psychological battery was completed. This extra information will allow us to examine confounding variables in considerably greater detail. If activity level is associated with lead level, we would expect that "pervasive overactivity" (Schachar, Rutter and Smith, 1981) should be clearly related to blood lead estimates. Finally, we hope that the repeat blood levels would allow for more stable estimates of body lead burden.

Lansdown, Yule, and Urbanowicz are now well through a study of a further 350 children in another British city. In addition to the refinements described in our second London study, we will have access to even better, more detailed measures of environmental exposure to lead. This should allow for a fuller examination of potential pathways whereby lead gets into children. If we can demonstrate differential relationships between lead level and development according to differential environmental exposure indices, we will have moved some way from examining correlations towards understanding the causal relationships between lead and development.

DISENTANGLING CONFOUNDING VARIABLES

Cross sectional research of the sort reported here - which is similar to most studies examining the relationship between lead and children's development - is bedevilled by the need to distinguish between correlation and causation. That there are correlations between low levels of body lead burden and a variety of indices of development is no longer seriously disputed. What is still far from certain is the nature of this relationship and, in particular, whether there is a simple (or even complex) <u>causal</u> relationship in which increasing lead levels <u>cause</u> poorer performances on tests. How can these important questions be resolved?

Within cross-sectional studies, one can attempt statistically to control for confounding variables. We have done this using analyses of covariance, partial correlations and step-wise regression analyses. In our data, these different techniques converged in showing closely similar results. However, they need not have done so. It is important to realize that each different statistical technique makes different assumptions about the nature of the data and the possible ways they might inter-relate.

In an analyses of variance, the children have to be categorized into groups according to their lead level. In the other statistical techniques, lead can be treated as a continuous variable and more information is utilized. However, social class has to be treated differently. Social class is essentially an ordinal scale, but not an interval one. That is, we know that a job rated as Social Class I carries more prestige than one rated as Social Class II and that one rated SC IV is more prestigious than one classified as SC V but we do not know whether the difference between SC I and SC II is the same as the difference between SC IV and SC V. When numbers are attached to labels it can sound scientific, but when the jobs are inserted, how much sense does it make to ask whether the difference between a judge and a school-teacher is the same as the difference between a milkman and a labourer? And yet, the <u>order</u> can be agreed on. If one treats social class as a continuous variable as in correlational analyses, one has to make the unwarranted assumption that it is both ordered and equal interval. If one uses dummy variable techniques as in some multiple regression analyses, then one acknowledges that social classes are not equal intervals but one also ignores the ordered nature of the material.

And all of this applies to one of the simplest, crudest indices used in social research. Where social class appears to be important, the measure is merely a rough indicator that some consistent difference in behaviour within families is responsible for whatever differences between groups has emerged. It is necessary then to enquire in much greater detail to find out the <u>mechanisms</u> which explain the differences between social groupings.

Rutter (1980) comments on this in relation to the immense difficulties in attempting to pinpoint the nature of any relationship between lead, intelligence and social factors. Even with good measures of social factors " .... there will always remain the possibility that the few points of IQ ...." which remain between groups, after controlling for background factors, will in reality be due to social or genetic factors not included, rather than to the lead levels which have been measured" (p.22). We accept that our pilot results have to be treated with caution in the light of our weak data on social factors. If more factors are to be investigated, much larger samples will have to be studied.

Are there any alternatives to larger and larger epidemiological studies? Fortunately, there are. Firstly, longitudinal studies in which both lead levels and developmental data are gathered repeatedly will allow the examination of changes over time. Statistical techniques designed for the analyses of longitudinal data will allow for clearer examination of the direction of causality. Secondly, experimental methods are always more powerful than epidemiological uses in establishing causality. Lead cannot be added to peoples diet, but the effects of its removal can be studied. The Lawther Committee (Department of Health and Social Security, 1980) has already recommended that any major reduction in lead levels should be studied. Thirdly, a subset of experimental investigations would be provided by chelation studies of the sort described by David (chapter 15). That activity level drops following the chelation of lead is an indication that lead was causally implicated. However, as Silbergeld (chapter 10) points out, chelation in rats does not usually remove lead once it is within brain cells. This poses important questions about the reversibility of the effects of lead and of its mode of action.

Bradford Hill (1977) described some requirements for establishing cause and effect relationships with respect to biological processes. Not all of these are relevant to the social sciences, but they provide a useful framework within which to summarize our views on the contribution of recent studies to the question of whether low level lead exposure causes developmental deficits.

He argued that causality is more likely where the association is strong. The studies we have reviewed point to a low, but statistically significant (i.e. a "real") correlation between lead level and IQ. As we noted, in the context of IQ, low correlations are more believable than large ones. Hill asked whether there was any consistency of the observed association. Earlier studies showed poor replication on IQ and neuropsychological measures, but they were beset with many design flaws, and, in any case, there were very few studies. Recent studies have been far better designed, and particularly with those reported in this volume, there is much greater congruence of results. Our replication of Needleman's behaviour rating study is especially noteworthy.

Is there a dose-response relationship? The evidence is not at all clear in relation to intelligence. We have suggested that there may be more than one threshold operating, others argue that there is no threshold at all. There is, as yet, insufficient data to decide. In relation to behaviour, then, the probability of a dose-response relationship is greater, but there is a need to control for the role of social factors and intelligence.

Undoubtedly, it is biologically plausible that if, very high levels of lead cause serious damage, lower levels may cause less damage. The animal research reviewed by Silbergeld (chapter 10) and Winneke (chapter 13) is particularly important in that connection. However the coherence of the human evidence is poor, and clear results are not yet evident.

In our view, there is a small, significant and socially important relationship between low level exposure and childrens' development. The nature of that relationship is becoming better understood as more sophisticated studies are undertaken of this important area.

ACKNOWLEDGEMENTS

This study was supported by a grant from the Medical Research Council (SPG 979/1160) to the first two authors. We are grateful to officers of the Inner London and Bexley Education Authorities and to the headteachers and teachers for their co-operation. We also thank the following colleagues for helpful comments and discussion on our work: Professors P. Lawther, M. Rutter, P. Graham, B. Clayton, and D Acheson; Drs. S. Pocock, D. Hand, M. Berger, T. Delves, Miss E. Benton and Mr. R. Waller. We wish to acknowledge the generosity of Drs. E. Taylor and S. Sandberg in making their unpublished data available to us. Miss J. Hunter assisted in the data analysis of the behavioural data.

DISCUSSION

Billick: There are several problems that arise from the use of blood lead. Firstly, differences of one to two micrograms are so small that I doubt whether the available analytical procedures can discriminate that accurately. Accordingly, there may be misclassification of subjects. Secondly, even over time periods as short as a few days, there may be extreme fluctuations in the blood lead of individuals. These are serious problems, which Needleman overcame in his study by using tooth lead. Would you comment on the relative advantages and disadvantages of blood lead as compared with tooth lead?

Yule: The use of tooth lead as an index does overcome the problem of day to day fluctuations.

but only at the rather great cost of a method limited to deciduous teeth that are spontaneously dropped. Tooth leads cannot be used with children whose teeth have yet to be shed; nor can it be used with older children who have already lost their deciduous teeth. With these age groups there has to be reliance on blood leads. While I agree that blood leads have the potential disadvantage of marked day to day fluctuations in level if the intake of lead alters markedly over time, this is less of a problem in practice than might be expected. The reason is that most children with raised lead levels have suffered chronic exposure from a relatively constant source. As a consequence of the constancy in intake, the blood lead levels tend to show quite high stability over time. Thus, Otto (1982) reported a very respectable test-retest correlation of 0.6 over a 2 year time period. With respect to your first point about very small differences in blood lead levels, we accept your reservation regarding our use of quartiles in the statistical analysis. Nevertheless, it constituted the best procedure for our data.

Lansdown: Billick is correct about the limitations imposed by a two microgram difference but our two extreme quartiles showed a difference of about nine micrograms which is more meaningful.

Billick: I agree that the use of extreme blood lead groups is a much better method than the continuum.

Yule: That solves one problem but only at the cost of a violation of the underlying assumptions of analysis of co-variance - a difficulty with many of the published studies.

David: In my study there were two groups of children who were not treated with penicillamine, the placebo group and the group treated with methylphenidate. The serial lead levels for those children showed quite insignificant changes over a three months period.

Question: I am surprised that you refer to the time factor as a problem with tooth leads. Spontaneous shedding of infant teeth can go on for 4 or 5 years, and with teeth extractions the period is even longer.

Yule: The time period for loss of teeth is limited. However, a greater problem concerns the effects on sampling of a reliance on spontaneously shed (or extracted) teeth. If analyses are restricted to a sample of children who have lost teeth, the sample is necessarily biased because children lose their teeth at varying ages. One cannot assume that those who lose teeth later are comparable with those who lose them early. We do not know whether these non-comparabilities are crucial to the study of lead effects. There is a great need to find out more about the factors that determine when teeth are shed.

Winneke: What happens to the dose-effect relationship for the behavioural parameters if occupation is taken into account?

Yule: There was no relationship whatsoever between social class and any of the individual behaviour items. That is a well replicated finding with the Rutter behaviour rating scale; the lack of any social class gradient seems to apply similarly to the Needleman scale. Because of the lack of an association with social class, it was justifiable to postpone multivariate analyses using social class until we have a larger sample.

Rutter: The lack of a social class association with individual itesm on the questionnaires does not necessarily mean that there would be no association between social class and total scores on the scales. After all, as you noted, the findings for individual items on the Conners' scale were not the same as those for the scale as a whole. However, let us assume for the moment that the total scores would not show an association with social class. If that were the case, it would raise an interesting possibility. The point is that the Needleman questionnaire items showed an association with IQ but not with social class. On the other hand, it is well established that IQ and social class are themselves inter-correlated, with that association due in part to genetic factors and in part to environmental influences in the family (Rutter and Madge, 1976). It follows that the proportion of the variance accounted for by the IQ-behaviour correlation must not apply to that part of the IQ that correlates with social class. Furthermore, it might be inferred that this also means that the IQ-behaviour correlation is not due to the genetic and familial influences that underlie the IQ-social class association. Some other variable, perhaps linked with lead toxicity, must be postulated. I appreciate that your data stem from a small pilot study and that, quite rightly, you are reluctant to press interpretations of the results too far. Nevertheless, could you comment?

Yule:

I understand the argument but I doubt that our sample is large enough to carry out the multivariate analyses necessary to test that hypothesis.

Carson:

It is generally held that the cognitive factor least affected by social class is mathematical performance. One might suppose, therefore, that attainments in mathematics would be most likely to be impaired by lead. Yet, your findings showed no effects of lead on maths.

Lansdown:

It is not that mathematical abilities are unassociated with social class. However, there is no good a priori reason why lead should not affect maths. It may be that the lack of any correlation between lead levels and mathematics scores in our study reflects the insensitivity of our test. The problem today in devising any adequate test for mathematics stems from the fact that the subject is taught quite differently from school to school, and even from school class to class. The content is different and not just the method of teaching; as a result, it is difficult to devise any test that is comparable across the general population of school children. What is more, recently published results suggest that the association between lead and verbal scores may be greater than that with performance scores. There is a close relationship between mathematics and spatial ability. It is possible, therefore, that there is less effect on mathematics because, for reasons as yet unknown, there is a reduced association between lead and spatial skills.

Miller:

One possible source of bias in our study concerns the heterogeneity of the population studied. Half the children had lived in the area for some time but half had moved in from other parts of London. Accordingly, there is a need to repeat the study with a different, and more stable, population - as we are doing now.

Nevertheless, the results of the research presented at this symposium, when considered as a whole, have made me revise my opinions on the blood lead levels at which adverse sequelae may arise. It seems that there may be effects below 30 micrograms per decilitre.

Edwards: The epidemiological studies undertaken with humans have produced reasonably consistent findings but, equally, all of them suffer from the inherent weaknesses produced by multiple overlapping variables. Each investigator has sought to unravel the associations by means of some form of multivariate analysis - usually analyses of covariance (in which one variable is held constant in order to examine the effects of another variable). Bradford Hill would, I think, have been very cautious about such a statistical approach. Moreover, this method gets one into difficult waters when estimating the strength of effects. You say that 0.21 is quite a large correlation, but once you square this to determine the force of the variance it drops to 5%, which seems very little. Also, you refer to the support provided by replication of findings in different studies, but surely each replication simply repeats the biases and errors in earlier investigations. With animal experiments, it is possible to introduce direct controls to eliminate the effects of confounding variables. Accordingly, I would have thought that they provide a more secure basis for Governmental policy.

Yule: Five per cent is, of course, a small proportion of the variance. Nevertheless, it would be large enought to have policy implications if one were sure that it was due to lead (and I am not cliaming that we can be sure of the size of the effect as yet). A large body of research has shown that there are multiple determinants of intelligence and lead could not be expected to do more than contribute a minor portion of the variance. I agree that animal studies are important in suggesting mechanisms, but ultimately these must be tested in man. Also, human studies may be necessary to delineate the particular patterns of lead sequelae. For example, Winneke's research (Chapter 13) suggested that different mechanisms may apply with different types of cognitive function. Surely, human studies and animal experiments are mutually complementary; both are necessary.

Comment from the floor:

With respect to Edwards' comments on multivariate analyses (such as analyses of covariance, stepwise multiple regressions and other similar procedures), I would like to emphasize that they were developed precisely for the purpose of dealing with the difficulties he mentioned. Moreover, they are reasonably robust in terms of the criteria required for their use.

Russell Jones:

The point is that these different types of research - epidemiological enquiries, neurophysiological studies, biochemical investigations and animal experiments - all point in the same direction. None of them conflicts with others.

Edwards:

All that I am saying is that if you demonstrate an association in human studies and if you replicate that effect in an animal experiment it would be unwise to regard this as trivial or irrelevant. Epidemiological studies are extremely complex and there is no way, as far as I can see, in which one can get comparable information in man as quickly as one can by using experiments in animals.

Lansdown:

I would have thought that that was an argument for replicating studies on humans rather than against. The sheer complexity that you mentioned demands human research. The fact that our study reproduced Needleman's behavioural profile in such a remarkable way seems to me to add a lot of weight to both sets of findings.

Needleman:

The findings of the two studies are indeed remarkably similar. The risk for poor functioning attributable to lead in your study was 63% whereas the same analysis in my study gave a figure of 69%.

Bryce-Smith:

Since animal studies and, to some extent, human studies demonstrate that the impairments associated with lead are most marked in the performance of the most demanding tasks, I wonder if there is a case for devising some more discriminating measures of learning ability and intelligence.

Yule: The human findings particularly point to the
                         need for good measures of sustained attention.
                         There are many theoretical models of attention,
                         but not very many replicable and easily
                         administered tasks that can be used with large
                         numbers of children.

REFERENCES

Baloh, R., Sturm. R., Green B. and Gleser, G. (1975) Neuro-
   psychological effects of chronic asymptomatic increased lead
   absorption. Arch. Neurol., 32, 326-330.
Bradford Hill, A. (1977). A Short Textbook of Medical Statistics.
   London: Hodder and Stoughton.
Conners, C.K. (1969) A teacher rating scale for use in drug
   studies with children. Amer. J. Psychiat., 126, 884-888.
David, O.J., Clark, J. and Voeller, K. (1972). Lead and
   Hyperactivity Lancet, 2, 900-903.
David, O.J., Hoffman, S. and Kagey, B. (1979). Sub-clinical lead
   levels and behaviour in children. Trace Substances in
   Environmental Health, 13, 52-58.
David, O.J., Hoffman, S., Sverd, J. and Clark, J. (1977). Lead
   and hyperactivity: lead levels among hyperactive children. J.
   Abnorm Child Pschol., 5, 405-416.
David, O.J., Hoffman, S., Sverd, J., Clark, J. and Voeller, K.
   (1976). Lead and hyperactivity: Behavioural response to
   chelation(a pilot study). Amer. J. Psychiat., 135, 1155-1158.
D.H.S.S. (1980). Lead and Health. The Report of the DHSS
   Working Party on Lead in the Environment (The Lawther
   Report) London: HMSO.
Erdina, K. and Winneke, G. (1978). Neuropsychological research
   on children with increased tooth lead content. Paper delivered
   at the Working Conference of the German Association of Hygiene
   and Microbiology 2/3 October, Mainz.
Ernhart, G.B., Landa, B. and Schnell, N.B. (1981). Subclinical
   levels of lead and developmental deficit - A multivariate follow-up
   reassessment. Pediatrics, 67, 911-919.
Jones, R.R. (1982). A Stronger Smell. World Medicine, 17(16),
   54-55.
Landsdown, R.G., Shepherd, J., Clayton, B.E., Delves, H.T.,
   Graham, P.J. and Turner, W.C. (1974). Blood lead levels,
   behaviour and intelligence: a population study. Lancet, 1,
   538-541.
Neale, M.D. (1958). Neale Analysis of Reading Ability Manual.
   London: Macmillan.
Needleman, H.L., Gunnoe, C., Leviton, A., Reed, R., Peresie,
   H., Maher, C., and Barrett, P. (1979). Deficits in pyschologic
   and classroom performance of children with elevated dentine lead
   levels. Neur. Eng. J. Med., 300, 689-695.
Needleman, H.L., Leviton, A. and Bellinger, D. (9182). Lead-
   associated intellectual deficit. Neur. Eng. J. Med., 306, 367.
Otto, D., (1982), Unpublished paper, presented at the Institute of
   Neurology, London, 7 April 1982.

Registrar   General   (1966).   Classification   of   Occupations.
    London:HMSO
Rogers, R. (1982). New Statesman, 9 April.
Rutter, M. (1967). A children's behaviour questionnaire for
    completion by teachers: preliminary findings. J. Child Psychol.
    Pychiat. 8, 1-11.
Rutter, M. (1980). Raised lead levels and impaired cognitive
    /behavioural functioning: a review of the evidence. Develp.
    Med. Child Neurol., 22, Suppl. 42.
Rutter, M., Cox, A., Tupling, C., Berger, M. and Yule, W.
    (1975). Attainment and adjustment in two geographical areas.
    I. The prevalence of psychiatric disorders. Brit. J. Psychiat.,
    126, 493-509.
Rutter, M., Graham, P., Chadwick, O. and Yule, W. (1976).
    Adolescent   turmoil: Fact   or   fiction.   J.   Child.   Psychol,
    Psychiat., 17, 35-56.
Rutter, M. and Madge, N. (1976), Cycles of Disadvantage: A
    review of research, London: Heinemann Educational.
Rutter, M., Tizard, J. and Whitmore, K. (Eds) (1970). Education,
    Health and Behaviour. London: Longmans.
Rutter, M. and Yule, W. (1968). Teachers Rating Scale B(2).
    London: Institute of Psychiatry.
Sandberg, S., Rutter, M. and Taylor, E. (1978). Hyperkinetic
    disorders in psychiatric clinic attenders. Devel. Med. Child
    Neurol., 20, 279-299.
Schachar, R., Rutter, M. and Smith, A. (1981). The
    characteristics of situationally and pervasively hyperactive
    children: Implications for syndrome defination. J. Child
    Psychol. Psychol. Psychiat., 22, 375-392.
Taylor, E. and Sandberg, S. (1982). Classroom behaviour
    problems and hyperactivity: A questionnaire study in English
    schools. (in press).
Thorley, G. (1982). Normative data on the Conner's Teacher
    Questionnaire in two British clinic populations (in Press).
Vernon, P.E. (1977). Vernon Graded Word Spelling Test. London:
    Hodder and Stoughton.
Vernon, P.E. and Miller, K.M. (1976). Vernon Graded Arithmetic-
    Mathmetics Test. London: Hodder and Stoughton.
Wechsler, D. (1974). Manual of the Weschsler Intelligence Scale for
    Children - Revised. New York: Psychological Corporation.
Yule, W., Lansdown, R., Millar, I.B. and Urbanowicz, M.A.
    (1981). The relationship between blood lead concentrations,
    intelligence and attainment in a school population: A pilot study.
    Develop. Med. Child Neurol., 23, 567-576.
Yule, W., Urbanowicz, M.A., Lansdown, R. and Millar, I.B. (1982)
    Teachers' ratings of children's behaviour in relation to blood
    lead levels (submitted for publication).

PENICILLAMINE IN THE TREATMENT OF HYPERACTIVE
CHILDREN WITH MODERATELY ELEVATED LEAD LEVELS

Oliver J. David, M.D., D.M.Sc.
Stanley Hoffman, Ph.D., Julian Clark, M.D.
Gary Grad, M.D., Jeffrey Sverd, M.D.

Department of Psychiatry
State University of New York
Downstate Medical Center
Brooklyn
New York
USA

This work was supported in part by The Office of Child Develop-
ment, Department of Health, Education and Welfare, Grant
OCD-CB-482, and by The National Institute of Environmental
Health, Grant No. ES00083 and Grant No. ES2359A.

Medication was supplied by Ciba Pharmaceutical Co., Summit, New
Jersey, and Merck, Sharp and Dohme, West Point, Pennsylvania.

INTRODUCTION

Many previous studies have shown correlations between elevated lead
burdens and aspects of neurological dysfunction. (David et al., 1972;
Perino and Emhart, 1974; Ladrigan et al., 1975; De La Burde and
Choate, 1975; David et al., 1976; Moore et al., 1977; Pihl and Parkes,
1977; Yourokos et al., 1978; Needleman et al., 1979; Yule et al.,
1981). Even where statistical significance is not reached, the trends
are usually in the expected direction (Kotok, 1972; Lansdown et al.,
1974; Rummo, 1974; McNeil and Ptasnik, 1975; Kotok et al., 1977).

Doubt remains, however, on the causal nature of these relationships. In science as a whole, the controlled experiment constitutes
the most powerful tool for testing whether or not one variable has a
causal influence on another. Animal experiments (chapter 10)
provide the only ethical means of determining whether or not
increases in body lead produce neuropsychological impairment.
But, it is possible to use the experimental method in humans to test
whether or not decreases in body lead are accompanied by improvements in neuropsychological functioning. This approach is made
feasible through the use of drugs (chelating agents) that serve to
mobilise lead and increase its excretion and hence its elimination
from the body. That is the method we followed in studying the
associations between moderately elevated lead levels and hyperactivity.

297

The hyperkinetic or attention-deficit disorder is a rather complicated syndrome which is chiefly characterized by problems in
selective attention and by inappropriate or poorly modulated overactivity (American Psychiatric Association, 1980). Other symptoms
that are frequently present include impulsivity, low frustration
tolerance and hyperexcitability. Often, too, there is cognitive
dysfunction (as shown by learning disabilities) and also disturbances of conduct. That is the syndrome we studied. It may arise
as a result of overt brain damage or as part of some general or
specific developmental disorder; however, such cases were excluded
from our investigation.

Nevertheless, even with this exclusion, the syndrome does not
constitute a condition with a single aetiology. It is likely that in
many cases genetic factors (Morrison and Stewart, 1974), and/or
perinatal complications (Pasamanick et al., 1956) play an important
role in causation. In other cases, there may be some other form of
covert cerebral insult or irregular brain maturation or maldevelop-
ment (Laufer and Denhoff, 1957). Recent work, too, implicates
psychosocial factors as significant, if not primary, contributors to
aetiology (Campbell, 1975). Thus, we are studying the effects of
lead exposure as one of several aetiological factors, and not
through any belief that it constitutes the main cause. Nevertheless, these other different aetiologies have been taken into account
in the design of the project and are used as one means of testing
the principal hypotheses.

PATIENTS AND METHODS

Behavioural Measures. The children included in this study were
referred to a child behaviour research and treatment unit at the
Downstate Medical Center complex. The behavioural measures
employed included Conners' (1969) teacher's rating scale (TRS);
two parent rating scales - the Werry-Weiss-Peters (WWP) hyperactivity check list (Werry, 1968) and Conners (1970) parent
symptom questionnaire (PSQ); together with a doctor's global
assessment. Since almost all the children had been referred by
schools, all of them were characterized as hyperactive on the TRS.
This scale, in wide use for the past ten years, measures five
behavioural factors, one of which describes the hyperactive
syndrome. Questions on this factor refer to the characteristics
previously noted and are scored from 1 (not at all present) to 4
(very often present). A child is deemed hyperactive if the score
on that factor exceeds 2.5. Findings on the conduct disturbance
factor are also reported as obviously they were germane to the
clinical assessment. However, scores on that factor were not used
as criteria for acceptance into the study.

If a parent did not characterize a child as hyperactive (that is a
score of 2 or more on the WWP), the child was admitted for study
only if there was a score greater than 2.5 on the TRS hyperactivity
factor, and if, after a month's observation, the treating child
psychiatrist made a diagnosis of hyperactivity. Accordingly, all

children were characterized as hyperactive by at least 2 of 3
observers, and the vast majority were described as hyperactive by
all three.

The doctor's global observation was based on the NIMH Assessment
Battery (1970) which has been in common use for the last dozen
years. It asks the physician to rate how mentally ill the patient is
at the time of assessment – using a scale extending from 1 (normal
– not at all ill) to 7 (among the most extremely ill patients).

Grouping and Exclusions.   Children with a diagnosis of psychosis
or who had evidence of significant neurologic disease were excluded
from the study, as were those with mental retardation and/or a
pervasive developmental disorder.

All other children with the hyperactive syndrome were included.
They were then subdivided according to whether or not there was a
history of some factor that was likely to have been causal.   All
such 'aetiological' groupings were made before treatment and without
knowledge of lead levels.   These assignments resulted in three
separate aetiological groups: (a) 'no known cause'; (b) non-lead
related 'highly probable cause'; and (c) lead-related 'highly
probable cause' – meaning a history of encephalopathic or pre-
encephalopathic lead toxicity.   Our experience in the chelation
treatment of children with a non-lead related highly probable cause
is reported elsewhere (David et al., 1976).   This chapter is
concerned only with hyperactive children without any known cause
for their condition and with those where there was a history of lead
poisoning.

Blood Lead Levels.   Two 5 ml specimens of blood were obtained
from each child at the beginning and end of the trial.   Blood-lead
levels were measured by the atomic-absorption spectrophotometry
method of Hessel (1968).   The standard deviations for this analysis
are ± 3.97 µg per 100 ml at a 30 µg per 100 ml concentration and
± 5.68 µg per 100 ml at a 60 µg per 100 ml concentration.   The
laboratory mean for 60 specimens containing 30 µg was 30.69 µg per
100 ml, and the mean on an unknown specimen containing 60 µg per
100 ml was 60.85.   To be included in the study, the children had
to have a raised blood lead level within the range of 25 to 55 µg on
the first sample.

RESEARCH DESIGN

The research design that was employed had two essential features.
Firstly, the therapeutic efficacy of methylphenidate and of penicillamine were compared.   Methylphenidate is a central nervous stimulant that has been widely used in the treatment of hyperactive
children.   Numerous studies have shown that, at least in the short
term, its use is associated with substantial behavioural improvements in many cases.   The precise mode of therapeutic action
remains a matter of dispute but it is clear that it has nothing
whatsoever to do with the metabolism of lead.   Accordingly, it was

hypothesized that methylphenidate might, on non-specific grounds, lead to some benefits in hyperactive children with raised lead levels. However, because the drug does not affect lead, such benefits should not be associated with any lead-related measures. In sharp contrast, penicillamine is a chelating agent whose main relevant therapeutic action concerns its effect in increasing the loss of lead from the body. It has been used extensively to treat lead intoxication but it has no known effects on hyperactivity as such. Accordingly, it was hypothesized that the benefits in hyperactive children should arise solely as a consequence of effects on lead levels. In short, the design involved the systematic comparison of two therapeutic agents, one of which has an effect on hyperactivity and the other of which has an effect on body lead.

The second feature of the design involved the comparison of each of the two active drugs with a chemically inert placebo. This comparison was necessary because it is known that, with all conditions, improvements may occur for a variety of non-specific reasons unconnected with the pharmacological action of the drugs employed. That is, often people get better because they expect to get better. Accordingly, the use of a drug-placebo comparison design enables the investigator to use the difference in effects between the two conditions (i.e. between the active preparation and its inert substitute) to determine whether or not the benefits were due to the specific chemical actions per se.

A rather different procedure was followed in the two aetiological sub-groups. For the hyperactive children with elevated lead levels and no known cause for their condition, there was random allocation into one or other of three treatment regimes. The first involved a comparison of active penicillamine and methylphenidate placebo; the second active methylphenidate and penicillamine placebo; and the third a comparison of the two placebos. There was no direct comparison of the two active agents. In all cases, the treatment evaluation period covered 12 weeks. Children assigned to the first regime were on active penicillamine for 4 weeks, on a penicillamine placebo for the middle 4 weeks and then back to active penicillamine for the last 4 weeks. In addition, they received methylphenidate placebo for the entire 12 week period. Those in the second regime received both active methylphenidate and penicillamine placebo for all 12 weeks; those in the third regime received both placebos for the entire period.

Almost all of the children with a history of lead poisoning were assigned to the first regime, that in which there was use of active penicillamine. However, this fact was not known to anyone involved in the treatment or evaluation of subjects. Furthermore, in order to aid the integrity of the double-blind assessment, an occasional assignment to the methylphenidate or placebo group was made. No one involved in the direct treatment or evaluation of any groups (i.e. treating physicians, parents or teachers) knew which medication was being taken nor to which 'aetiologic' group the subject belonged.

Subjects were given research numbers as they were accepted for treatment in a stratified random fashion. That is, there was a series of random numbers for each aetiologic group that corresponded to a random arrangement of the three treatments. Medication bottles were similarly numbered so that a subject received medication from a bottle corresponding to his research number. There were two bottles for each subject, one containing active penicillamine or its placebo, the other active methylphenidate or its placebo. Each subject took two medications: penicillamine or its placebo and methylphenidate or its placebo. Bottling of the medication was done by the drug companies that supplied the medications, using a master plan prepared before the study began. Each bottle contained enough medication for the maximum dosage possible for any subject. A research assistant gave out the medication weekly and counted any medications not used at the next visit.

Dosage Schedule. Penicillamine or its placebo was prescribed at a fixed dosage of 250 mgm twice a day if the child weighed less than 60 lbs, and 250 mgm three times a day if 60 lbs or more. Methylphenidate or its placebo was prescribed on a flexible dosage schedule. The starting dose of both was set low, 5-10 mgm/day, to minimize side effects, and allowed to rise to a maximum of 40 mgm/day as per the recommendation of the treating physician.

Population Description. The population is described in Table 1. Only those subjects who completed the twelve week treatment protocol are included in this report. It will be seen that the groups tested were rather similar to each other in respect to age, sex, race and socio-economic groups.

The penicillamine treated group was twice as large as the other groups as a consequence of three separate factors: a) a high dropout rate for the placebo group; b) a chance preponderance in the random assignment of children to the penicillamine group in the first two years; and c) eight children who were initially treated with methylphenidate or placebo in one year were assigned directly to the penicillamine treatment regime the following year. None of the evaluators were aware of the non-random assignment of this small subgroup and its deletion would not affect the significance of any of the findings.

RESULTS

Blood Lead Changes. Table 2 shows that there were non-significant decreases in blood lead levels over the 12 week treatment period in those children taking methylphenidate or placebo. However, the fall in blood lead was much greater (and statistically significant) in the group receiving active penicillamine. Between group comparisons of change scores demonstrated the obvious efficacy of penicillamine as a chelating agent, together with the absence of this effect for both methylphenidate and placebo. An analysis of variance comparing all subjects on active penicillamine with all those on methylphenidate or placebo showed a highly significant difference ($F = 11.38$; d.f. $= 2.60$; $p < 0.005$).

TABLE 1.　Demographic characteristics of four groups of children

	N	SEX M/F	AGE mean ± S.D.	RANGE	ETHNIC GROUP Black	Hispanic	Caucasian	S.E.S.* $\bar{X}$ Hollingshea
Penicillamine No known/minimal cause	31	29/2	7.4 ± 3.0	5.2 – 11.7	25	5	1	4.3
Penicillamine History of Lead Poisoning	14	13/1	8.6 ± 1.6	5.9 – 11.4	9	4	1	4.2
Methylphenidate No known/minimal cause	12	11/1	7.4 ± 1.4	4.3 – 10.0	7	4	1	4.3
Placebo No known/minimal cause	11	10/1	7.8 ± 1.7	4.4 – 10.2	8	1	2	4.7

* Socioeconomic status

TABLE 2. Within and between group comparisons of blood-lead concentrations

TREATMENT GROUP	ETIOLOGIC GROUP	N	BASELINE mean ± S.D.	WEEK 12 mean ± S.D.	COMPARISON OF CHANGE WITHIN GROUP	COMPARISONS OF CHANGE AMONG 4 GROUPS	
						a vs. d	c vs. d
Penicillamine	No known/ minimal cause (a)	29	28.5 ± 7.9	19.8 ± 6.7	$t=9.44$ $df=28$ $p<.001$	$t=4.02$ $df=38$ $p<.001$	$t=0.15$ $df=19$ not significant
	History of Lead Poisoning (b)	13	35.0 ± 10.0	25.7 ± 8.6	$t=4.11$ $df=12$ $p<.01$	b vs. d $t=2.71$ $df=22$ $p<.02$	a vs. c $t=3.94$ $df=37$ $p<.001$
Methylphenidate	No known/ minimal cause (c)	10	28.4 ± 6.6	26.6 ± 6.2	$t=1.31$ $df=9$ not significant		
Placebo	No known/ minimal cause (d)	11	26.3 ± 3.4	24.3 ± 5.1	$t=1.76$ $df=10$ not significant		

Within and among group changes measured by 2 tail t-tests

TABLE 3.   Within and between group comparisons of teacher rating scale factor IV (hyperactivity)

TREATMENT GROUP	ETIOLOGIC GROUP	N	BASELINE mean ± S.D.	WEEK 12 mean ± S.D.	COMPARISON OF CHANGE WITHIN GROUP	COMPARISONS OF CHANGE AMONG 4 GROUPS
Penicillamine	No known/minimal cause (a)	26	2.2 ± .49	1.5 ± .68	t=5.51 df=25 p<.001	a vs. d: t=3.37 df=33 p<.01 / c vs. d: t=2.99 df=19 p<.01
	History of Lead Poisoning (b)	14	2.3 ± .47	2.0 ± .58	t=2.16 df=13 p<.05	b vs. d: t=1.87* df=21 p<.05 / a vs. c: t=0.72 df=36 not significant
Methylphenidate	No known/minimal cause (c)	12	2.2 ± .45	1.5 ± .65	t=3.70 df=11 p<.01	
Placebo	No known/minimal cause (d)	9	2.2 ± .55	2.4 ± .42	t=0.75 df=8 not significant	

* 1 tail t-test; all other change measured by 2 tail t-tests

BEHAVIOURAL CHANGES

Teacher Evaluations. Table 3 demonstrates how the teachers rated the children's hyperactivity at baseline and at the week 12 treatment evaluation. All children treated with penicillamine improved significantly on the hyperactivity factor. This within-group finding was also present in the between-group comparisons. That is children treated with penicillamine improved significantly when compared to a placebo-treated group. As expected, the methylphenidate group also improved significantly both within- and between-treatments. There were no differences, however, between the methylphenidate and penicillamine regimes. When it is recalled that methylphenidate is the treatment of choice for this condition, irrespective of aetiology, the perspective appropriate for the evaluation of this finding may be appreciated. An analysis of variance for the hyperactivity factor, comparing all children on penicillamine with those on methylphenidate and with those on placebo was significant (F = 6.31; df 2.58; p < .01). The more complex behavioural factor 'conduct disorder' showed trends in the direction of improvement for those on penicillamine and methylphenidate, but none of the differences was statistically significant.

Parent Evaluations. The parental WWP scale measure of hyperactivity showed a significant within-group improvement for all children taking methylphenidate or penicillamine (Table 4). The between-group comparisons between methylphenidate and placebo, and between the penicillamine treated group with a history of lead poisoning showed only non-significant trends in favour of the active medication. The larger group treated with penicillamine (no known cause), however, showed a significant improvement (p < .01) when compared to the placebo group. An analysis of variance comparing the three treatment groups showed significant differences (F = 3.36; df 2.63; p < .05). The results for hyperactivity as assessed on the PSQ are shown in Table 5 and for conduct disorder in Table 6. Hyperactivity showed a dramatic and statistically significant within-group improvement in those children treated with either penicillamine or methylphenidate. The small but insignificant improvement registered by the children on placebo probably accounts for the absence of any between-group significance and an insignificant overall analysis of variance. The conduct disorder factor, however, did show significant improvement (within- and between-groups) for those children on penicillamine; but not for those on methylphenidate. The latter is congruent with methylphenidate-treated children generally; that is, hyperactivity systematically improves but other symptoms do so much less consistently. An analysis of variance comparing the three treatment groups on the PSQ conduct factor gave a significant difference (F = 4.64; df 2.56; p < .01).

Doctor Evaluation. Table 7 shows that most children were initially rated by doctors as moderately ill (i.e. a rating of approximately 4). Those children treated with either penicillamine or methylphenidate improved significantly on the doctor-ratings. Between-

TABLE 4.   Within and between group comparisons of parent completed Werry Weiss Peters hyperactivity list

TREATMENT GROUP	ETIOLOGIC GROUP	N	BASELINE mean ± S.D.	WEEK 12 mean ± S.D.	COMPARISON OF CHANGE WITHIN GROUP	COMPARISONS OF CHANGE AMONG 4 GROUPS a vs. d c vs. d	
Penicillamine	No known/minimal cause (a)	31	2.4 ± .93	1.5 ± .74	t=6.15 df=30 p<.001	a vs. d t=2.42 df=40 p<.01	c vs. d t=1.40* df=19 p<.10
	History of Lead Poisoning (b)	14	2.2 ± .88	1.4 ± .93	t=3.42 df=13 p<.01	b vs. d t=1.60* df=23 p<.10	a vs. c t=0.48 df=39 not significant
Methylphenidate	No known/minimal cause (c)	10	2.8 ± .78	2.0 ± 1.04	t=3.33 df=9 p<.01		
Placebo	No known/minimal cause (d)	11	2.1 ± 1.04	2.0 ± 1.02	t=0.15 df=10 not significant		

* 1 tail t-test; all other change measured by 2 tail t-tests

TABLE 5.   Within and between group comparisons of parent symptom questionnaire
factor III (impulsive-hyperactive)

TREATMENT GROUP	ETIOLOGIC GROUP	N	BASELINE mean ± S.D.	WEEK 12 mean ± S.D.	COMPARISON OF CHANGE WITHIN GROUP	COMPARISONS OF CHANGE AMONG 4 GROUPS	
Penicillamine	No known/ minimal cause (a)	30	1.3 ± .68	0.7 ± .67	t=4.26 df=29 p<.001	a vs. d t=1.21 df=38 not sig- nificant	c vs. d t=0.46 df=17 not sig- nificant
	History of Lead Poison- ing (b)	11	1.4 ± .43	0.8 ± .47	t=5.16 df=10 p<.001	b vs. d t=1.35 df=19 not sig- nificant	a vs. c t=0.70 df=37 not sig- nificant
Methylphenidate	No known/ minimal cause (c)	9	1.7 ± .73	1.3 ± .64	t=2.23 df=8 p<.05		
Placebo	No known/ minimal cause (d)	10	1.2 ± .68	1.0 ± .65	t=0.81 df=9 not significant		

All change measured by 2 tail t-tests

TABLE 6. Within and between group comparisons of parent symptom questionnaire factor I (conduct disorder)

TREATMENT GROUP	ETIOLOGIC GROUP	N	BASELINE mean ± S.D.	WEEK 12 mean ± S.D.	COMPARISON OF CHANGE WITHIN GROUP	COMPARISONS OF CHANGE AMONG 4 GROUPS
Penicillamine	No known/minimal cause (a)	29	0.9 ± .72	0.6 ± .59	t=2.52 df=28 p<.01	a vs. d t=2.05 df=37 p<.05 c vs. d t=0.57 df=17 not significant
	History of Lead Poisoning (b)	11	1.1 ± .65	0.5 ± .36	t=4.11 df=10 p<.005	b vs. d t=3.16 df=19 p<.01 a vs. c t=1.52 df=36 not significant
Methylphenidate	No known/minimal cause (c)	9	0.7 ± .73	0.8 ± .56	t=-0.32 df=8 not significant	
Placebo	No known/minimal cause (d)	10	0.7 ± .46	0.9 ± .80	t=-0.92 df=9 not significant	

Within and among group changes measured by 2 tail t-tests

TABLE 7.   Within and between group comparisons of physician completed clinical global impressions

TREATMENT GROUP	ETIOLOGIC GROUP	N	BASELINE mean ± S.D.	WEEK 12 mean ± S.D.	COMPARISON OF CHANGE WITHIN GROUP	COMPARISONS OF CHANGE AMONG 4 GROUPS a vs. d c vs. d
Penicillamine	No known/minimal cause (a)	28	4.0 ± .51	3.1 ± 1.13	t=4.34 df=27 p<.001	a vs. d t=4.07 df=34 p<.001 a vs. c t=2.99 df=15 p<.01
	History of Lead Poisoning (b)	13	3.9 ± .76	3.3 ± 1.25	t=1.67* df=12 p<.10	b vs. d t=2.67 df=19 p<.02
Methylphenidate	No known/minimal cause (c)	10	4.0 ± .94	3.2 ± .92	t=-1.92* df=9 p<.05	c vs. d t=0.14 df=35 not significant
Placebo	No known/minimal cause (d)	8	3.4 ± .92	4.1 ± .64	t=-3.00 df=7	

* 1 tail t-test; all other change measured by 2 tail t-tests

group comparisons similarly indicated significant improvement. An overall analysis of variance comparing the three treatment paradigms was significant (F = 6.50; df 2.56; p < .01).

DISCUSSION

The findings reported here need careful consideration in terms of both their scientific and public policy implications. The results clearly demonstrate that certain hyperactive children with elevated lead levels are significantly improved behaviourally after a trial of chelation medication. It is relevant that, although the lead levels were raised they were no so high as to give rise to the traditional clinical signs of lead intoxication. THe most salient conclusion to be drawn from these findings is that the lead levels, which are lowered as a result of chelation, probably play a causal role in the children's behavioural disturbance. Thus, the lead levels in the 25 to 55 µg/dl range should be regarded as toxic. This operationally defined behavioural improvement was apparent on the evaluation of the parent, teacher and doctor, all of whom were blind as to medication. For the most part, improvement concerned symptoms associated with the hyperactive syndrome. However, similar trends in other spheres of behaviour were also noted. The improvement on overactivity was both statistically significant and clinically noteworthy. In terms of clinical efficacy, it should be noted that at the end of the three month treatment evaluation, penicillamine-treated children were indistinguishable from those treated with methylphenidate, the present day treatment of choice.

The hyperactive children who improved on penicillamine included both those with no known cause for their hyperactivity and those with a history of encephalopathic or pre-encephalopathic lead poisoning. The few children who had elevated lead levels but, in addition, non-lead related aetiology for their hyperactivity, did not improve on chelation (David et al., 1976). Non-lead related aetiologies included low birth weight (less than 2000 g), ABO or Rh incompatability requiring an exchange transfusion, eclampsia or severe pre-eclampsia, and meningitis. The above findings demonstrate that penicillamine does not exert an effect on hyperactivity independent of its action as a lead-chelating agent.

Obviously, this study does not provide an unqualified recommendation to use penicillamine in hyperactive children with increased lead levels. It is true that their behaviour improved significantly over 12 weeks; however, we do not know whether or not this improvement would be sustained over a longer time period. It is possible, perhaps even probable, that when chelation is stopped there is a re-equilibrium between blood or soft tissue lead and bone lead. Furthermore, while the dosage of penicillamine used here was virtually trouble-free with respect to unwanted side-effects, this might not remain true if the treatment period were to be substantially prolonged. Other studies specifically designed to test the practicality of penicillamine in the treatment of these children are warranted. Meanwhile, the ideal way to cope with the problem of lead-induced CNS dysfunction is to prevent the lead from getting to children in the first place.

Major reforms in environmental codes, particularly as they bear on lead in paint and lead in the atmosphere, have been promulgated in the United States. Undue absorption of leaded paint through pica is generally associated with grossly elevated lead levels and correspondingly severe neurological sequelae. Lead in air is particularly relevant to the problem of minimally elevated lead levels. It is generally agreed that most airborne lead is derived from exhaust emissions. In the US where catalytic convertors, requiring non-leaded petrol, have been in increasing use since the early 1970s, the amount of lead in air has noticeably decreased. This has been accompanied by a concommitant and very significant decrease in blood lead levels in the entire population (Chapter 3). In 1972-73, when this study began, approximately half the hyperactive children examined (an inner city population) had elevated lead levels (David et al., 1972). Over the last decade the number of hyperactive children with elevated lead levels has decreased considerably. At present scarcely 5 per cent of children screened have lead levels above the 25 µg/mdl level required for entrance into this study. An absolute decrease in the number of hyperactive referrals has also occurred, although it is not known whether or not this is a consequence of lower environmental lead levels.

However, the maintenance of low lead levels in the environment requires continuing effective regulation and vigilance (Marshall, 1982). It is our belief that if the level of lead in the environment is allowed to rise, an increase in lead-induced CNS dysfunction will almost certainly follow. We should dwell on the concommitant toll of personal misery, family anguish and increased societal cost and unrest before we allow such a course to become established.

DISCUSSION

Burney: Could you comment on the drop-out rate in your study, as I note that you lost up to a sixth of the penicillamine group. Also, could Dr. Silbergeld comment on the apparently marked benefits from penicillamine. From the animal data that would seem unexpected.

David: The drop-out rates in any clinical trial tend to be quite high, no matter how effective the medication. In fact we lost as many children on methylphenidate as on penicillamine. However, there were differential drop-out rates in that the placebo group dropped out in droves. Most of the penicillamine drop-out probably occurred during the four to eight week placebo treatment period. The parents came to us to obtain treatment for their children's troubled behaviour at school, and if this was not ameliorated, many of them just left (although they had previously agreed to participate in the study).

Silbergeld: There are two points regarding penicillamine effects. First, effects of penicillamine on circulating levels of lead may be quite important. Second, penicillamine may reverse the effects of lead on haem synthesis which, in turn, may ameliorate the neuro-behavioural problems through the putative effects of ALA on GABAnergic transmission.

Raab: What were the numbers in your original groups and what proportions dropped out? Were you able to obtain any ratings on the drop-outs and, if so, did they differ from those who completed the trial?

David: If we restrict attention to the single run children (i.e. excluding those who entered the trials twice), there were about 35 to 40 in the penicillamine group at the outset, approximately 25 in the methylphenidate groups, and about the same number or slightly more in the placebo group. We had follow-up ratings on only some of the drop-outs. When analyses were undertaken with respect to the total population, the within-group differences were much the same, but the between-group differences were somewhat less strong. This may be because the point before people drop-out is when they feel reasonably well treated. Thus, the missing children in the placebo group are likely to be those whose behaviour had already deteriorated but whose behavioural reports recording this were not available because they had dropped out of the study. Even so, in spite of that, the differences were still statistically significant for the between group comparisons on the teacher rating of hyperactivity and the parental scored hyperactivity list.

Rutter: It is important to recognise that the validity of the hyperactive syndrome is not universally agreed, and it is clear that the behaviours designed by the syndrome can arise from social as well as physical causes.   I would like to comment also on the inter-pretation of the findings on the benefits associated with the administration of penicillamine. There are two rather separate

points here. Firstly, there is the possibility
that the benefits were not real. As you
pointed out, clinical trials are exceedingly
difficult to undertake and are plagued by all
sorts of practical problems. Nevertheless, the
fact that there was both a differential drop out
and an unbalanced allocation between groups
raises worries that the results may be
artefactual, although of course it does not
necessarily invalidate the findings. The
second issue concerns the mechanism by which
the benefits were brought about - assuming
that the benefits were real. As you noted,
penicillamine has a variety of pharmacological
actions, and in order to test whether the
reduction in blood lead constituted the key
action, the usual approach would be to
undertake a within-group analysis. That is to
say, there is variation within your
penicillamine group both in terms of reduction
in blood lead and in terms of changes in the
children's behaviour. If the one is related to
the other with the children who showed the
greatest reduction in blood lead also showing
the greatest improvement in teacher's scores,
that would greatly strengthen the interference
that it was the reduction in blood lead that
produced the improved behaviour.

David: that would be an extremely difficult analysis in
view of the fact that there was a very limited
range with respect to both the diminution of
blood leads and changes in teacher's scores.
Of course, there was some individual variation
but the possibility of finding a statistically
significant correlation between the two sets of
changes is remote.

Bryce-Smith: It is often said in this country that it would
be unethical to administer penicillamine to
nominally asymtomatic children in view of the
hazardous side-effects. Did you observe any
adverse side effects that might argue agains
the more general use of penicillamine? In that
connection, there are alternative ways of
detoxification, or, at least, of antagonising
lead effects. For example, dietary
manipulation and the provision of a calcium and
phosphate supplement may both be helpful.
They would be ethically much more acceptable;
have you considered alternative approaches?

David: Although I did not encounter any significant
                problems at the dosage I was using, I would
                be very loth to recommend the more general
                use of penicillamine. It is not an innocuous
                medication. I would not treat a lead level per
                se, unless significant dysfunction had been
                noted in that child. Of course, there are real
                difficulties in determining whether of not there
                has been lead-induced dysfunction. Lead may
                produce impairments that we can not recognize
                such as a drop of potential IQ of 130 to an
                actual IQ of 100. Nonetheless, I would not
                recommend the use of penicillamine in the
                context of uncertain dysfunctions. If someone
                can come up with an effective way of lowering
                lead levels without using the medicaments
                (such as EDTA) that are presently available,
                that would be a significant advance. I know
                that some of the dietary supplements in fact do
                have an effect but I am not sure that they
                have sufficient effect for the purpose.

Question: Were the children in your study given
                psychotherapy or nutritional guidance and, if
                so, were the controls treated differently?

David: The controls and the experimental groups were
                treated in the same fashion. No specific
                psychotherapy was given; psycotherapy is a
                very poor treatment for hyperactivity.
                Behaviour modification may be effective
                sometimes but it was not used in this study.
                Nutritional supplementation was not suggested.

Gallacher: Although your trial was double-blind, I
                presume that everybody involved knew that
                the experiments concerned lead. That,
                together with the differential drop-out, raises
                the possibility of the inadvertent introduction
                of bias. I appreciate the difficulties involved
                in any work of this kind, and especially with
                clinical trials using chelating agents.
                Nevertheless, this is an important issue –
                because there have been several studies where
                the possibility of the preselection of subjects
                has been either openly admitted or seems
                highly likely. In the light of this, how
                confident are you in generalizing your results
                to the general population?

David: This was a deliberately preselected population
                in terms of the requirement that the children
                meet the criteria for both hyperactivity and

raised lead levels. This was not a matter of bias; rather, it was a necessary step in order to determine whether the experimental lowering of lead levels brought about a reduction in hyperactivity. Accordingly, the findings can be applied only to hyperactive children with raised lead levels; it is not intended that they be extended to the general population.

So far as the question of possible bias in the assessment of effects is concerned, the use of a random assignment double-blind protocol is the most effective means of eliminating experimental bias. The teachers knew that the children were being treated for a behavioural problem, but they had no idea that the children were being treated with a lead chelating medication. Similarly, the parents, although they were aware of the lead presence, did not know which medication their child was on; the placebo looked exactly like the active preparation. Obviously bias can never be ruled out entirely but the study controlled for it.

It terms of the genralizability of our findings, it is clear that hyperactivity may be caused by many factors other than lead. Similarly, all children with elevated lead burdens do not show hyperactivity. There is an enormous range of lead effects and individual variations in host susceptibility are very important. At an international symposium held in Paris in 1974, Guinee and co-workers reported on 2,500-3,000 New York children with blood lead levels in the 60 - 100 micrograms range. 100 µg is a level that may cause death or is often associated with catastrophic effects on the brain, as shown by an encephalopathy. Yet, forty per cent of the children studied with this lead level showed no symtoms at all! Thus, at the same the lead level there is one child who is apparently healthy and another who is dead. As in so many illnesses, the presence of a toxin alone is not sufficient. Biologic variability (in terms of host resistance and sensitivity) is a crucial factor. Moreover, as lead levels get lower, biological variability is going to become increasingly important.

Russell-Jones: There seems to be a contrast between American and British clinicians in the ways in which they approach the syndrome of hyperactivity.

I would like to ask Professor Rutter whether he routinely screens his hyperactive patients for lead and, if he finds a high blood lead level, what therapeutic regime he institutes?

Rutter: Wheras I do screen for raised lead levels in all cases of developmental delay or mental retardation, I do not do so routinely with hyperactive children unless there are other grounds (such as pica) for suspecting possible lead intoxication. My reasons are fourfold: firstly, hyperactivity is an extremely common symtom; secondly, lead levels above 35 µgm/dl are now quite rare in the children I see; thirdly, the evidence that raised lead levels are specifically associated with hyperactivity (rather than with behavioural disturbance in general) is quite weak; and fourthly, I doubt the wisdom of chelating children with only slightly raised lead levels. So far as the treatment regime I use for high blood lead levels is concerned, if is some years since the situation arose, although in the past I have used chelation.

REFERENCES

American Psychiatric Association, 1980; Diagnostic and Statistical Manual of Mental Disorders (3rd ed.); 41–45.

Campbell, S.B., Mother-child interaction, 1975; A comparison of hyperactive learning disabled, and normal boys, Am. J. Orthopsychiatry 45: 51–57.

Conners, C.K., 1969; A teacher rating scale for use in drug studies with children, Am. J. Psychiatry 126: 884–888.

Conners, C.K., 1970; Symptom patterns in hyperkinetic, neurotic, and normal children. Child Dev. 41: 667–682.

David, O.J., Clark, J., Voeller, K., 1972; Lead and Hyperactivity. Lancet 1: 900–903.

David, O.J., Hoffman, S., McGann, B., Sverd, J., Clark, J., 1976; Low lead levels and mental retardation. Lancet 1: 1376–1379.

David, O.J., Hoffman, S.P., Sverd J., Clark, J., Voeller, K., 1976; Lead and Hyperactivity. Behavioural Response to Chelation: A Pilot Study. Am. J. Psychiatry 133: 1155–1158.

De la Burde, B., Choate, M.S., 1975; Does asymptomatic lead exposure in children have latent sequelae? J. Pediatr. 87: 638–642.

Guinee, International Symposium, Paris, 1974.

Hessel, D.W., 1968; A simple and rapid quantitative determination of lead in blood. Atmoic Absorption Newsletter 7: 55–56.

Kotok, D., 1972; Development of children with elevated lead levels: a controlled study. J. Pediatr. 80: 57–61.

Kotok, D., Kotok, R., Heriot, T., 1977; Cognitive evaluation of
    children with elevated blood lead levels. Am. J. Disabil. Child.
    131: 791-793.
Landrigan, P.J., Whitworth, R.H., Baloh, R.W., Staehling, N.W.,
    Barthel, W.F., Rosenblum, B.T., 1975; Neuropsychological dys-
    function in children with chronic low level lead absorption.
    Lancet 1: 708-712.
Lansdown, R.G., Shepherd, J., Clayton, B.E., Delves, H.T.,
    Graham, P.J., Turner, W.C., 1974; Blood-lead levels, behavior,
    and intelligence. A population study. Lancet 1: 538-541.
Laufer, M.W., Denhoff, E., Solomons, G., 1957; Hyperkinetic
    impulse disorder in children's behavior problems. Psychomosom.
    Med. 19: 38-49.
Marshall, E., 1982: EPA May Allow More Lead in Gasoline. Science
    215: 1375-1378.
McNeil, J.L., Ptasnik, J.A., Croft, D.B., 1975; Evaluation of long
    term effects of elevated blood lead concentrations in asymptomatic
    children. Arhiv. Hig. Rada. Toksikol. 14: 97-119.
Moore, M.R., Meredith, P., Goldberg, A., 1977; A retrospective
    analysis of blood lead in mentally retarded children. Lancet 1:
    717-719.
Morrison, J.R., Stewart, M.A., 1974; Bilateral inheritance as
    evidence for polygenicity in the hyperactive child syndrome. J.
    Nerv. Ment. Dis. 158: 226-228.
Needleman, H.L., Gunnoe, C., Leviton, A., Reed, R., Peresie,
    H., Maher, C., Barrett, P., 1979; Deficits in psychologic and
    classroom performance of children with elevated dentine lead
    levels. New Engl. J. Med 300: 689-695.
National Institute of Mental Health, 1970. Manual for the ECDEU
    Assessment Battery, Rockville, Maryland.
Pasmanik, B., Rogers, M., Lillienfeld, A., 1956; Pregnancy
    experience and behavior disorders in children. Am. J.
    Psychiatry 112: 613-618.
Perino, J., Ernhart, C.B., 1974; The relation of subclinical lead
    level to cognitive and sensorimotor impairment in black pre-
    schoolers. J. Learn. Disabil. 7: 26-30.
Pihl, R.O., Parkes, M., 1977; Hair element content in learning
    disabled children. Science 198: 204-206.
Rummo, J.H., 1974, (Ph.D. Thesis). Intellectual and behavioral
    effects of lead poisoning in children. University of North
    Carolina, Chapel Hill, N.C., Ann Arbor, Michigan, University of
    Michigan, Microfilms.
Werry, J.S., 1968; Developmental hyperactivity. Pediatric Clinics
    of North America 5: 581-599.
Yourokos, S., Lyberatos, C., Philippidou, A., Gardikas, C.,
    Tsom, A., 1978; Increased blood lead levels in mentally retarded
    children. Arch. Environ. Health 33: 297-300.
Yule, W., Lansdown, R., Millar, I.B., Urbanowicz, M.A., 1981:
    The relationship between blood lead concentration, intelligence
    and attainment in a school population: A pilot study. Dev. Med.
    Child Neurol. 23: 567-576.

Lead Versus Health
Edited by M. Rutter and R. Russell Jones
© 1983 John Wiley & Sons Ltd.

ELECTROPHYSIQLOGICAL EVIDENCE OF CHANGES IN CNS
FUNCTION AT LOW-TOMODERATE BLOOD LEAD LEVELS
IN CHILDREN

David Otto,[1,2] Vernon Benignus,[1,2,3] Keith Muller,[4] and
Curtis Barton[1,3].

1.   US   Environmental   Protection   Agency   Research
      Triangle Park, NC 27711.

2.   Biological Sciences Research Centre.

3.   Department Of Psychology.

4.   Department of Epidemiology, University of North
      Carolina, Chapel Hill, NC 27514.

What is the biological threshold of adverse central nervous system
effect in children? The Centres for Disease Control (1978)
designated 30 µg/dl blood lead (PbB) and 50 µg/dl erythrocite
protorphyrin as the upper "safe" limits of body burden, threshold
values that are widely accepted in clinical practice today.
However, considerable psychometric data (Needleman et al, 1979;
Yule et al 1981, Lansdown et al, Chapter 14) and
electrophysiological data (Benignus et al, 1981; Landrigan et al,
1976; Otto et al, 1981; Seppalainen et al, 1972, 1975, 1980) from
the peripheral and central nervous system of children and adults
suggestive of lead-related alterations of brain function at PbB levels
below 30 µg/dl have been accumulating. Moreover, much of the
data suggests a continuum of nervous system effects across a broad
range of body lead burdens with no obvious threshold of effect
(David et al, 1979; Landrigan et al, 1980). If the continuum model
of lead effects is correct, then no arbitrary theshold limit of body
burden can be considered absolutely safe in children. The
objectives of this paper are to review recent electrophysiological
data from our laboratory (Benignus et al, 1981; Otto et al, 1981,
1982) that are consistent with the continuum view; and to discuss
some limitations in the interpretation of this data.

METHODS

One hundred children (53 boys) aged 13 to 75 months were studied.
These children came primarily from low-income Black families, a
subset of the population that is known to be at increased risk for
lead poisoning (Mahaffey et al, 1982). Parents of about half the
children worked in a lead battery fabrication plant. Lead dust from
work clothes was an inadvertent source of contamination in some
homes (Dolcourt et al, 1978). Peeling lead paint was the source of
elevated PbB levels in other children.

This study was a part of a comprehensive neurobehavioural evaluation that included a neurological examination; measurement of maternal and child IQ, language development, and motor activity; together with assessment of mother-child interaction in the home. Results of these assessments have been reported elsewhere (Milar et al, 1980, 1981).

Twenty-eight children (19 boys) from the original sample were re-evaluated two years later to determine if the observed relationship between slow brain potentials and body Pb burden persisted over time. Insufficient funds were available to re-assess all children from the original sample. The percentage of battery factory children used in the original and follow-up evaluations was very similar - 44% and 43% respectively. The age range at follow-up was 35 to 95 months.

Blood lead (PbB) levels were measured from venipuncture samples obtained on the day of evaluation. Lead determinations were made in the Heavy Metals Laboratory of the University of North Carolina, a participant in the Centre for Disease Control Proficiency Testing Program. PbB levels were analyzed by flame atomic absorption spectrometry according to Delves (1970). PbB levels ranged from 6-55 µg/dl in the initial evaluation and 14-39 µg/dl in the follow-up study. Only three children had PbB levels above 30 µg/dl at re-evaluation. Demographic characteristics, PbB levels and IQs of children in the initial and follow-up samples are summarized in Table 1.

Electrophysiological recording procedures have been described previously (Otto et al, 1981). In brief, EEG was recorded from the vertex, left and right parietal regions of the scalp referred to linked mastoids. Vertical eye movements were recorded for artifact editing. Trials with eye, muscle, or amplifier artifacts were eliminated from signal averages computed off-line. Analyses of EEG power spectra coherence and interhemispheric gain were computed from parietal leads as described by Benignus et al (1981). In order to engage the attention of very young children during electrophysiological testing, cartoons were shown by 8 mm projector (initial study) or video tape recorder (follow-up). The basic testing paradigm was a passive sensory conditioning task in which a brief tone (conditioned stimulus) was paired with a short blackout of the cartoon (unconditioned stimulus). The interval between tone onset and video blackout was 1.5 seconds.

The conditioned electrophysiological response was computed as the mean EEG voltage during the one second interval preceeding blackout. EEG was recorded during 35 trials in the initial study and 100 trials during follow-up. At least ten artifact-free trials were required for individual subject data to be included in slow wave (SW) analyses. Data from 65 children were used in the initial EEG spectrum analyses, from 41 children in the initial SW analysis, and from 28 children in the follow-up analysis. Subjects were rejected for medical, technical and behavioural problems. Only 13

children under 36 months of age satisfied criteria for inclusion in
the   SW   analysis.
TABLE 1.   DEMOGRAPHIC CHARACTERISTICS OF INITIAL
TWO-YEAR FOLLOW-UP SAMPLES.

A.   INITIAL EVALUATION SAMPLE (N = 75)*

AGE IN MONTHS

	13 - 35	36 - 59	60 - 75	SAMPLE MEAN (STANDARD ERROR)
N (MALE)	35 (19)	31 (17)	9 (2)	
PbB	29.8	28.5	27.8	29.0 (1.6)
IQ	89.2	79.7	90.8	85.5 (1.7)
SES	69.0	67.3	54.8	66.7 (1.5)

B.   TWO-YEAR FOLLOW-UP SAMPLE (N = 28)

AGE IN MONTHS

	35 - 66	67 - 95	STANDARD MEAN (STANDARD ERROR)
N (MALE)	16 (11)	12 (8)	
Original PbB	31.4	33.8	32.5 (2.4)
Follow-up PbB	21.5	20.5	21.1 (1.4)
Original IQ	90.1	83.4	87.1 (2.5)
Follow-up IQ	80.5	85.7	82.8 (1.8)
SES	67.3	62.7	65.2 (1.5)

abbreviations: N = sample size; PbB = blood lead level;
                IQ = intelligence quotient; SES = socio-economic
                status.

* Subjects used in EEG spectra and/or slow wave analyses.

Stepwise multivariate procedures were used for statistical analysis.
In order to maximise the power of a priori tests, SW analyses were
limited to one recording site (vertex).   A regression model was
chosen since the distributions of most variables were continuous.
The first step was an overall test of the linear effects of demographic variables (age, sex, SES, and IQ).   Linear, quadratic, and

cubic effects of age and PbB were then tested using orthogonal polynomials.

TABLE 2.   RESULTS   OF   MULTIVARIATE   REGRESSION ANALYSES   OF   SLOW   WAVE   VOLTAGE   FOR INITIAL   AND   TWO-YEAR   FOLLOW-UP ASSESSMENTS.

Source	df (num, den)	F	P
Initial assessment			
Demographics	3, 37	2.32	.10
Age	3, 37	0.39	.76
PbB	3, 37	3.11	.038
linear	1, 37	5.51	.025
quadratic	1, 37	3.21	.09
cubic	1, 37	0.07	.79
Age x PbB	4, 35	5.40	.0018
linear x linear	1, 35	17.03	.0003
linear x quadratic	1, 35	0.23	.64
quadratic x linear	1, 35	0.32	.58
quadratic x quadratic	1, 35	0.81	.38
Follow-up assessment			
Overall test	6, 24	3.30	.009
All trials (1-100)			
Age	1, 24	0.36	.56
Mean PbB*	1, 24	7.16	.014
Age x Mean PbB	1, 24	2.66	.12
Early trials (1-40)			
Age	1, 24	0.48	.50
Mean PbB*	1, 24	0.15	.71
Age x Mean PbB	1, 24	0.35	.56
Late trials (41-100)			
Age	1, 24	2.65	.12
Mean PbB*	1, 24	6.61	.017
Age x Mean PbB	1, 24	7.22	.013

*Mean PbB was calculated for each child as the average value of initial and follow-up PbB values [(PbB1 + PbB2)/2]. This value provides a crude estimate of the mean body burden during the period between the initial and follow-up assessments.

Fig. 1.   Summary averages of slow cortical potentials recorded during sensory conditioning in children with elevated body lead burden. Children have been arbitrarily divided into younger (left column) and older (right column) age groups at blood lead levels above (dashed line) and below (solid line) 30 μg/dl. Averages in the top row were recorded from 41 children during the initial evaluation. Averages in the bottom two rows were recorded from 28 children two years later. Temporal changes in slow wave voltage during early (middle row) and late (bottom row) trials are also shown.

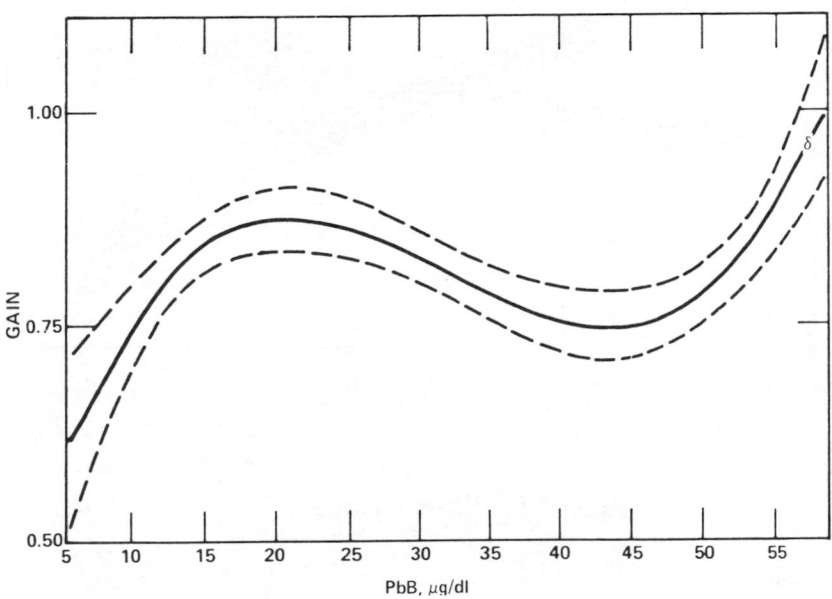

Fig. 2.   Predicted slow wave voltage and 95% confidence
                 bounds as a function of original blood lead levels for
                 children at the extreme age ranges represented in
                 the initial evaluation (upper box) and the follow-up
                 evaluation (lower box). These plots depict the
                 linear of PbB and age.

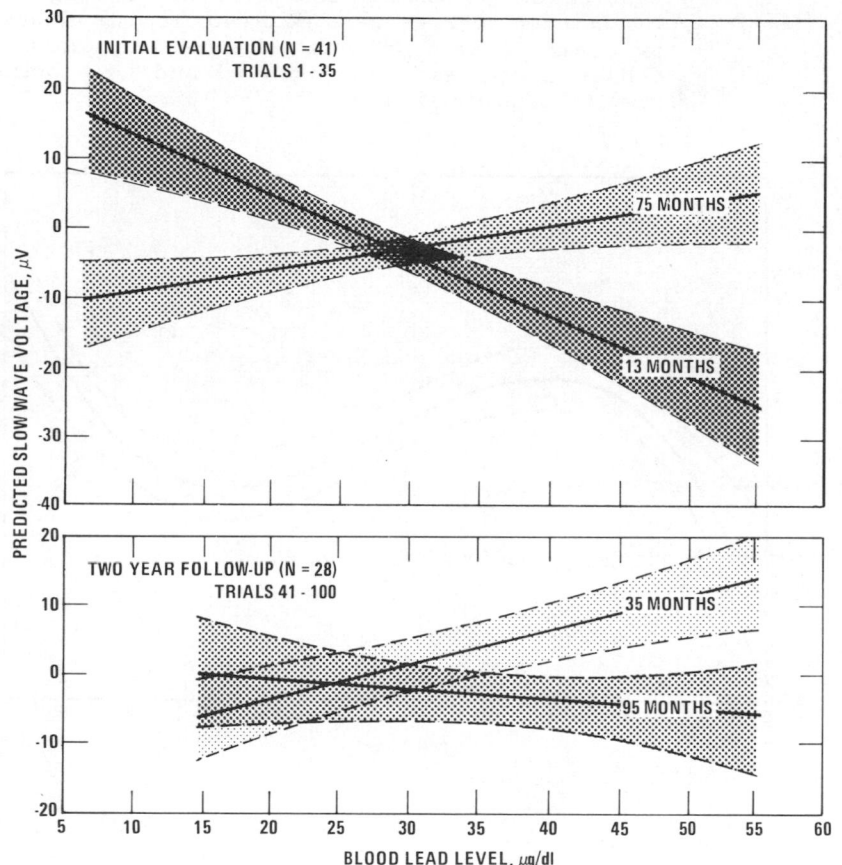

RESULTS

No significant main effects of demographic variables were observed. Summary averages of slow cortical potentials recorded during initial and follow-up assessments are shown in Fig. 1. Regression analyses of slow wave (SW) voltage (Table II) revealed a significant age-by-PbB interaction in both the initial and follow-up samples. The nature of this relationship may be characterized as follows: SW voltage varied as a linear function of PbB, but the slope of this function changed with age. Fig. 2 illustrates this interaction. Results of the initial evaluation indicated that SW voltage in children under five years of age tended to be positive at PbB levels below 30 μg/dl, but to be negative at PbB levels above 30 μg/dl. Children over five years of age showed an opposite pattern: negative voltage at low PbB levels, but less negative or positive voltage at elevated PbB levels.

Results of the initial assessment presented in Table 2 differ slightly from the original report (Otto et al, 1981, Table 3). A careful validation of all data used in the original analysis revealed a sizable error in the PbB value of one subject and several minor errors in ages and SES. The same multivariate regression analyses were rerun with corrected values. The use of corrected values reduced the error variance and increased the level of significance of several tests, although the same age linear and PbB linear interaction was obtained. The main effect of PbB, which was the only marginal in the original analysis (p = .08), reached significance in the re-analyses (p = .038).

During the initial assessment, 35 sensory conditioning trials were recorded from each subject. After editing the data for artifacts resulting from eye or body movement, too few trials remained for meaningful assessment of temporal changes during conditioning. In the follow-up evaluation, 100 trials were recorded for each child to permit a limited analysis of temporal changes. Individual averages of trials 1-40 and 41-100 were constructed to compare SW voltage during early and late conditioning. The asymmetrical breakdown of trials was necessary to obtain approximately equal numbers of early and late trials since more artifact problems occured during late trials. The middle and bottom rows of Fig. 1 show summary averages of early and late trials, respectively. The voltage of early and late trials was inversely correlated (r = .46, p < .02), suggestive of a polarity inversion during conditioning. This apparent inversion between early and late trials accounts in part for differences in the slopes of age functions for initial and follow-up data depicted in Fig. 2.

The effects of age and PbB on EEG power spectra and hemispheric laterality were also explored in the initial and follow-up assessments. Methods and results for the initial spectrum analyses are described in Benignus et al. (1981). No significant effects of PbB on power spectra or coherence measures were observed, although the relative amplitude of synchronized EEG between left and right hemispheres (gain spectra) increased relative to PbB

Fig. 3.   Estimated cubic trend line and 95% confidence
               bounds for EEG spectra gain between left and
               right hemispheres (P3 and P4) in the δ band
               as a function of blood lead (PbB) level. Age
               was held at a mean value of 36.8 months.
               (Reprinted from Benignus et al, 1981, p 245).

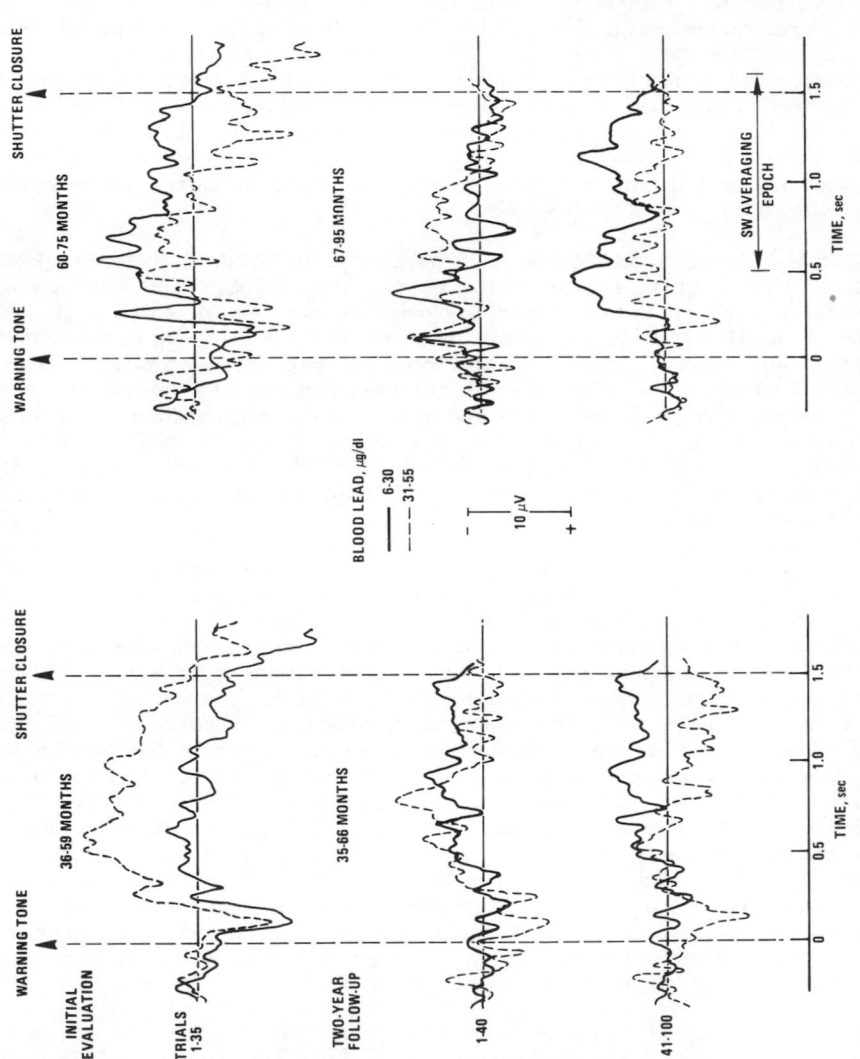

levels. A significant cubic trend for gain between the left and right parietal lobes was found as shown in Fig.3. This effect was observed in all frequency bands (δ, θ, α, and β) at the time of initial assessment, but, no significant difference associated with PbB was found at follow-up.

DISCUSSION

This study offers provocative evidence of altered central nervous system function at blood lead levels below 30 µg/dl, the threshold above which children are presently considered to have an elevated body burden (Centers for Disease Control, 1978). SW voltage recorded from the scalp of young children during sensory conditioning varied as a linear function of PbB within an observed range of six to 55 µg/dl. The slope of this function, moreover, varied systematically with age. When a subset of the children was retested two years later, the same linear relationship of SW voltage, age and PbB was observed. EEG spectrum gain, an orthogonal measure of CNS function, was also found to vary as a function of PbB during the initial evaluation, although this measure did not vary significantly with PbB in the follow-up analysis. These data imply (1) that there is no clearly defined PbB threshold below which SW voltage is unchanged; and (2) that the altered brain wave patterns associated with asymptomatic body Pb burdens in young children persist for at least two years, despite a substantial reduction of the mean PbB level during the test-retest interval.

These data are consistent with a continuum model of lead neurotoxicity - i.e., that CNS deficits are proportional to body lead burden. According to the continuum model, CNS function is affected in a graded manner across the entire range of exposure - i.e., there is no absolutely safe criterion level of lead burden below which the developing nervous system will be unharmed. Evidence has been accumulating over the past four decades of the untoward sequelae of early asymptomatic lead exposure (see reviews by U.S. Environmental Protection Agency 1977, Rutter 1980, Bornschein et al 1980). Mental retardation, minimal brain dysfunction, attention-deficit disorders, and a variety of subtle learning disorders have been linked with exposure levels that do not produce overt symptoms of Pb poisoning and that are unlikely to be detected. Evidence of IQ and/or attentional deficits in children at PbB levels below 40 µg/dl have been reported by Needleman et al (1979), Winneke et al (1982 a,b) Yule et al (1981) and Lansdown et al (Chapter 14), although a variety of methodological questions have been raised (e.g. Ernhart et al, 1981) that cloud the interpretation of these data. These problems include the use of PbB measures as an index of body lead burden, extrapolation from tooth-Pb to blood-Pb measures, and possible confounding effects of other variables such as socioeconomic status, parental IQ, and child-rearing practices. Despite these problems, the aggregate of data from recent neurobehavioural studies suggests that lead absorption in children produces a continuum of CNS impairments of increasing severity relative to the amount of Pb absorbed.

Failure of previous studies to demonstrate a linear relationship between PbB and neurobehavioural outcome may be the consequence of using statistical analyses that are relatively insensitive for evaluating the effects of continuous variables such as toxicant body burdens. In the present study a regression model was chosen because the distributions of critical variables (age, PbB, and EEG measures) were continuous. Any arbitrary grouping of data (such as 6-30 and 31-55 μg/dl PbB), as required in a traditional analysis of variance, results in a loss of information. For instance, any EEG changes that might be present within a specific exposure group (e.g. 6-30 μg/dl) would be obscured by averaging all data within that group. If this grouping had been used in the present study and a significant difference had been observed between the "elevated PbB" and "normal PbB" groups, our conclusions might have been quite different. In all likelihood we would have interpreted our data in support of the prevailing view that PbB levels above 30 μg/dl are associated with increased prevalence of CNS abnormalities. The statistical model chosen thus has profound implications for the conculsions drawn from a particular data set. In particular, the ANOVA model tends to suggest an arbitrary "threshold" view of toxicant effects based on the comparison of discrete means, while the linear regression model tends to suggest a "continuum" view based on the utilization of a continuous range of exposure values.

Although the regression model permits a more efficient use of available data relative to the ANOVA model, limitations in the interpretation of results should be noted. Demonstration of a linear relationship in the absence of higher order effects is a case in point. For example we observed a significant <u>linear</u> relationship of SW voltage and PbB within an observed range of six to 55 μg/dl. However, we cannot arbitrarily pick the lower limit or any other value within the observed exposure range and conclude that a significant impairment exists at or below that point. In order to identify a "threshold point" within the exposure continuum, a discontinuity (or inflection point) must be demonstrated. A linear relationship over the observed range implies no such inflection point. Tests for quadratic and cubic trends were, in fact, made (Table 2) to look for such inflection points. No significant higher order effect was found in the SW voltage analysis, although a cubic relationship of EEG spectrum gain and PbB was observed (Benignus et al 1981). The prominent inflection point in this cubic function provided the basis for concluding that CNS effects of Pb exposure were observed below 15 μg/dl.

Finally, we would like to reiterate several other caveats in the interpretation of our data (Otto et al, 1981, p 237-8):

> The use of blood lead level as an index of body burden is problematic. PbB level is an accurate measure of the amount of Pb circulating in the body at the time of sampling, but an isolated observation reveals little about the exposure history of the

individual. A high value could reflect an uncharac-
teristic, episodic elevation in PbB level, while a low
value could belie dangerously high exposures at an
earlier (and extremely vulnerable) period of
development. If PbB values obtained in the present
sample were systematically low across the entire range
of observations, a fixed error would be present in
the predictor model and CNS effects would be
attributed to artificially low body burdens.
Alternatively, if random sampling errors were
encountered in PbB measures - a more likely
possibility - the variance would presumably increase
relative to the amount of error. That is, a
systematic underestimate of PbB levels would tend to
yield a nonconservative error, while random PbB
fluctuations would tend to produce a conservative
error.

Another caveat concerns the nature of the measures.
The paradigms used are experimental, normative data
for young children do not exist, and the lack of
concurrent behavioural measures limits the assessment
of functional significance. Therefore, the present
data must be considered preliminary until the results
have been replicated.

In summary, we have observed statistically significant changes in
two different parameters of CNS function (slow wave voltage and
EEG gain spectra) within a range of low-to-moderate blood lead
levels (6 to 55 µg/dl) in young children. The SW voltage change
appears to persist for at least two years despite a substantial
decrease in PbB levels. These results challenge the
widely-accepted view that 30 µg/dl is a "safe" threshold below
which no adverse effects will occur in children. On the other
hand, the limitations of PbB as an index of body burden and the
experimental nature of the CNS measures employed must be clearly
understood. Efforts to replicate and validate these findings in an
independent sample are in progress.

ACKNOWLEDGEMENT

Supported by NIEHS Grant No. ES-01104, USPHS Grant No.
HD-03110, EPA Contract No. 68-02-1702, and MCH Project 916. The
extensive co-operation of J. Dolcourt, L. Grant, C. Milar, P.
Mushak, and S. Schroeder and technical assistance of L. Boone, J.
Nichols, J. Prah and K. Seiple are gratefully acknowledged.

FOOTNOTE

Although this research has been funded in part by the U.S.
Environmental Protection Agency, it has not been subjected to the
Agency's required peer and policy review and therefore does not
necessarily reflect the views of the Agency and no official
endorsement should be inferred.

REFERENCES

Benignus, V., Otto, D., Muller, K. and Seiple, K. Effects of age and body lead burden on CNS function in young children: II EEG spectra. Electroenceph. Clin. Neurophysiol., 1981, 52:240-248.

Bornschein, R., Pearson, D. and Reiter, L. Behavioural effects of moderate lead exposure in children and animal models. Part 1: Clinical studies. CRC crit. Rev. Toxicol., 1980, 8:43-99.

Centres for Disease Control. Preventing lead poisoning in young children. J Pediatr, 1978, 93:709-720.

David O., Clark, V. and Hoffman, S. Childhood lead poisoning: A re-evaluation. Arch. Environ. Health, 1979, 34:106-111.

Delves, H. A micro sampling method for the rapid determination of lead by atomic absorption spectrometry. Analyst, 1970, 95:431-438.

Dolcourt, J. Hamrick, H., O'Tuama, L., Wooten, J. and Barker, E. Increased lead burden in children of battery workers: Asymptomatic exposure resulting from contaminated work clothing. Pediatrics, 1978, 62:563-566.

Ernhart, C., Landa, B. and Schnell, N. Subclinical levels of lead and developmental deficit - A multivariate follow-up reassessment. Pediatr., 1981, 67:911-919.

Landrigan, P., Baker, E., Feldman, R., Cox, D., Eden, K., Orenstein, W., Mathev, J., Yankel, A. and Von Lindern, I. Increased lead absorption with anaemia and slowed nerve condition in children near a lead smelter. J. Pediatr., 1976, 89:904-910.

Landrigan, P., Baker, E., Withworth, R. and Feldman, R. Neuroepidemiological evaluations of children with chronic increased lead absorption in H. Needleman (ed.) Low Level Lead Exposure: The Clinical Implications of Current Research. Raven Press, New York, 1980, pp. 17-33.

Mahaffey, K., Annest, J. and Murphy, R. National estimates of blood lead levels: United States, 1976-1980. Association with selected demographic and socio-economic factors. N. Engl. J. Med., 1982, 307:573-579.

Milar, C.R., Schroeder, S.R., Mushak, P., Dolcourt, J.L., and Grant, L.D. Contributions to the Caregiving Environment to increased lead burden of children, 1980, 84:339-344.

Milar, C., Schroeder, S., Mushak, P. and Boone, L. Failure to find hyperactivity in preschool children with moderately elevated lead buden. J. Pediatr. Psychol., 1981, 6:85-95.

Needleman, H., Gunnoe, C., Leviton, A., Reed, R., Peresie, H., Maher, C. and Barrett, P. Deficits in psychologic and classroom performance of children with elevated dentine lead levels. N. Engl. J. Med, 1979, 300:689-695.

Otto, D., Benignus, V., Muller, K. and Barton, C. Effects of age and body lead burden on CNS function in young children. I. Slow cortical potentials. Electroenceph. Clin. Neurophysiol., 1981, 52:229-239.

Otto, D., Benignus, V., Muller, K., Barton, C., Seiple, K., Prah, J. and Schroeder, S. Effects of low to moderate lead exposure on slow cortical potentials in young children: Two year follow-up study. Neurobehav. Toxicol. Teratol., 1982, in press.

Rutter, M. Raised lead levels and impaired cognitive/behavioural functioning: A review of evidence. Dev. Med. Child. Neurol., 1980, 22 (Suppl.): 1-26.

Seppalainen, A.M. and Hernberg, S. Sensitive technique for detecting subclinical lead neuropathy. Br J Indus. Med., 1972, 29:443-449.

Seppalainen, A.M. Sakari, T., Hernberg, S. and Kock, B. Subclinical neuropathy at "safe" levels of lead exposure. Arch. Environ. Health, 1975, 30:180-183.

Seppalainen, A.M., and Hernberg, S. Subclinical lead neuropathy. Am. J. Indus. Med., 1980, 1:413-420.

U.S. Environmental Protection Agency. Air Quality Criteria for Lead. EPA-600/8-77-017, U.S. Govt. Printing Office, Washington, D.C.Dec 1977.

Winneke, G., Hrdina, K.-G., and Brockhaus, A. (1982a) Neuropsychological studies in children with elevated tooth-lead concentrations. Part I: Pilot study, Int. Arch. Occup. Environ. Health, 1982a, (in press).

Winneke, G., Kramer, U., Brockhaus, A., Ewers, U., Kujanek, G., Lechner, H, and Janke, W. Neuropsychological studies in children with elevated tooth-lead concentrations. Part II: Extended study. Int. Arch. Occup. Environ. Health, 1982b, (in press.)

Yule, W., Lansdown, R., Millar, I., and Urbanowicz, M. The relationship between blood lead concentrations, intelligence, and attainment in a school population: A pilot study. Develop. Med. Child Neurol., 1981, 23:567-576.

PART 5
Conclusions

LOW LEVEL LEAD EXPOSURE: SOURCES, EFFECTS AND
IMPLICATIONS

Michael Rutter

Department of Child and Adolescent Psychiatry
Insititute Of Pyschiatry
De Crespigny Park
Denmark Hill
London SE5

INTRODUCTION

The problems involved in the assessment of the effects of low level
lead exposure in human beings are extremely complex. The findings and concepts involve a wide range of scientific disciplines including chemistry, pharmacology, neurobiology, psychology and
epidemiology (Needleman, 1980). Because none of us has skills in
all of these areas it is not possible for anyone to provide a comprehensive summary statement - let alone one that would meet with
universal agreement! Accordingly, I will make no attempt to do so.

Moreover, as the discussion following earlier chapters make clear
there are inevitable doubts and uncertainties surrounding the findings from all of the empirical investigations. It is important to
realise, of course, that this is not an unusual state of affairs in
science. Studies in the real world have to deal with complex situations and with many influences of different kinds that are difficult
to disentangle. No one study ever finally resolves the scientific
questions in these circumstances and it would be scientifically fool-
ish, as well as politically irresponsible, to wait for the perfect
study to be undertaken. Rather, we have to consider the weight
of the evidence when viewed as a whole. We have to ask:- To what
extent are the limitations in the research ones that are likely
seriously to bias the findings? What are the conclusions if attention
if focused on the best of the studies? And, with particular reference to the timing of this symposium, do the investigations undertaken during the last two years strengthen or weaken the suggestion that low level lead exposure may be damaging to health?

In those connections it is important that we do not exaggerate the
difficulties. They are real enough but it would be quite wrong to
suppose that we know nothing. To the contrary, there are some
findings that are reasonably well established. However, we need to
differentiate between the factual evidence, the scientific inferences
based on that evidence, and the value-laden policy implications that
stem from the inferences. In my remarks, I will try to indicate
which is which.

LEAD IN THE ENVIRONMENT

Let me begin, as did the symposium, with the issues involved in the assessment of environmental lead pollution. It is obvious from all of the available evidence that the amount of lead in the environment today is far above that in ancient times. Dr. Patterson's elegant measurements (see chapter 2) suggest that the increase has been very great indeed. There is room for argument on the exact figures but the general message is not in dispute. It is also agreed that this increase is likely to be due to non-natural sources - that is from technological changes of one kind or other. The increase in environmental lead began many, many years before lead began to be added to petrol in 1923 and, hence, the initial huge rise cannot possibly be attributed to lead in petrol. Rather, it was the result of a host of other hazards, many of which are no longer relevant. But, that does not necessarily mean that petrol is not responsible for most of the pollution today. I will return to the evidence on that point in a moment. However, let me note first that the fact that the environment now contains a lot of lead does not necessarily mean that that matters. The fact that it is not 'natural' is not in itself grounds for action. Rather, we need to assess the actual risks.

That there are risks is all too evident from what is known about the neurotoxicity of lead, from the occasional cases of overt lead poisoning, and from the American surveys of a few years ago showing the substantial numbers of children with blood leads and, more recently, dentine leads above acceptable limits by any standard. The more difficult question concerns the particular level of body lead at which the risks become appreciable.

However, with respect to that issue, it is clear from the data presented by Drs. Annest and Billick (see chapters 3 and 4) that there has been a very substantial fall in blood lead levels in the USA during the last dozen years or so. Also, the findings from the EEC survey and from other British investigations show that the current blood lead levels in British children are well below those that applied in the US a few years ago when the concern over environmental lead first came to the fore. Thus, only one child in the Lansdown et al investigation (see chapter 14) had a blood lead as high as the average for Needleman's high dentine lead group (see chapter 12). Indeed, only a mere handful had blood lead levels as high as the average in Needleman's low lead group! The whole concept of low level lead exposure has had to change.

Of course, we need to ask whether this fall is a real one - could the drop be due to changing standards in laboratory measurement? In Dr. Annest's study (chapter 3) this possibility was examined systematically with the answer that the fall was real and not explicable in terms of changing standards.

The next question is: What has happened to bring about this very considerable fall in children's levels of blood lead? Drs. Annest and Billick were careful to point out the difficulties in coming to an answer to that question. It seems likely that some of the fall stems from actions taken to control lead contamination in canning and some from reductions in the use of high lead paints. But, equally, it is highly probable that much of the fall has been a consequence of the phasing out of lead in gasoline in the USA.

THE CONTRIBUTION OF LEAD IN PETROL

That leads to the further question of what proportion of lead intake in children stems from the lead in petrol. It is clear that estimates of this figure have varied widely. The Lawther report (Department of Health and Social Security, 1980) came to the conclusion that, in the population as a whole, the lead in petrol contributed only about 10 per cent of the body burden of lead - although, also, they emphasised that in 'hot spots' with particularly high levels of air lead, "such air lead concentrations may well make air lead the major contribution to uptake for some individuals" (p. 84). The report's estimate of 10% has been much criticised but it is necessary to recognise that it was based on a detailed analysis of empirical findings. The Committee noted the huge amounts of lead emitted into the atmosphere each year in the exhaust gases from petrol-engined vehicles; also, they pointed to the extremely high concentrations of air-borne lead at major traffic intersections (some 12 $\mu g/m^3$ on the M4 motorway compared with less than 0.1 $\mu g/m^3$ in most rural areas). Nevertheless, although the Committee pointed to the important hazards from airborne lead in certain areas, they concluded that, even in city dwellers the lead derived from vehicle emissions accounted for only "between 10 and 20% of blood lead" (p. 55). The main reasons for that conclusion were a) the empirical demonstration that the concentration of airborne lead decreases rapidly and markedly with distance away from roads (so that concentrations fall to about 20% of their kerbside value at a distance of 50 metres); b) that the reduction of the lead content of petrol in Germany from 0.4 to 0.15 g/l was associated with a marked reduction in kerbside concentrations of lead but with a lesser change in areas away from main roads; c) the evidence that inhaled lead contributes far less than ingested lead to the overall body burden of lead; and d) the repeated observation that most clinical cases of lead poisoning in children are associated with pica. Subsequent research has given no reason to doubt those four sets of findings. But, what has been called in question are the inferences based on them.

At the other end of the spectrum, Drs. Russell Jones and Stephens (Chapter 8) suggest that as much as 70 per cent, or even more, of body lead is likely to be derived from petrol. Their chapter usefully brings together the extensive body of evidence that points to the high probability that lead in petrol is a major contributor both to the overall level of lead in the environment and also to the lead that finds its way into the human body through a variety of different routes. In particular, they outline some of the main research findings that suggest that lead in petrol is a serious

contaminator of food and that, in most circumstances, the route of
ingestion constitutes a greater hazard in the population as a whole
than the route of inhalation.   I find those arguments convincing for
reasons that I explain below.   However, my opinion, like that of
most reviewers of this body of evidence, is that the available
empirical data are not sufficient to permit any quantitative estimate
of the contribution of lead in petrol to food, and hence that there
is no basis for precise estimates of the contribution to the overall
body burden of lead.   There are too many unknowns and too many
untested assumptions, for claims on quantification to be credible.
Nevertheless, I do think that the evidence strongly indicates that
lead in petrol is a much greater contributor than was suggested by
the Lawther Committee.

Four main sets of findings are relevant.   The first two sets concern
the routes by which airborne lead may enter the body and the
second two sets aim to provide more direct assessments of the
connections between changes in petrol lead and changes in blood
lead.   The Lawther Committee's estimate of a 10% contribution was
based on the implicit assumption that inhalation constituted the main
route by which petrol lead entered the body.   The findings
regarding lead contamination of dust and of food raise serious
doubts with respect to the validity of that assumption.

To begin with, there are the various studies suggesting that lead-
polluted street dust may be a more important vector for children
than for adults (see chapters 7 and 8; Duggan & Williams, 1977;
Mahaffey, 1978).   Young children play in the dirt, suck their
fingers, and eat sticky sweets to which dust readily adheres.
Clearly, this provides the possibility for substantial direct ingestion
of contaminated dust in early childhood – a route of negligible
relevance among adults.   But, to what extent does this actually
take place?   Several pieces of evidence indicate its likely
importance.   First, there is the finding that substantial amounts of
lead are indeed present on the hands of children - especially city
children (e.g. Vostal et al, 1974; Roels et al, 1980).   Second, it
has been found that whereas adult blood lead levels are not
consistently associated with the amount of lead in the soil,
children's blood lead levels are related to soil concentrations (e.g.
Barltrop et al., 1975; Jansen et al, 1978; Schmitt et al, 1979; Stark
et al, 1982; Yankel et al, 1977).   Third, peak lead levels tend to
be found during the toddler age period when children are both most
exposed to dust and tend to such their hands (see chapter 7).
Fourth, studies of children with raised blood lead levels have been
found to have higher hand-lead levels, to play more in the soil and
to suck their fingers more often than children with low lead levels
(e.g. Charney et al, 1980).   Moreover, in preschool children
household dust levels have been found to correlate significantly
with blood lead levels (Walter, Yankel and von Lindern, 1980).
Fifth, inter-group correlations show that in children, but not
adults, blood lead levels are more strongly associated with
hand-lead levels than with air-lead levels (Roels et al, 1980).
Duggan's conclusion (chapter 7) that the ingestion of urban dust

via dusty hands probably gives rise to a significant intake of lead
during early childhood seems justified. The correlations between
traffic density, air lead and dust lead indicate that in many
circumstances much of the lead in dust is likely to derive from
petrol (Chamberlain et al, 1978; Duggan and Williams, 1977;
Harrison, 1979; Jansen et al, 1978) although also it may derive from
paint (Ter Haar and Aronow, 1974; Stark et al, 1982) or from lead
smelters (Roels et al, 1980).

The second set of studies concern the effects of airborne lead in
the pollution of food (see chapter 8). The general view, until
recently, has been that this is of minor importance because it
mainly affects plants growing near major highways (which constitute
a small proportion of produce), because much of the air deposition
of lead is washed off by rain, and because most of the remainder is
removed during preparation, washing and cooking (Department of
Health and Social Security, 1980). These assumptions now seem
questionable. In the first place, it is clear that petrol combustion
produces very small particles of lead that can carry very long
distances indeed (Chamberlain et al, 1979). Although, of course, it
is well established that air lead levels are very much higher in
areas of high traffic flow (Department of Health and Social
Security, 1980), nevertheless the dispersion of fine lead particles is
widespread. Secondly, with at least some (but not all) plant
surfaces it has proved quite difficult to remove lead particles by
ordinary washing techniques (Arvik and Zimdahl, 1974; Lagerwerff
et al, 1973); Schuck and Locke, 1970).

However, the most important reason for querying the assumption
that airborne lead contributes little to the lead in food is of a
rather different kind in that it focuses attention on the cumulative
effect of minor lead deposition in <u>all</u> areas, rather than on the
major deposition in the few high risk areas. The argument runs as
follows. Because improved techniques have shown that the levels of
lead in the environment during prehistoric times were a tiny
fraction of those today (see chapter 1), it would seem that the
'natural' level of lead in the environment is very low and hence that
most of the lead in food is likely to derive from industrial sources.
That poses the questions of where the extraneous lead comes from
and how it gets into the food. So far as plants are concerned, the
lead may be found in the plant cells themselves or on the surface of
the plant. It seems that there is very little lead absorption from
plant surfaces into the plant structure (Koeppi, 1981). However,
because lead from air deposition may stick to the surface quite
tenaciously it appears that at least half the total lead in plants
derives from airborne sources (Crump and Barlow, 1980). Because
it is clear that most (probably about 80-90 per cent) of airborne
lead comes from petrol (Nriagu, 1979), it follows that the bulk of
surface lead stems from petrol. Nevertheless, one experimental
study (Ter Haar, 1970) showed that variations in air lead make
little difference to the lead concentration of the edible portions of
many crops. The amount of lead that plants can take in from
contaminated soil remains somewhat uncertain (and certainly varies

by plant and according to soil conditions) but it appears that most lead accumulates in the roots with limited transfer to fruits and leaves (Koeppi, 1981; Zimdahl, 1976).   On the other hand, in experimental studies controlling for air levels; it has been found that high levels of lead in soil are associated with substantial translocations to plant tissues, at least in the roots (Spittler and Feder, 1979).   The extent to which petrol lead contributes to soil pollution varies greatly according to circumstances; in some it constitutes an important contributor but in others a quite minor one.

It is obvious that arguments on the overall contribution of petrol lead to food are circumstantial.   It is apparent that airborne lead can and does contaminate plants to a substantial extent and it is likely that this makes a substantial contribution to the lead in food. It is not possible to quantify the contribution but it is implausible that it is as trivial as previously assumed.

The third set of studies are not concerned with how petrol lead enters the body but rather seek to estimate its contribution to the body burden of lead through the study of change.   The pertinent findings in this connection stem from the recent American studies (see chapters 2 and 3) showing close parallels over the last decade between the timing and extent of the reduction of lead in gasoline and the marked drop in blood lead levels in the population as a whole.

The size of the drop, its timing, and the pattern of seasonal variations, together with the very high correlation over time between gasoline lead consumption and blood lead levels, all point to the probability that the phasing out of lead in gasoline was a major contributor to the important drop in blood levels.   Of course, it is likely that other factors also played a significant role, and the evidence pointing to the contribution of gasoline has some puzzling features.   Thus, the fall in blood lead values began shortly before the introduction of regulations on lead-free gasoline.   However, here, the change to smaller cars and to fuel with a lower octane level is likely to have been influential.   Also, it is curious that the fall has not been greater in cities than in rural areas.   Insofar as dust ingestion by children and inhalation by all age groups represent routes of intake, a greater fall in cities might be expected.   However, insofar as airborne lead enters the body as a result of food contamination, rather than through inhalation, perhaps a large urban-rural differential should not be anticipated. It should be added that the lesser reduction in petrol-lead in Germany resulted in only a 10 per cent fall in the blood leads of adults (Sinn, 1980; 1981), and that there has been an apparent (but not certain) slight fall in blood leads in the UK over the last decade in spite of a lack of change in the proportion of lead in petrol (Oxley, 1982).   Although, in their chapters, Drs. Annest and Billick suggest that regulations on lead-free gasoline have made a major contribution to the fall in blood lead values, they point out that public health campaigns other than these regulations have also

played a role, and that the data do not allow any precise quantitative estimate of the contribution of petrol engine emissions to the
overall body burden of lead. Nevertheless, it seems most unlikely
that that contribution is as low as 10 per cent. Indeed, statistical
modelling suggests that the data are consistent with a 46%
contribution (I.C.F., 1982).

Lastly, there is the preliminary evidence from the Italian isotopic
lead experiment (Facchetti, 1979). Because petrol additives were
derived from lead with a known, and different, isotopic ratio it was
possible to trace the lead stemming from such additives and hence
to determine its relative contribution to the overall lead in both the
environment and the body. The reported findings indicate that the
isotopic ratio changes in air lead closely paralleled those in petrol
lead; this was strikingly so in Turin but it was marked even in the
countryside. These findings confirm that petrol is responsible for
a very high proportion of the lead in air. Ths isotopic ratio
charges in blood lead were smaller and it was calculates that about
24 per cent of the blood lead in the adult population of Turin (the
test area) came from petrol. This figure does not represent the
total contribution of petrol lead bacause: a) it is likely that the
Turin inhabitants will have eaten food contaminated by petrol lead
from areas outside Turin (and hence not included in the isotopic
change); and b) the fall in blood isotopic ratio was still continuing
after that of airbourne lead had reached a plateau. Also most of
the data apply to adults and it is not known whether comparable
figures would be obtained for children. As the authors of this
study point out, there must be caution in the interpretation of their
findings because of the limited sampling, uncertainties on the
contribution of petrol not included in the isotope change, and the
lack of data on dietary lead. However, it seems probable that all
of these features mean that the figure of 24% is an under, rather
than an over-estimate of the contribution of petrol.

Taken as a whole, the evidence clearly indicates that petrol
accounts for a substantial proportion of the overall variance in
environmental lead. Moreover, it may well be that petrol contributes more to the body burden of lead in early childhood than it
does in adult life. The empirical facts do not allow any precise
estimate of the size of that contribution and, in the present state of
knowledge, not much is to be gained by attempts to derive any
such figure. The Lawther Committee estimate of 10 per cent
appears much too low in the light of recent evidence, but it is not
possible to determine how much higher the figure should be.

There are too many unknowns and too many inconsistencies for this
to be a sensible enterprise on the basis of existing data. Because
some workers have argued to the contrary (see chapter 8), it may
be worthwhile to note just a few of the main types of problems.
The most important is that the calculations depend on estimates of
the contributions of other known sources; it is then suggested that
the major proportion left unaccounted for must be due to petrol lead
because we know of no other source. That is always a hazardous

line of reasoning and it is so here. Secondly, there is a lack of
any direct study of the contribution of petrol lead to food. Taking
the parallel with the approach used by Drs. Annest and Billick,
one method would be to determine if changes over time in the level
of lead in food covary with changes in petrol lead emission. One
Danish study that did just that (Solgaard et al, 1978) produced the
surprising finding that as petrol lead emission was increasing there
was a decrease in food leads. In view of the concerns expressed
by Dr. Patterson (chapter 2) regarding the serious errors in
measurement of low levels of leads, the finding cannot necessarily
be taken at face value. But, still, it provides a puzzle. Thirdly,
as already noted, there is both uncertainty and disagreement on the
relative importance of uptake from soil and surface deposition as
contributors to plant lead (as well as uncertainty on the importance
of petrol lead as a soil pollutant). Fourthly, very substantial
amounts of lead may be added to food as a result of the canning
process (Settle and Patterson, 1980; Tolan and Elton, 1973; U.S.
Food and Drug Administration, 1975) and of cooking in water with a
high lead content (Little et al, 1981; Moore et al, 1979; Smart et al,
1981). Estimates of the average dietary intake of lead from these
sources vary (and of course, they will differ according to circumstances) but it seems likely that, especially for babies with a high
intake of tinned foods, the figure may be higher than sometimes
supposed. Fifthly, both the Annest and Billick findings are limited
by their lack of data on non-gasoline sources of environmental lead
and hence by their inability to assess the impact of other lead
exposure mitigation programmes. Also it is puzzling that Billick
found air lead higher in the summer than in the winter whereas
several other studies (U.S. Environmental Protection Agency, 1982)
have shown the reverse. Sixthly, as discussed in chapter 8, much
of the research on the relative importance of soil uptake and of
atmospheric deposition with regard to the lead content of plants
derives from the use of radioactive ^{210}Pb added to soil as a tracer
of soil uptake processes. The findings are imformative and useful
but the chemical form and plant availability of added ^{210}Pb are not
identical to those of the stable lead in the soil (Harrison, 1982).
As a result some caution is needed in the extrapolation of findings
from the one to the other.

Lastly, the Frankfurt findings (Sinn, 1980; 1981) suggest a lesser
effect from the lead in gasoline than that indicated by the American
findings (chapters 2 and 3). Of course, too, caution is needed in
extrapolating to Europe from American data when blood lead levels
in the U.S.A. tend to be so much higher than those in the U.K.
One might ask in addition why blood lead levels are higher in the
U.S.A., which has introduced regulations that have markedly
reduced lead in gasoline, than in Britain which has yet to do so.
The literature is full of puzzles and inconsistencies of this kind. It
is possible to find explanations for most of them and in their
chapter Russell Jones and Stephens put forward their reasons for
rejecting findings that seem not to support the hypothesis that
petrol lead is the major contributor to the overall body burden of
lead. They may well be correct in their arguments but it has to be
said that different explanations are also possible.

Nevertheless, in my view, although these difficulties prevent any accurate estimate of the contribution of petrol to body lead, they fall far short of any serious detraction from the general thesis that it is a major, probably the major, contributor. Certainly, it is apparent that the removal of lead from petrol - or, rather, the prohibition of the addition of lead to petrol would result in a significant and worthwhile reduction in environmental lead. It is important, too, to appreciate that much of the intake of lead from petrol does not occur through inhalation but through the ingestion of lead polluted food and dust. The implication is that living in a rural area away from motorways may not help as much as once was thought.

But, there have to be serious reservations about the whole business of coming to any one overall estimate, because it is bound to be wrong for many people (see U.S. Committee on Lead in Human Environment, 1980). The point is that the estimate crucially depends on the ambient sources of lead and that this varies from individual to individual. Of course, the figures will vary with the degree of atmospheric pollution from petrol - those for rural New Zealand are scarcely likely to be the same as those for central London where the atmospheric lead concentration is 100 times as high. Similarly, the contribution of petrol will be greater for those living near a busy major highway than for those with homes in a rural area, but even within the former group the role of petrol will be much greater for toddlers than for adults. However, at least as important, the figures will vary according to other sources of lead. In some situations, it has been clear that lead smelters have constituted the main source of lead uptake, to the extent of being a serious health hazard (Landrigan et al, 1975; Yankel et al, 1977). In others it has been apparent that the children of lead workers gain most of their lead from contaminated clothing brought into the home - again to the extent of causing serious lead intoxication (Baker et al, 1977). If during the 1970s you were living in south-west Scotland in a house with lead plumbing and soft water, your main source of lead would have been drinking water - as indicated by Dr. Moore's studies (chapter 5). But this is not a significant problem in London. If you are a young child with pica living in a house with crumbling high lead paint, then undoubtedly the ingestion of paint will be the main source.

The implication is that the removal of lead from petrol is one public health action that would reduce environmental lead, but there are others of more importance to some children (although perhaps less important in the population as a whole). These need equal attention. Moreover, such evidence as is available suggests that the sources may vary according to body lead level. Studies of children with moderate or relatively high levels of body lead indicate that in most cases the lead intoxication stems from pica (especially the eating of lead paint peelings), from cosmetics, or from other more 'personalised' sources of lead ingestion or exposure. This is shown by the very high rates of pica in clinic studies of children treated for frank lead poisoning (Lin-Fu, 1973) by lead isotope studies in

young children with both high lead levels and pica (Ter Haar and
Aronow, 1974), but the associations between paint hazards and
faecal lead excretion (Hammond et al, 1980) and also by Needleman's
finding that, whereas nearly a third of his high lead group showed
pica, only one in nine of his low lead group did so (see chapter
12). The environmental lead that stems from petrol probably
constitutes but a minor contribution to lead exposure in most
individual cases of moderate or high lead toxicity (although it may
add to the body lead burden by virtue of children's ingestion of
polluted dust). However, it constitutes a much more major cause of
lower level lead exposure, which is only very weakly associated
with pica. The implication is that the Lawther Committee were right
to argue that, as well as progressively taking lead out of petrol,
there should be vigorous action to deal with non-airborne sources
of lead contamination in the environment. On the other hand, it
now seems that they very substantially underestimated the risks
from lead in petrol.

EFFECTS OF LEAD ON BEHAVIOUR AND INTELLIGENCE

Let me turn now to the central issue of whether relatively low
levels of lead exposure in childhood may lead to intellectual
impairment or disturbances of behaviour. The research prior to
1980 has been extensively reviewed several times (e.g. Rutter,
1980; U.S. Committee on Lead in the Human Environment, 1980;
U.S. Environmental Protection Agency, 1977) and it appears that
the factual findings are reasonably straightforward. That is to
say, the great majority (but not quite all) investigations have found
slight but significant differences between the intelligence and
behaviour of childen with high lead levels compared with those of
children with low lead levels (whether assessed on the basis of
blood or tooth measurements). These findings are not in any
reasonable doubt but there has been much dispute on the interpretations to be placed on them. Three issues have dominated that
debate: first, the uncertainty as to whether the statistical associations reflect a causal effect such that high lead produces a drop in
IQ or an increase in inattentive disruptive behaviour; secondly, the
uncertainty on the level of lead exposure at which such effects may
occur; and, thirdly, doubts on the reliability and validity of both
the measures of body lead burden and measures of neuropsychological impairment. In my own 1980 review I concluded that: "it is
very likely that psychological impairment occurs in some asymptomatic children with repeated blood lead levels in the 40 to 80 μg/100
ml range, and that it is possible (although much less certain) that
impairment sometimes occurs at levels lower than 40"(p.21). Before
reappraising the evidence as a whole, it is appropriate to note
briefly the new evidence that has become available during the last
two years.

New Evidence. Much of that research is reported in other chapters
of this volume. Thus, Needleman (Chapter 12) described further
analyses based on his epidemiological study in Massachusetts.
These demonstrated that the associations between lead level and

psychological impairment were not explicable in terms of pica as a confounding variable; in addition, associations between lead level and neurophysiological measures were reported. Also, new data on systematic classroom observations were provided. These showed that inattentive behaviour was more frequent in the high lead than in the low lead group - validating the earlier teacher's ratings. While, necessarily, these further findings do not resolve all doubts regarding the causal interpretation, they make that hypothesis more plausible.

Winneke's (chapter 13) new data from his Stolberg study add very greatly to those from his earlier pilot study in Duisburg. It is clear that considerable care was taken over measurement and methodology, and that rigorous control over confounding variables was provided. The findings, once again, showed significant associations between tooth lead levels and various measures of psychological functioning. Three aspects of Winneke's research warrant special emphasis. First, the associations on some of the key measures remained even after possibly confounding social variables had been taken fully into account. It should be noted, too, that the 4½ point verbal IQ difference (after correction) between his high lead and low lead groups, although statistically non-significant, was very closely comparable to that reported by Needleman. The finding emphasises both the high consistency of findings across studies and also the need for a very large sample size if small effects are to be detected. Second, these associations apply to lead levels well below the supposedly safe limit of 35 µg/dl attributed to Lawther report recommendations (Department of Health and Social Security, 1980). Third, the differential pattern of findings after controlling for confounding variables has implications for the possible mechanisms by which raised lead levels predispose to psychological impairment (a point discussed more fully below).

Lansdown et al (chapter 14) reported the findings from a new study in London undertaken as a result of the Lawther committee's advice that further research was particularly needed to investigate the possibility of psychological sequelae as a result of low level lead exposure. Their results are important in terms of a) the demon- stration of the associations between psychological measures and lead at quite low levels, far below the 35 µg/dl cut off; b) the replica- tion of Needleman's findings with respect to the particular behavioural measures used; and c) the finding of a dose-response gradient. Nevertheless, as they point out, caution in the interpretation of these results is needed because the sample size was relatively small, the lead measure was confined to a single blood sample, and their measure of the children's psychosocial environment was relatively crude.

In many respects, David's chelation study (chapter 15) provides the most convincing evidence to date on the behavioural improvements associated with an experimental reduction in lead levels. The importance of this evidence lies in the especial value of studies of change as a means of investigating causal relationships. It is very difficult, when dealing with children and families who have come to the clinic to seek help, to ensure the degree of control that is desirable to test causal hypotheses. As a consequence there are limitations in the design of this study (the drop-outs from treatment, the departures from a strictly randomized design, and the lack of evidence on whether the within-group changes in blood level correlated with behaviour change) that leave some doubts on the causal interpretation of the findings. Even so, the results certainly point to the possibility of a causal effect.

Finally, Otto and his colleagues (chapter 16) gave findings relating computer analyzed EEG data to blood lead levels in the range 6 to 55 μg/dl in a group of young children from a socially disadvantaged background. Earlier results from this study had been reported previously (Benignus et al, 1981; Otto et al, 1981,) but the chapter added new data based on a reassessment of a subsample of 28 children for whom further EEG recordings were available two years later. The particular importance of this work lies in its demonstration that there is a dose response relationship between blood lead levels and measures of neurophysiological functioning. The fact that multivariate analyses showed a significant effect of lead on slow wave voltage at the follow-up, as well as initially, gives one some confidence that the effect is likely to be meaningful one. However, as Otto et al point out, there are no normative data for these EEG measures in young children and their functional significance remains uncertain. Moreover, the EEG findings showed a complicated relationship with age; also the pattern of results at the follow-up were not directly comparable with those obtained earlier. Clearly, Otto and his colleagues are right to emphasise the caveats in the interpretation of their data. On the other hand, the study was carefully conducted and the findings are provocative in their implications of effects at quite low levels of blood lead.

In addition to the research reported in earlier chapters of this volume, there have been other studies published during the last two years that are relevant to the investigation of the neuro-psychological sequelae of low level lead exposure. Probably, the most important of these are the investigations undertaken by Ernhart, by Thatcher and by Milar. Perino and Ernhart (1974) had previously compared 30 asymptomatic children with lead levels in the 40 to 70 μg/dl range with 50 children showing levels in the 10 to 30 range. They reported that blood lead levels were significantly related to children's scores on the McCarthy Scales (a measure of intellectual performance), and even after taking account of parental intelligence and the children's birth weight. In their further study, Ernhart and her colleagues (1981) re-examined 63 of the original sample of 80, with further psychological and lead assessments. The blood lead values correlated moderately well (0.46) with those obtained five years earlier but the mean level had dropped from 32.5 to 26.9 with a restriction in the range. As in the original analysis, the mean IQ of the low lead group (93.9) was significantly higher than that of the moderate lead group (81.6). Moreover, the concurrent blood lead measure still showed a

significant association with IQ after partialling out the effects of
sex, parental IQ and parental education. The proportion of the IQ
variance explained (7.7%) was substantially less that (17.6%)
observed before controlling for confounding variables and much less
than that (20.8%) accounted for by parental IQ, although more than
that (5.2%) attributable to parental education. No associations were
found between lead levels and five individual items of Conners
scale.

The authors concluded that: "the few statistically significant
findings of this study are due to methodologic difficulties inherent
in this area of research". However, that seems an unwarranted
inference for several rather different reasons. Firstly, it is
standard scientific practice to place most weight on the best
measures. In this connection, it is relevant that it was the more
reliable and valid general cognitive index that showed a lead effect,
and some of the individual subscales that did not. Secondly, also
it is standard practice to pay attention to the overall pattern of
findings. In that connection, it is pertinent that, of the 4
McCarthy subtests that showed a significant association with lead
before correction for confounding variables, two did so afterwards
(and the two that did not show a non-significant trend in the same
direction). Thirdly, in the original analysis, weight was placed on
the finding that the parent IQ - child IQ correlation in the
moderate lead group (.10) was lower than that in the low lead
group (.52), suggesting that lead toxicity may have interfered with
the usual indication of heritability. In their re-analysis, the
difference (.33 versus .48) was no longer statistically significant.
However, the direction of difference was similar in spite of the fact
that the analysis was inappropriately based on the children's
pre-school lead levels (which, after correction, did not correlate
with the follow-up IQ) rather than their current levels (which did
correlate with IQ). Fourthly, although Ernhart (1982) argued,
citing Reichardt (1979), that with analysis of covariance "results
are inescapably undercorrected" (p. 219), that is not so.
Reichardt's thoughtful discussion of the problems of controlling for
confounding variables with non-equivalent groups emphasizes that
"there are ample sources of overadjustment bias" (p. 164). He
does make the point that, with a single covariate, errors in the
measurement of the covariate tend to lead to under-correction
biases. But, equally, he goes on to show that the situation is
rather different when multiple covariates are used (as they were in
the Ernhart et al study) - "the bias in the analyses can either be
an overadjustment or an underadjustment" (p. 174).

The more appropriate conclusion from Ernhart et al's (1981)
empirical findings is that their results are in reasonably good
agreement with those of other investigators. That is, they show
that blood lead levels in the 27 to 49 µg/dl range (mean = 32.4)
when compared with those in the <26 range (mean = 21.3), show a
significant association with IQ even after controlling for confounding
variables. However, an important part of the raw lead level/IQ
association is due to confounding variables rather than lead per se

and, after correction, the IQ effect is quite small, although not insignificant in its implications.

The second new investigation not covered in earlier chapters is Thatcher et al's (1982) hair lead study of 149 rural school-age children in the U.S.A., subjects being recruited through newspaper advertisements. Hair was taken from the nape of the neck as close to the scalp as possible and sent to the Food and Drug Administration Laboratory in Washington, D.C., for analysis. Wechsler Intelligence Scale and Wide Range Achievement Test scores were used to divide the population in quartiles. Hierarchical regression analyses showed that hair lead was significantly associated with IQ after regressing out the possible confounding effects of age, sex, race and socioeconomic status. In general, this appears a well conducted study but it suffers from the lack of control over sampling biases, limited data on social factors and no indexing of the hair lead data against blood lead measures. Nevertheless, the findings are consistent with those of other studies and are of particular interest with respect to their derivation from a rural population.

The other important study not included in this volume is that by Milar and his colleagues (1980; 1981) based on the same sample as that used by Otto et al (1981; also chapter 16). Milar et al (1980) found that their high lead and low lead groups differed substantially in the quality of their caregiving environment at home - a difference that needs to be taken into account in any analysis of the relationship between lead exposure and psychological functioning. In addition, a detailed investigation (Milar et al, 1981) was made of the children's activity level using a standardized observation of playroom behaviour, as well as the Werry-Weiss-Peters and Conners parental rating scales. No differences according to lead level were found for any of the measures of hyperactivity (even before correcting for the family background characteristics). The study was well conducted but the negative finding is difficult to interpret in that differences would be expected on the basis of the home background features associated with high lead levels, quite apart from the lead exposure. The results are important but it may well be that the lack of difference reflects the lack of validity of the hyperactivity measures in the age group studied, as an index of the attentional deficits hypothesized to be associated with lead exposure. Of the 88 children studied, 54 were under the age of 3 years. Also, it should be noted that the attentional deficits linked with lead exposure in the Needleman and in the Lansdown et al studies (chapters 12 and 14 referred to the children's behaviour at school, rather than at home. Further research is needed to determine the reasons for these apparently discrepant findings.

In summary, the new evidence since 1980 has been generally consistent in pointing to significant effects at the low levels of lead exposure (below 40 µg/dl) where there was most doubt on the basis

of the earlier studies (see Rutter, 1980). Also, the recent investigations have been able to demonstrate that the effects tend to be
maintained (although substantially reduced) after control for
possible confounding variables. However, in addition, they
confirmed earlier findings in their indication that the effects on
psychological functioning tend to be relatively small.

It should be added that, also, there have been advances in
experimental studies of lead exposure in animals. Much of the
earlier research investigated the effects of lead at levels so high
that it was scarcely surprising that adverse sequelae were found
and, often, the effects of lead exposure were seriously confounded
with the effects of severe undernutrition (see Bornschein et al,
1977 and 1980; Mahaffey and Michaelson, 1980). This, together with
species- differences in response (see chapter 10), made many
workers reluctant to place much weight on animal research as a
means of understanding effects on humans. As pointed out in
earlier chapters, caution in the extrapolation of findings from rats
to humans is still essential. On the other hand, recent studies
have both used the lower levels of lead exposure and have dealt
with many of the methodological problems in the earlier research.
The result has been the beginnings of an accumulation of evidence
that measurable effects on neural development and on behaviour may
be evident with blood levels in the 20 to 40 µg/dl range as well as
at higher levels (see e.g. Bull et al, 1979; Grant et al, 1980;
Kimmel et al, 1980; McCauley et al, 1979).

Measurement Issues. As noted above, earlier reviews have pointed
to the problems stemming from doubts on the quality of the
available measures of both body lead burden and of
neuropsychological functioning. It is important to recognize that
the main doubts have been concerned with the amount of random
error in these measures, rather than the presence of systematic
bias. Accordingly, in so far as errors have been present, they
will have tended to result in an under-rather than an over-estimate
of the effects of lead. Nevertheless, the concern over measurement
issues is real and important. With respect to blood leads, the main
worry has stemmed from the fact that these reflect only the very
recent ingestion of lead, and do not provide a satisfactory guide to
the overall body burden. This constitutes a major drawback when
studying the effects of acute lead exposure but, in practice, it has
proved to be much less of a problem when studying chronic
exposure (the much more usual situation). As discussed in other
chapters, blood lead levels up to 5 years apart have shown
correlations in the 0.4 to 0.6 range. Accordingly, single blood lead
estimates have provided a better index of lead exposure than
sometimes supposed. Even so, it it obvious that multiple
assessments spread over time are to be preferred.

The problems with dentine lead and tooth lead are rather different
as they do reflect the body burden of lead as accumulated over
time. Here, the concerns have been over problems of
inter-laboratory agreement on techniques and measures, over the

lack of concordance between different tooth samples, and over possible biases stemming from the factors that influence when children shed teeth. The first technical problem is now less than it was a few years ago, although the measurement techniques have not yet reached the standards achieved for blood lead. The problem of discordance between teeth samples remains but, for the moment, the procedure of reliance on cases where good concordance has been achieved between at least two samples seems the most appropriate. The nature and extent of biases associated with variations in the timing of loss of teeth are, as yet, largely unexplored.

Hair, too, has been used for lead analyses (Gibson, 1980; Grandjean, 1978. It has the major advantage of ease of access and sample stability, but the considerable disadvantage of possible external contamination by the atmosphere,hand dirt, and hair preparations. Less is known on the validity of hair lead analyses than on tooth and blood measures and the potential has yet to be assessed adequately.

It may be concluded that progress is being made on matters of measurement of body lead and that, although some difficulties remain, the standards of measurement are adequate for the purposes of assessment of the neuropsychological sequelae of increased lead exposure – at least in the upper ranges of so-called low level exposure.

The problems involved in neuropsychological assessment are discussed more fully elsewhere (Chadwick and Rutter, 1983; Yule and Rutter, 1983). In brief, the main concerns are: i) doubts as to just what is being measured on some of the less well standardized and validated tests; ii) the unreliability of many individual subtests; iii) the difficulties that stem from using a large number of measures, which are likely to give rise to at least a few statistically significant differences as a result of chance alone (because of the multiple comparisons); and iv) the poor sensitivity of most screening tests. There is no one entirely satisfactory solution to these problems, but reasonable confidence can be placed on the overall scores of the well standardized broad range IQ tests (such as the Wechsler scale), particularly if these are supplemented by appropriate tests of more specialized neuropsychological functions and if appropriate multivariate procedures are used to assess statistical significance when multiple tests are used. Many of the more recent studies meet thes criteria, and it is evident that now the means are available to reach sufficient standards of measurement – with respect to both lead and neuropsychological functioning – for the research findings to be meaningful.

CAUSAL HYPOTHESES

There are several different types of evidence that may be used to evaluate causal hypotheses about lead effects. Dr Lansdown and his colleagues, in their chapter, helpfully drew attention to Bradford Hill's (1977) list of requirements for inferring a cause and

effect relationship from data of this kind. Let me, too, turn to his
guidelines in order to consider the problems in or objections to the
causal hypothesis.

Consistency. Firstly, there is the question of the consistency of
the observed association - has it been repeatedly noted in different
investigations using different research strategies? The short
answer on that point is 'yes, the observed associations have been
reasonably consistent', and this lends some support to the causal
inference.

Biological Gradient. Secondly, there is the matter of a biological
gradient or dose response curve. In other words, if there were a
causal relationship it would be expected that low levels of lead
would have minor effects, moderate levels of lead should have
rather greater effects, and high levels of lead should have the
greatest effect of all. As Dr Winneke noted (chapter 13), this is a
particularly important point, as the failure to find a dose-response
relationship undoubtedly would cast serious doubt on the causal
hypothesis. With respect to most investigations there is some
evidence of a dose-response relationship within each study. The
problem is that there is a lack of consistency with respect to the
biological gradient if results are compared across studies. For
example, the difference in IQ in the investigation by Needleman and
his colleagues (chapter 12 was of much the same order as that
found by Lansdown et al (chapter 14 or by Winneke (chapter 13)
dealing with much lower levels of lead; moreover the size of the
difference in lead levels in different studies seems to bear little, if
any, relationship to the difference in IQ between high and low lead
groups found.

There is no doubt that this does pose somewhat of dilemmma.
Nevertheless, personally, I am somewhat less inclined to place
weight on the lack of a dose-response relationship across studies
than I was two years ago. I think that there are at least three
major possible explanations for the disparity between the
within-sample and across-sample results. The first consideration is
that the comparisons across studies have not used the same
standard. What has been defined as 'low lead' group in one
investigation has been a 'high lead group in others. Thus, the
mean blood lead level for Needleman et al's (1979) low lead sample
was 23.8 µg.dl, wheras in Lansdown et al's study (chapter 14) the
high lead group was definedin terms of a level above 13 µg.dl!
Dose response gradients can be compared across studies only if like
is being compared with like - that is if the low-level or control
group is comparable in all cases - which manifestly it is not in the
lead studies. The Lawther Committee attempted to circumvent that
problem by comparing the within-group IQ difference with the
within-group lead level difference (Department of Health and Social
Security, 1980). But, as they pointed out, that exercise demanded
assumptions of equivalence across different IQ tests, different age
groups and different measures of lead level - a very dubious
procedure indeed.

The second issue stems from the fact that it is known, with both intelligence and behaviour, that there are numerous other powerful influences. Moreover, the strength and patterning of these other influences is likely to vary greatly from sample to sample. The effects of lead at different doses can be compared meaningfully only if such non-lead factors are constant across investigations which, obviously, has not been the case. Because lead is never more than a minor contributor to the overall variance (a point discussed further below), a consistent dose-response relationship across studies is not to be anticipated.

Thirdly, there is not a very close degree of comparability between different approaches to the measurement of lead. There is a reasonable association between blood leads, dentine leads and tooth leads but there is no easy and straightforward way of translating one into another. Generally high levels of agreement are now obtainable between different laboratories for blood lead levels, provided that the laboratories have good experience in these estimations and take the necessary precautions. But it is apparent that the quality of measurement has not been uniformly high in all published reports (Vahter, 1982). Moreover, the analysis of dentine lead and tooth lead have been developed more recently and there is not agreement, as yet, on the most effective technique.

Probably the only reasonable conclusion to be drawn at the moment is that methodological difficulties invalidate dose-response comparisons across studies in terms of currently published data. The research strategy remains a potentially valuable one but it has yet to be exploited effectively. In the meanwhile, we are forced to rely on the regularity of dose-response relationship within studies. Those data are sparse but, on the whole, they are consistent with the causal argument.

Biological Plausibility. Thirdly, there is the equally important matter of biological plausibility. That is to say, do the research findings indicate a likely biological mechanism by which the causal effect could be mediated. The crucial issue with respect to lead is whether, at levels of lead short of those associated with clinical signs and symptoms, there is evidence of impaired biological functioning. The evidence on this point needs to be subdivided into that deriving from human studies and that stemming from animal experiments, The human evidence is more directly applicable but it is more sparse and less certain in its implications. Nevertheless, there are findings suggestive of biological impairment. In adults, Seppäläinen (1978; Seppäläinen et al, 1975; Seppäläinen and Hernberg, 1980) found that nerve conduction velocities were impaired in subjects with blood leads greater than 50 µg/dl - an observation in keeping with the well established effect of high doses of lead as a cause of peripheral neuropathy. Other investigators (e.g., Araki and Honma 1976; Feldman et al, 1973; Landrigan et al, 1975) have found impaired peripheral nerve conduction velocities at somewhat lower levels in both children and adults.

In a computer assisted spectrum analysis of the EEG in a subsample
of Needleman's study, Burchfiel et al (1980) found that high lead
children had significantly increased amounts of low-frequency delta
activity and significantly decreased amounts of alpha. The results
are important in their implication that, at relatively low levels of
lead exposure, there are neurophysiological changes that could
serve as a mediating mechanism for the psychological and
behavioural symptoms attributed to lead. However, that argument
would be stronger if it could be shown that the neurophysiological
features were themselves related to the psychological deficits. The
published findings are consistent with that possibility but the
association has not been tested directly as yet. It should be added
that caution is required in extrapolating from the findings –
because they are based on a small select sample, because the
statistical significance of the multivariate analyses varied according
to the test used (being significant on one but not on the other)
and because there is uncertainty regarding the functional meaning
of the EEG changes.

Nevertheless, the results seem to be broadly in keeping with those
of Otto and his associated (Otto et al, 1981; Benignus et al, 1981;
also chapter 16) in their investigation of 1-6 year old children with
blood lead levels in the 7-59 µg/dl range, most of whom were from
low income black families. Using a passive conditioning paradigm to
elicit slow brain potentials, it was found that the slow wave voltage
during sensory conditioning varied as a linear function of blood
lead level – that is there was no detectable threshold and effects
were evident at levels below 30 µg/dl. Power spectra analyses of
the EEG in the same group of children showed a curvilinear
relationship between lead levels and the relative amplitude of
synchronized EEG – such that there was a sharp increase in gain
below 15 µg/dl, a levelling off, a slight decrease between 30 and
40 µg/dl and then a sharp rise above 40 µg/dl. Follow-up data two
years after the initial assessment (Chapter 16) again showed a
significant effect of lead on slow wave voltage but did not confirm
the earlier power spectra findings. In view of the lack of
knowledge on either the physiological meaning or the functional
significance of these changes, no firm conclusions on biological
mechanisms are possible. However, these three groups of studies
are consistent in showing neurophysiological patterns that have a
systematic association with lead levels – an association that is
apparent both above and below the cut-off 30-35 µg/dl sometimes
claimed to represent a safety limit.

The evidence from animal studies is succinctly reviewed by Dr
Silbergeld in chapters 10 and 11. It is apparent that a variety of
rather different effects have been found to be associated with lead.
One of the best documented effects concerns inhibition of the haeme
biosynthetic pathway – an effect that is measurable at levels of lead
below 30 µg/dl (Chisolm et al, 1975). In addition, lead has effects
on several neurotransmitters and has been found to delay brain
development in rat pups exposed to quite modest levels of lead in
the neonatal period (Bull et al, 1979; McCauley et al, 1979). The

behavioural effects of raised lead levels has been demonstrated in terms of adverse effects on learning. Nevertheless, the precise functional significance of the various neurochemical and other effects associated with raised lead levels remains uncertain. The animal experiments provide a convincing case that there are important biological consequences of lead exposure at levels well below those associated with clinical signs and symptoms of lead poisoning. Furthermore, the findings are important in their failure to find any clear threshold below which ill-effect are not found. In most of the investigations, the levels of lead studied were above 30 μg/dl (although direct extrapolation from blood levels in rats to those in humans is an uncertain business), but in some investigations changes were recorded below that level and, in many more, abnormalities were found in animals not showing any overt behavioural changes. We may conclude that increased levels of body lead can and do cause impairment of biological functioning at levels below those associated with recognizable signs and symptoms attributable to lead toxicity.

What remains somewhat uncertain, however, is whether such impairment is responsible for any of the psychological or behavioural changes associated with levels of blood lead below 30 μg/dl in children. That it could be is clear, whether in fact it is so remains less certain. Dr David's important chelation study (Chapter 15) raises difficult issues here. At first sight, it seems to suggest that the fall in blood lead associated with treatment had had direct behavioural benefits, and it may have done. However, the animal evidence suggests that it is unlikely that the chelation had reduced brain lead. So why had the slight drop in blood lead had such a rapid effect in behaviour? Indeed, was the improvement in behaviour even a result of the reduction in blood lead and, if it was, would it persist? We do not know. Nevertheless, the findings are provocative and if the mechanisms remain obscure this provides a good reason for the issue to be investigated further.

Thus, the evidence considered as a whole is compatible with the suggestion that low level lead exposure might cause some form of biological impairment, but that is about as much that can be said. In short, the biological plausibility evidence provides some support for the causal inference, but more research is required to determine the links between impairment of biological systems and the psychological sequelae, particularly at the levels of lead currently applicable to children in the UK.

Other Traumata. Another important issue is the extent to which the causal inference is in keeping with what is known about the ways in which biological systems function generally and what is known about the effects of other traumata or agents thought to act in a comparable manner. The main difficulty, here, with respect to the effects of low level lead exposure concerns the general finding that with other traumata there is a fairly high threshold for persisting psychological sequelae following brain injury. This is a consistent finding, for example, with respect to head injury in

childhood (Rutter, Chadwick and Shaffer, 1983) and the same seems
to apply to the effects of perinatal complications (Drillien, Thomson
and Burgoyne, 1980). If generally there is a high threshold, how
could there be such a low threshold with lead exposure, as some of
the research findings seem to suggest?

So far, there is no satisfactory resolution to this dilemma.
Nevertheless, it is important to recognise that the lead findings are
not only ones to raise queries on the general validity of the high
threshold of psychological sequelae following brain damage (see
Rutter, 1982). For example, our own studies of children with
localized head injuries showed that reading backwardness was
surprisingly common even among the children with only slight local
traumata to the brain and no generalized damage (Chadwick et al,
1980; Shaffer et al. 1980). Or, again, there are the findings
linking neurological soft signs with an increased risk of psychiatric
disorder (Shaffer, O'Connor, Shafer and Prupis, 1983) and those
linking neurometric measures with learning disabilities (Prichep,
John, Ahn and Kaye, 1983). The problem in the interpretation of
both the soft sign and neurometric findings lies in the uncertainty
regarding the meaning of the clinical signs of neurodevelopmental
impairment or the computer-analysed neurophysiological measures
(Taylor, 1983). Obviously, is cannot be assumed that they reflect
brain dysfunction but they may well do so. Until these
contradictory findings on threshold can be explained satisfactorily,
there must be some doubt on the reality of the damaging effects
from low level lead exposure.

On the other hand, it is quite possible that the mechanisms
involved are rather different. After all, the head injury findings
and those concerned with perinatal complications largely represent
the reaction of the organism to a severe acute trauma whereas the
lead exposure findings concern the reaction of the organism to a
mild trauma but a very chronic one. It is quite possible that
sequelae are more likely following relative mild chronic damage than
rather more severe acute damage. Moreover, it is probable that
chronic lead exposure will cause more sequelae when it is associated
with psychosocial adversity. For example, this seems to be the
case with both malnutrition (Cravioto and Arrieta, 1983) and
perinatal complications (Rutter, 1981). Or, again, experimental
studies with animals suggest that the effects of lead toxicity are
much greater in the presence of under-nutrition (Mahaffey and
Michaelson, 1980). Findings from a re-analysis of Winneke's data
(Winneke, personal communication) and the preliminary findings
(Yule, personal communication) from a new larger study by
Lansdown et al (see chapter 14), that became available just as this
book was going to press, both suggest that the neurophysiological
effects of lead may be greater in (or even largely confined to)
socially disadvantaged children than in those from a more middle
class background. Obviously, this possibility needs to be
investigated further. If confirmed, it might go some way towards
explaining why studies have varied somewhat in their estimates of
lead effects.

It is important both scientifically and practically to recognise the possibility that much of the effects of low level lead exposure may result from an <u>interaction</u> between the effects of lead as such and the effects of other variables such as malnutrition or social disadvantage. But, of course, much of the concern about the damage that may follow low level lead exposure involves effects in the less affluent sections of society. The possibility that the effects of lead come not from some 'pure' form of permanent damage to the brain but rather through the effects of lead as part of a more complex set of interacting factors in no way absolves us from the responsibility of dealing with the one biological toxin (namely lead) that forms part of that set of interacting influences. it would be quite wrong to assert that the apparent discrepancy between the effects of brain injury (which seem to operate at only a relatively high threshold) and those of lead (which seem to operate at a much lower threshold) has been explained. But, equally it would be seriously misleading to suppose that the existence of this discrepancy nullifies the findings on lead. It does not, and, moreover, there are various plausible explanations as to why there should be a discrepancy. Further research is needed to test these hypotheses but, in the meanwhile, the research findings do not necessarily constitute an objection of the hypothesis that low level lead exposure leads to psychological sequelae.

<u>Strength and Specificity of the Association</u>   The last two considerations that stem from Bradford Hill's list of requirements for cause and effect relationships concern the strength and specificity of the association. There is no doubt, that causal inferences are much more likely to be correct when the associations are both strong and specific. Thus, the hypothesis that cigarette smoking predisposes to cancer of the lung is powerfully supported by the fact that the association is a strong one (the death rate from cancer of the lung among cigarette smokers is 9 to 10 times that in non-smokers, and the rate in heavy cigarette smokers is even greater still), and by the fact that the association is specifically with cancer of the lung and not with cancer generally. When associations are weak and general there must always be doubt about the causal hypothesis. Perhaps, it is this fact more than any other that has made many people sceptical about the reality of the supposed pyschological sequalae to low level lead exposure.

Although claims have been made that lead tends to predispose to particular types of cognitive deficit, the findings are quite contradictory and it seems more probable that lead leads to a relatively widespread cognitive impairment rather than to a disability of some specific type. So far as the behavioural effects are concerned, there is too little evidence at the moment to draw any firm conclusions. The most attention has been paid to sequalae that take the form of attentional deficits or hyperactivity. Accordingly, the evidence is greatest in terms of sequelae of this kind but we do not yet know whether this is simply a function of the fact that it is these behaviours that have mainly been looked at or, rather, whether it is these behaviours that are the ones most likely to be affected by lead exposure. It would be premature to rule out the possibility of a more specific consequence of lead toxicity, but the balance of evidence suggests that relatively general effects are more likely to be the case. Accordingly, we need to consider whether this casts serious doubt on the causal hypothesis. It does not. The point is that the evidence with respect to other forms of trauma to the brain are reasonably consistent in showing that the effects tend to impair a wide range of brain systems rather than just one (Rutter, 1981). We may conclude that, far from throwing doubt on the causal hypothesis, the generality of effects is entirely consistent with what might have been anticipates from what is known concerning brain function and malfunction.

However, one further issue regarding specificity needs to be considered. Dr Winneke (chapter 13) noted that most studies have found effects on verbal intelligence to be greater than those on performance wheras with other brain traumata it tends to be the other way round. That is so and it creates a problem. But two points need to be made. Firstly, the mechanisms may be different - we cannot assume that lead acts on intelligence and attention as a consequence of brain damage as such (a point considered further below). Secondly, the tendency for brain traumata to have the greatest impact on performance skills is not so with all traumata and, probably it is not so in the case of damage occurring in infancy (see Eiser, 1981; Woods, 1980) - a point of some importance in relation to lead exposure.

What, then, about the weakness of the association? To begin with, we do need to be quite clear that the association is indeed a weak one. All, but all, of the studies are consistent in showing that low level lead exposure is associated with deficits in the order of three to five points of IQ and with moderate increases in the proportion of children showing attentional deficits or hyperactivity. The occasional individual claims that low level lead exposure is responsible for much of the delinquency and educational retardation in our society can be firmly dismissed. There is not the slightest indication from the empirical findings that that is the case. But, to what extent does the weakness of the association throw doubts on the causal hypothesis? Perhaps, the most crucial point is that there is no way that strong associations could be found. This is because we know that there are many powerful genetic and environmental influences on intelligence and behaviour. Lead could add to these but it could not be expected to replace them. Accordingly, weak associations are not necessarily inconsistent with the causal hypothesis. To the contrary, they are to be expected.

Nevertheless, there are two main objections related to the weakness of the associations that have to be considered seriously. The first is the possibility that both the increase in body lead levels and the intellectual impairment or abnormal behaviour are the result of pica. The argument here is that the tendency to eat unsuitable or inedible substances (such as dirt or peeling paint) is itself part of a behavioural disturbance commonly found in children with lower levels of intelligence. That is indeed the case (Bicknell, 1975). Also it is known that a regrettably high proportion of old houses have peeling paint with a high lead content. If, as a result of pica, children eat this paint then lead levels will inevitably rise. But the association with the intellectual impairment and behavioural disturbance would not be due to the lead toxicity but rather would be a consequence of the kinds of children who eat peeling paint. There is no question that this is a definite possibility. the fact that pica was so strongly associated with high dentine lead in the Needleman study indicates that much of a children's lead exposure in that study was likely to be the result of pica rather that of airborne lead deposited on food or absorbed through the lungs.

On the other hand, Needleman's further analyses (see chapter 12) have shown that raised lead levels are associated with lower IQ and with inattentive behaviour even after controlling for the effects of pica. In other words, although the argument concerning pica has a degree of validity, the empirical findings suggest that it does not constitute the whole story. Even after the effects of pica are taken into account, the association between high lead and pychological sequalae remain.

The second issue concerns the possibility that the associations between lead and phychological impairment are due to some other uncontrolled social variable. That is a real possibility. One can never be sure that one has measured all relevant variables and it is clear that there are variables of possible importance that have not been included in most studies undertaken so far. For example, only a few investigations have obtained measures of parental IQ – probably the most powerful predictor of children's intelligence (through both genetic and environmental mechanisms). Also, it would be valuable to have more sensitive and discriminating measures of family adversity and psychopathology as these constitute the best predictors of children's disturbed behaviour. It is good that some of the studies now being undertaken will include those measures. As a consequence, their findings will do much to resolve the question of whether the associations with lead are merely artefacts stemming from the prior associations between lead and social disadvantage. But, even on the evidence available to us now, it would not seem likely that social variables will explain away the whole of the apparent effects of lead on psychological functioning. This is because in the studies undertaken so far, many of the effects of lead have remained even after the introduction of statistical controls for appropriate social variables and because the associations hold the investigations with the greatest social controls. We cannot be sure that the effects of lead are 'real' but the balance of evidence suggests that they are.

As the philosopher, Sir Karl Popper, pointed out, the way of science does not consist of any 'proof' of a hypothesis; rather, it consists of a series of failures to disaprove the hypothesis. By this standard, it is evident that the best of the most recent studies have indeed failed to disprove the hypothesis that low level lead exposure leads to psychological impairment. Inevitably, for the reasons that I have discussed at some length, there are doubts but, as a result of the further research that has been conducted over the last few years, these doubts are less than they were some time ago. The implication is that it would be both safer in practice, and scientifically more appropriate, to act as if the hypothesis were true rather than to do nothing on the assumption that it might be false. However, before considering what that means in terms of policy, attention needs to be paid to two other issues that have underlain the whole of the discussion up to this point, namely, the threshold of effects and the nature of effects.

THRESHOLD EFFECTS

Throughout the literature on lead effects, investigators have been concerned with the very important question of the level of body lead at which adverse sequalae occur. It has long been known that lead is a neurotoxin and that lead poisoning in children can cause encephalopathy and death (Thomas and Blackfan, 1914). That well demonstrated fact is not disputed by anyone. There is considerable individual variations in the blood lead levels at which encephalopathy occurs but, in general, such effects may start at about 100 µg/dl (although some individuals do not develop symptoms until the levels are two or three times as high - see U.S. Environmental Protection Agency, 1977). Overt encephalopathy is rare at blood lead levels below 100, but clinical signs of lead poisoning may be seen in the 60 to 100 µg/dl range and pyschological studies undertaken before 1980 indicated that cognitive sequalae could be seen with blood lead levels in the range above 40 µg/dl (Rutter, 1980). At that time there were very few studies of children with levels below 40 and it was possible to conclude only that "There are pointers that there may be psychological risks with lead levels below 40 µg/100 ml, but the evidence on this point is inconclusive so far" (p. 23). The Lawther report (Department of Health and Social Security, 1980) similarly pointed to the lack of convincing evidence of effects below about 35 µg/dl. Unfortunately, that appropriately cautious conclusion was put in a context that has been read by many people as implying there was positive evidence that there was an absence of effects below 35. That would have been scientific nonsense, and of course, it was not the view of the Working Party. A paucity of evidence on ill-effects (which was the case in 1980) is an entirely different matter to the presence of good evidence that there are no ill-effects (which was not the case). Accordingly, it never could have been justified to assume that levels below 35 µg/dl were safe.

However, as I have indicated, since 1980 there have been several studies that have examined effects in the range below 35 µg/dl. All of them have demonstrated effects and none had produced evidence that there is a threshold below which there is safety. Of course, it is likely that effects are less frequent and less severe at lower levels of lead exposure, and it may be that there is a point at which ill-effects are so extremely rare that they can be discounted for all practical purposes. However, if there is such a threshold it has yet to be determined. At present, all that one can conclude is that it now seems much more likely than hitherto that there are effects at levels below 35 µg/dl and that we cannot specify any range of safety. The animal evidence points to the same conclusion.

NATURE OF EFFECTS

Because high doses of lead may lead to abortions and still births there have been claims that low levels of exposure may have the same effect, albeit in lesser degree (see review by Wynn and Wynn, 1982). But animal studies have shown that this is not necessarily the case. Thus, neither Bull et al (1979) not Kimmel et al (1980) found any effect of slightly raised lead levels (about 36 µg/dl) on the ability of rats to conceive, to carry a litter to term, or to deliver the young; moreover, there was no effect of lead on the rate of foetal malformations. It is not that there are no effects of lead on reproduction; there are, as Dr Silbergeld's review (chapter 11) demonstrates. These are important and demand our attention, but it should not be assumed that the mechanisms at low dosage are the same as those at high dosage.

In the same way, because it is known that lead is a neurotoxin and because poisoning leads to encephalopathy and death, with obvious gross neuropathological changes evident on post-mortem examination of the brain, there is a tendency to assume that lower levels of lead exposure have similar (but lesser) effects leading to minor degrees of brain damage. In the same way, because high lead exposure can cause serious intellectual impairment following recovery from encephalopathy, often it is supposed that lower levels of lead exposure will have comparable (but lesser) effects serving to impair intellectual capacity. The animal studies that concern moderately high blood lead levels (say 40-80 µg/dl) are compatible with that viewpoint.

As Dr Silbergeld pointed out (chapter 10), once lead is deposited in the brain it is quite difficult to remove. For that reason, and because of the particular neurotixic actions of lead at moderately high blood levels, she argued that the effects were 'irreversible', although she also noted that the concept of reversibility has many different meanings. In my view, several rather different points need emphasis with respect to the permanence or otherwise of lead effects on neuropsychological function (Rutter, 1981; 1982). Firstly, even if the structural effect is permanent this does not mean that the functional effects will be so as well. It is a commonplace observation that children make the most remarkable recoveries following quite serious brain injuries. This is because most organs have a substantial effective 'reverse capacity', because different parts of the brain may take over functions ordinarily served by damaged parts, and becauase children learn ways to compensate for their handicaps. Secondly, recent research has shown that, contrary to previous views, brain tissues may regrow after injury (although this does not necessarily restore function). Thirdly, because it is probable that the effects of high lead exposure are mediated through actual damage to the brain, it does not follow that this constitutes the mechanism for lower levels of lead exposure. Indeed, if Dr David's chelation findings (chapter 15) are confirmed there is the strong implication that it <u>cannot</u> constitute the mechanism. The point is that the rapid behavioural improvement found suggests that this must reflect some transient action of lead circulating in the blood rather than any permanent effect of lead in the brain tissues.

In this connection, too, Dr Winneke's suggestions (chapter 13) are pertinent. He put forward the hypothesis that, at least at the relatively low levels found in his study, lead exposure did not act by impairing intellectual capacity as such. Rather, he argued for an effect on emotional reactivity that, in turn might secondarily lead to both cognitive and behvioural sequale. Of course, as he recognised, the suggestion is speculative at the moment. However, its importance lies less in whether or not it is true in its specifics than in its reminder to us that we do not as yet know how low level lead exposure causes neuropsychological effects and that we would be wise to keep an open mind to the possibility that the mechanisms involved at lower levels of lead may not be the same as those implicated at higher levels. After all, the animal research strongly suggests that some chemical systems are affected by quite low levels of lead whereas others require rather higher levels before effects are detectable. The question of the mechanisms underlying the functional deficits associated with lead has not yet received a satisfactory answer; it warrants further serious study.

POLICY IMPLICATIONS

Lastly, I need to say just a word or two on the policy implications of these findings. The symposium has been about empirical research rather than policy. Nevertheless, all of us need to be aware that the scientific findings do have crucial policy implications. The issues involved in coming to policy decisions, of course, go way beyond the evidence on psychological effects of low level lead exposure. In the first place, they involve value judgements. We have to decide, as a society, how much we are prepared to pay in order to remove the risks and hazards in our environments. Those are not easy questions even in affluent society, in that if we spend more money on this, we tend to have to spend less money on that. On the other hand, there are certain public health actions that are relatively inexpensive, so that the value judgements, in turn, are relatively straightforward. But, also there is a second issue which we ignore at our peril. All too often in the history of modern society, we have removed one hazard only to replace it with another as bad or worse than the first. We need to be clear that this is not theoretical possibility - it is a very real one with ever present concerns.

Non-barbiturate sedatives and hypnotics were introduced because doctors became aware of the problems of dependency and addiction associated with the regular use of barbiturates. One of the results was the introduction of what seemed to be a range of safe and harmless drugs that had many of the benefits of barbiturates without the disadvantages. As we all know, thalidomide was one of those 'safe' drugs. I do not need to dwell on what happened as the story is all too familiar. Similarly, over recent years there has been concern about the possible ill-effects from the amount of sugar in our diet but are we certain that the sugar-substitutes in such wide use are free from harmful effects?

The same questions need to be applied to the situations involving lead. If we do not use lead in the manufacture of petrol, are we sure that the new alternative processes are not going to introduce some other hazard of which we, as yet, remain unaware? So far as I can judge, the elimination of lead from the manufacture of petrol need not result in the introduction of new risks but, still, the question is an important one. If new processes are introduced in the place of lead additives to petrol it will be essential to check their safety and to monitor their effects. The American biologist, Lewis Thomas (1979), has posed the dilemmas in his usual witty but cynical fashion in his essay entitled, 'On Meddling'. He makes the point that all too often we tinker with biological and social systems, taking some action to deal with a risk we recognise only to discover some years later that the action we took made other things worse. Of course, this should not be taken as a recipe for inaction. After all, we are meddling with the environment all the time. But it does introduce a note of necessary caution which reminds us that virtually all effective actions have their disadvantages and we need to weigh these carefully in coming to our decisions on how to intervene in taking preventive or therapeutic actions.

With all these issues in mind, then, what are the policy implications of the empirical findings discussed in this volume? As I have made clear, there is no direct and necessary connection between empirical findings and policy, and hence, my conclusions inevitably reflect my own value judgements as well as my scientific appraisal of the evidence. The research findings tell us that there is a probability (although not certainty) that low level lead exposure may have important adverse psychological effects. These effects are not large and it is clear that there are many other more important influences on psychological functioning. Moreover, it is probable that there are considerable individual differences to susceptibility - related to age, ethnicity, nutrition, social variables and other factors as yet imperfectly understood. But, the risk seems to be substantially more than a trivial one and, at least in some individuals, the effects are likely to be of practical importance in causing impairment of functioning. The implication is that we now know enough to warrant taking such public health actions as are likely to reduce lead pollution in the environment, provided such actions do not have other hazards and provided they are not prohibitively expensive.

I place the emphasis on prevention before the event rather than treatment after the event, not just because prevention is preferable to cure (although it is), but because actions need to be chosen in terms of their efficacy and safety. As Dr David (chapter 15) made clear, the use of chelating agents to remove lead from the body is a major intervention which is not without some risks. No one doubts that those risks are justifiable in the case of overt lead poisoning and, too, they may be warranted when moderately high lead levels are associated with symptoms. But, it is much more dubious whether it would be appropriate to chelate children with slightly raided lead levels and behavioural or cognitive difficulties that are less directly and less certainly caused by lead. Clearly, it would not be sensible to embark on a policy of treating the relatively large number of children who fall into that category.

Instead, we need to turn to policies of prevention. As numerous reviews have pointed out, there are a variety of effective preventive policies at our disposal. Dr Moore (chapter 5) told the important story of lead-contaminated water in south-west Scotland. It provides a model of the ways in which scientists and policy-makers can work together. Research findings identified the risk factor (i.e., lead in drinking water) and demonstrated that its solvency was affected by the pH of the water. This pointed the way to a mode of intervention (namely altering the pH). The policy was implemented and further research confirmed that, to a worthwhile extent, it had been effective. The story also reminds us that preventive policies need to be concerned, not only with opportunities to prevent the toxin getting into the environment, but also with opportunities to prevent existing environmental toxins from entering the body. Water provided one example of effective prevention but, as we all know, there are numerous others. As the Lawther report (Department of Health and Social Security, 1980) emphasised, effective steps can and should be taken with respect to lead in paint and in cosmetics or hair preparations; to the use of lead in the food-canning process; to lead used in glazing and in pewter; and to safety precautions in industry. These steps are well known and, for the most part have been, or are being, implemented already to some extent. It is desirable to intensify the preventive programmes where they are less than fully effective but, also we need to search for other public health policies that might be both cost-effective and without hazards.

The removal of lead from petrol would seem to be one of those worthwhile and safe public health actions. The evidence suggests that the removal of lead from petrol would have quite a substantial effect in reducing lead pollution and the costs are quite modest by any reasonable standard. Other countries, such as the United States, have already taken action and there is every reason that Britain should do likewise. In my view, the reduction of lead in petrol to an intermediate level is an unacceptable compromise without clear advantages and with definite disadvantages. But, equally, it is very apparent that the lead in petrol constitutes but only one of many sources of lead pollution. In the concern to deal with the hazards from petrol we should not overlook these other hazards that demand equal attention. But, also, a concern that other actions are needed, which indeed they are, should not blind us to the value of the one immediate step that could and should be taken - namely, the removal of lead from petrol.

Of course, it might be argued that the lowering of the permitted level of lead in petrol to 0.15 g/l ought to be enough. In itself, that would have a substantial effect in reducing blood lead levels in the population at large. Do we need to go further? Indeed, I am aware that the U.S. Environmental Protection Agency has been urged by representatives of the lead industries to rescind the regulations on lead in gasoline on the grounds that it "would help improve the economic condition of the lead industry which is seriously depressed" (Cole, 1982) and that the impact on health would be negligible. How far do we need to go in reducing the lead in the environment?

Of course, the only honest answer to that question is that we do not know that, still, we are quite unclear on the level of body lead at which risks to health appear. Nevertheless, we have no alternative but to make an educated guess in order to come to some decision on what action to take. Moreover, as I indicated in my introduction (chapter 1), we need to recognise that, effectively, no decision (i.e., a wait-and-see policy in the hope that better evidence will become available) is equivalent to a decision not to act. Accordingly, we need to weigh carefully the likely risks that will follow the various decisions that could be taken.

Often society has the problem that small amounts of potential toxins are essential to health in spite of the fact that large amounts may be damaging. In these circumstances, a careful balance is essential between doing too much and not doing enough. That situation does not arise with lead. So far as is known, there are no health benefits from small amounts of lead and hence there would be no health risks attached to the complete removal of lead from the environment (were that practicable, which it is not). So we can put that concern on one side.

It now seems fairly clear that the blood lead level of 35 µg/dl does not constitute a safety limit but, perhaps, there is such a limit at some (as yet unknown) lower level. Perhaps. Certainly, it would not be justified to rule out the possibility of a threshold, although there is no evidence at the moment that one exists. However, before we act on the assumption that there is some safety limit, several crucial considerations must be weighed in the balance. Firstly, the study by Dr Winneke (chapter 13) strongly suggests that there may be ill-effects from quite low levels of lead. If his results are valid, it is apparent that the reduction of lead in petrol to 0.15 g/l would not be enough. Indeed his study was undertaken in a country (Germany) that had already taken the step of reducing the lead in petrol to 0.15 a few years previously. Lansdown et al's study (chapter 14) points in the same direction.

Secondly, it is known that there is considerable individual variation
in susceptibility to lead - a variation that applies to most toxins.
Dr Duggan's chapter (7) suggests that 2 to 3 year olds may be at
particular risk because of their tendency to put objects into their
mouths.   Other work points to the interaction between lead and
malnutrition (Mahaffey and Michaelson, 1980) and it is quite likely,
too, that the effects of biological hazards are intensified in the
presence of social disadvantage.   But, even considered in isolation,
there is marked individual variation in the level of body lead at
which adverse sequelae appear.   Accordingly, one person's safety
limit is in someone else's danger zone.   It is for that reason that,
when establishing the safety limit for the dosage of drugs, the limit
is set well below that at which ill-effects generally appear.

Thirdly, it is necessary to take account of geographical variations.
As the Lawther report noted, not only are there 'hot spots' in
which traffic conditions mean that the lead in petrol engine
emissions constitute a particular hazard, but also there are areas
where the risks from petrol have to be added to those from water
or lead smelters or some other adventitious source.   We need to set
the safety limit at a level that will be safe for people living and
working in those circumstances, and not just for 'Mr Average'.

Fourthly, it is known that lead levels as low as 20 μg/dl have
effects on haeme biosynthesis, that this effect may be more marked
in children than adults and that it is possible that these may be
implicated in the neuropsychological sequalae (Angle and MacIntyre,
1978; Roels et al, 1976 - see also chapter 10).   It is not known
that the effects on haeme biosynthesis at levels as low as 20 μg/dl
'matter' in terms of any impairment of health,   Reductions in
haemoglobin levels do not occur until much higher burdens of lead
are reached.   On the other hand, the fact that there is a
demonstrated alteration in biological functioning ought to serve as a
warning that there are possible implications for health even at these
low lead levels.

It is for those reasons that we have to set a limit for lead well
below that at which adverse effects commonly appear.   Unless there
is a very substantial gap between the overall population limit and
the usual threshold (if there is one) of toxicity, some individuals
will suffer.   The costs of setting the safety limit too high,
therefore, are that some children will be damaged unnecessarily.

What are the risks of setting the limit 'too low'?   As we have seen,
there are no health risks.   The only consequence is that there will
have been some industrial expenditure that was not strictly
necessary.   These costs are not great and have been undertaken
already in the United States.   As I have noted, pleas have been
made in the U.S. to rescind the gasoline regulations in order to
help the lead industry.   Of course, that is an issue - a cynic might
argue that it is comparable to the need to wage war from time to
time in order to maintain the armaments industry!   Of course, the
effects of war and of keeping petrol are of an entirely different

lead in order and should not be equated. Nevertheless, most people are likely to feel concern over the argument that one section of the population should be at a potential health risk in order to protect the employment of some other section of the population. The answer to the question on industrial costs must depend on value judgements rather than on science. On the matter, each of us has to take out own decision. However, what is important is that we are all clear on the grounds for such decisions and on the cost-benefits involved.

So far, most of my remarks have been concerned with the risks associated with the presence of lead in the environment. What, then, are the likely benefits that should follow reductions in the level of environmental lead? As I have emphasised at several points, we need to be quite clear that the benefits will be small. The reduction of lead will not bring about major improvements in the health and development of British children as a whole. If we claim that, we are raising false expectations and we run the real danger of a backlash when those hopes are unfulfilled. They will be unfulfilled in the context of a society as a whole because the ill-effects of low level lead exposure are relatively slight, because there is an as yet ill-understood marked individual variation in response to lead and, most of all, because we know that there are many other more powerful influences on cognition and behaviour. On the other hand, as I have observed, a marked reduction in the level of environmental lead is likely to make an important difference to some children. Moreover, it is necessary to recognise that a small change in the mean IQ or average behaviour of the population as a whole will have a much greater effect at the extremes of the distribution. The statistical reasons why this should happen were noted previously (Rutter, 1980), but Dr Needleman's findings (chapter 12) have gone on to demonstrate that this also occurs in practice. Accordingly, actions to cut down the amount of lead pollution of the environment should be worthwhile; there is quite sufficient justification for action now.

REFERENCES

Angle, C.R. and McIntire, M.S. (1978). Low level lead and inhibition of erythrocyte pyrimidine nucleotidase. Environ. Res., 17, 296-302.

Araki, S. and Honma, T. (1976). Relationships between lead absorption and peripheral nerve conduction velocities in lead workers. Scand.J.Work. Environ.Health, 2, 225-231.

Arvik, J.H. and Zimdahl, R.L. (1974). Barriers to the foliar uptake of lead J. Environ. Qual., 3, 369-373.

Baker, Jr., E.L., Folland, D.S., Taylor, T.A., Frank, M., Peterson, W., Lovejoy, G., Cox, D., Housworth, J. and Landrigan, P.J. (1977). Lead poisoning in children of lead workers: home contamination with industrial dust. New. Engl. J. Medicine, 296, 260-261.

Barltrop, D., Strehlow, C.D., Thornton, I. and Webb, J.S. (1975). Absorption of lead from dust and soil. Postgraduate Medical Journal, 51, 801-804.

Benignus, V.A., Otto, D.A., Muller, K.E. and Seiple, K.J.
(1981). Effects of age and body lead burden on CNS function in
young children. II. EEG spectra. Electroenceph. Clin.
Neurophysiol., 52, 240-248.

Bicknell, D.J. (1975). Pica: A Childhood Syndrome. IRMMH
Monograph No.3. London: Butterworths.

Bornschein, R.L., Michaelson, I.A., Fox, D.A. and Lock, R.
(1977). Evaluation of animal models used to study effects of
lead on neurochemistry and behaviour. In Lee, S.D. (ed)
Biochemical Effects of Environmental Pollutants. Ann Arbor,
Mich.: Ann Arbor Science (pp 441-460).

Bornschein, R., Pearson, O. and Reiter, L. (1980). Behavioural
effects of moderate lead exposure in children and animal models.
C.R.C. Crital Reviews in Toxicology, 8,43-152.

Bradford Hill, A. (1977). A Short Textbook of Medical Statistics.
London:Hodder & Stoughton.

Bull, R.J., Lutkenhoff, S.D., McCarty, G.E. and Miller, R.G.
(1979). Delays in the postnatal increase of cerebral cytochrome
concentrations in lead exposed rats. Neuropharmacology, 18,
83-92.

Burchfiel, J., Duffy, F., Bartels, P.H. and Needleman, H.L.
(1980). Combined discriminating power of quantitative
electroencephalography and neuropsychologic measures in
evaluation CNS checks of lead at low levels. In Needleman, H.
(ed) Low Level Lead Exposure: the clinical implications of
current research. New York: Raven Press. Pp 75-90.

Chadwick, O. and Rutter, M. (1983). Neuro-psychological
assessment. In Rutter, M. (ed) Developmental Neuropsychiatry.
New York: Guildford Press (in press).

Chadwick, O., Rutter, M., Thompson, J. and Shaffer, D. (1981).
Intellectual performance and reading skills after localized head
injury in childhood. J. Child Psychol. Psychiat., 22, 117-139.

Chamberlain, A.C., Heard, M.J., Little, P. and Wiffen, R.D.
(1979). The dispersion of lead from motor exhausts. Phil.
Trans. Roy. Soc. Lond. A., 290, 577-589.

Chamberlain, A.C., Heard, M.J., Little, P., Newton, D., Wells,
A.C. and Wiffen, R.D.,μ (1978). Investigations into lead from
motor vehicles. Report AERE-R9198. Harwell Laboratories,
England. November 1978.

Charney, E., Sayre, J. and Coulter, M. (1980). Increased lead
absorption in inner city children: where does the lead come
from? Pediatrics, 65, 226-231.

Chisolm, J.J., Barrett, M.R. and Harrison, H.V. (1975).
Indicators of internal dose of lead in relation to derangement in
hemo synthesis. John Hopkins Med. J., 137.

Cole, J.F. (1982). Testimony to the U.S. Environmental Protection
Agency.

Cravioto, J. and Arrieta, R. (1983). Malnutrition in childhood. In
Rutter, M. (ed) Developmental Neuropsychiatry. New
York:Guildford Press (in press).

Crump, D.R. and Barlow, P.J. (1980). A field method of assessing
lead uptake from plants. Sci., Total Environ., 15, 269-274.

Department of Health and Social Security (1980). Lead and Health:

The report of a DHSS Working Party of Lead in the Environment (Lawther Report). London, HMSO.

Drillien, C.M., Thomson, A.J.M. and Burgoyne, K. (1980). Low-birthweight children at early school-age: a longitudinal study. Develop. Med. Child Neurol., 22, 26-47.

Duggan, M. and Williams, S. (1977). Lead-in-dust in city streets. Sci., Total Environ., 7, 91-97.

Eiser, C. (1981) Psychological sequelae of brain tumours in childhood: a retrospective study. Brit.J. Clin. Psychol., 20, 35-38.

Ernhart, C.B. (1982) Lead and petrol. Lancet, ii, 209-210 (letter to the editor).

Ernhart, C.B., Landa, B. and Schell, N.B. (1981) Subclinical levels of lead and developmental defict - a multivariate follow-up reassessment. Pediatrics, 67, 911-919.

Facchetti, S. and Geiss, F., with the collaboration of Gaglione, P., Colombo, A., Garibaldi, G., Spallanzani, G. and Gilli, G. (1982). Isotopic Lead Experiment: Status Report, July, 1982. Commission of the European Communities Joint research Centre, Ispra.

Feldmam, R.G., Haddow, J., Kupito, L. and Schwachman, H. (1973). Altered peripheral nerve condition velocity: chronic lead intoxication in children. Amer, J. Dis. Childhd, 125,39-41.

Gibson, R.S. (1980) Hair as a biopsy material for the assessment of trace elememt status in infancy: a review. J. Human Nutr., 31. 405-416.

Grandjean, P. (1978) Lead concentration in single hairs as a monitor of occupational lead exposure. Int. Arch. Occup. Environ. Health, 42,69-81.

Grant, L.D., Kimmel, C.A., West, G.L., Martinez-Vargus, C.M. and Howard, J.L.(1980) Chronic low-level lead toxicity in the rat.II. Effects on postnatal physical and behavioural development. Toxicology and Applied Pharmacology, 56, 42-58.

Hammond, P.B., Lerner, S.I., and Hong, C.G., (1980) New perspectives on lead. Amer, J. Ind. Med. 1, 401-404.

Harrison, R.M. (1979) Toxic metals in street and household dusts. Sci. Total Environ. 11, 89-97.

Harrison, R.M., (1982) Environmental aspects of lead pollution. Evidence to the Royal Commission on Environmental Pollution, May 1982, London.

I.C.F. Incorporated. The Relationship Between Gasoline Lead Emissions and Lead Poisoning in Americans. Prepared for the Office of Policy and Resource Management Office of Policy Analysis, Washington, D.C. : I.C.F., 1982.

Jansen, S.J., Carnow, B.W. and Namekata, T. (1978) Morton Grove Lead Study: An Investigation of the contribution of airborne lead from automobile exhaust to blood lead levels in suburban children. Report P6-280717 to the U.S. Environmental Protection Agency.

Kimmell, C.A., Grant, L.D., Sloan, C.S. and Gladen, B.C., (1980) Chronic low-level lead toxicity in the rat. 1. Maternal toxicity and perinatal effects. Toxicology and Applied Pharmacology, 56, 28-41.

Koeppi, D.E. (1981) Lead: Understanding the minimal toxicity of
    lead in plants. In: Lepp, N.W. (ed) Effect of Heavy Metal
    Pollution on Plants, Vol.1. Applied Science Publication, pp.
    55-76.
Lagerwerff, J.V., Armiger, W.H. and Specht, A.W. (1973) Uptake
    of lead by alfalfa and corn from soil and air. Soil Sci., 115,
    455-460.
Landrigan, P.J., Gehlback, S.H., Rosenblum, B.F., Shoulta, J.M.,
    Candelaria, R.M., Barthel, W.F., Liddle, J.A., Smrek, A.L.,
    Staehling, N.M. and Sander, J.D.F. (1975) Epidemic lead
    absorption near an ore smelter: the role of particulate lead. New
    Eng. J. Med., 292, 123-129.
Little, P., Fleming, R.G. and Heard, M.J. (1981) Uptake of lead
    by vegetable foodstuffs during cooking. Sci. Total Environ., 17,
    111-131.
Lin-Fu, J.S. (1973) Vulnerability of children to lead exposure and
    toxicity. New Eng. J. Med., 289, 1229-1233; 1289-1293.
McCauley, P.T., Bull, R.J., and Lutkenhoff, S.D. (1979)
    Association of alterations in energy metabolism with lead-induced
    delays in rat cerebral cortical development. Neuropharmacology,
    18, 93-101.
Mahaffey, K.R. (1978) Environmental exposure to lead. In Nringu,
    J.O. (ed) The Biogeochemistry of Lead in the Environmental.
    Elsevier: North-Holland Biomedical Press 1.
Mahaffey, K. and Michaelson, I.A. (1980) Interaction between lead
    and nutrition. In Needleman, H.L. (ed) Low Level Lead
    Exposure: The clinical implications of current research. New
    York: Raven Press.
Milar, C.B., Schroeder, S.R., Mushak, P. and Boone, L. (1981)
    Failure to find hyperactivity in preschool children with
    moderately elevated lead burden. J. Pediat. Psychol., 6, 85-95.
Milar, C.B., Schroeder, S.R., Mushak, P., Dolcourt, J.L. and
    Grant, L.D. (1980) Contributions of the caregiving environment
    to increase lead burden of children. Amer. J. Ment. Defic. 84,
    339-344.
Moore, M.R., Hughes, M.A. and Goldberg, D.J. (1979) Lead
    absorption in man from dietary sources. The effect of cooking
    upon lead concentrations of certain foods and vegetables. Int.
    Arch. Occup. Environ. Health, 44, 81-90.
Needleman, H.L. (ed) (1980) Low Level Lead Exposure: The
    Clinical Implications of Current Research. New York, Raven
    Press.
Needleman, H., Gunnoe, C., Leviton, A., Reed, M., Peresie, H.,
    Maher, C. and Barrett, P. (1979) Deficits in psychological and
    classroom performance of children with elevated dentine lead
    levels. New Eng. J. Med., 300, 689-695.
Nriagu, J.D. (1979) Global inventory of natural and anthropogenic
    emissions of trace metals to the atmosphere. Nature, 279,
    409-411.
Otto, D.a., Benignus, V.A., Muller, K.E. and Barton, C.N.(1981).
    Effects of age and body lead burdens on CNS function in young
    children.I. Slow cortical potentials. Electroenceph. Clin.
    Neurophysiol., 52, 229-239.

Oxley, G.R (1982) Blood lead concentrations: apparent reduction over approximately one decade. Int. Arch. Occup. Env. Health, 49, 341-343

Perino, J. and Ernhart, C.B. (1974). The relation of subclinical lead level to cognitive and sensorimotor impairment in black preschoolers. J. Learn. Dis., 7, 26-30.

Prichep, L., John, E. R., Ahn, H. and Kaye, H. (1983). Neurometric techniques. In Rutter, M. (ed) Developmental Neuropsychiatry. New York: Guilford press (in press).

Reichardt, C.S. (1979). The statical analysis of data from nonequivalent group designs. In Cook, T.D. and Campbell, D.T. (eds) Quasi-Experimentation: Design and Analysis Issues for Field Setting. Chicago: Rand McNally (pp 147-205).

Roels, H.A., Buchet, J-P. Lauwerys, R.R., Bruaux, P., Claeys-Thoreau, F., Lafontaine, A. and Verduyn, G. (1980). Exposure to lead by the oral and the pulmonary routes of children living in the vicinity of a primary lead smelter. Environ. Res., 22, 81-94.

Roels, H., Buchet, J-P., Lauwerys, R., Hubermont, G., Bruaux, P., Claeys-Thoreau, F., Lafontaine, A. and van Overschelde, J. (1976). Impact of air pollution by lead on the heme biosynthetic pathway in school-age children. Arch. Environ. health, 31,310-316.

Rutter, M. (1980). Raised lead levels and impaired cognitive/behavioural functioning: A review of the evidence. Develop. Med. Child Neurol., 22, Supplement No. 42.

Rutter, M. (1981). Psychological sequelae of brain damage in children. Amer. J. Psychiat., 138, 1533-1544.

Rutter, M. (1982). Developmental neuropsychiatry: Concepts, issues and prospects. J. Clin. Neuropsychol. (in press).

Rutter, M., Chadwick, O. and Shaffer, D. (1983). Head injury. In Rutter, M. (ed) Developmental Neuropsychiatry. New York: Guilford Press (in press).

Schmitt, N., Philou, J.J., Larsen, A.A., Hannadek, M. and Lynch, A.J. (1979). Surface soil as a potential source of lead exposure for young children. Can. Med. Assoc. J. 121, 1474-1478.

Schuck, E.A and Locke, J.K. (1970). Relationship of automotive lead particulates to certain consumer crops. Environ. Sci. Technol., 4, 324-330.

Seppalainen, A.M. (1978). Diagnostic utility of neuroelectric measures in environmental and occupational medicine. In Otto. D. (ed) Multidisciplinary Perspectives in Event-Related Brain Potential Research. EPA - 600/9-77-043 (Pp 448-452) Washington, DC: US Government Printing Offices.

Seppalainen, A.M. and Hernberg, S. (1980). Subclinical lead neuropathy. Amer. J. Occup. Med., 1, 413-420.

Seppalainen, A.M., Tola, S., Hernberg, S. and Kock, B., (1975). Subclinical neuropathy at 'safe' levels of lead exposure. Arch. Environ. Health, 30, 180-183.

Settle, D.M. and Patterson, C.P. (1980). Lead in albacore: guide to lead pollution in Americans. Science, 207, 1167-1176.

Shaffer, D., Bijur, P., Chadwick, O. and Rutter, M. (1980).

Head injury and later reading disability. J. Amer. Acad. Child
Psychiatry, 19, 592-610.

Shaffer, D., O'Connor, P.A., Shafer, S.Q. and Prupis, S. (1983).
Neurological 'soft signs': Their origins and significance for
behavior. In Rutter, M. (ed) Developmental Neuropsychiatry.
New York: Guildford Press (in press).

Sinn, W. (1980). Relationship between lead concentrations in the
air and blood lead levels of people living, and working in the
centre of a city (Frankfurt blood lead study)- I. Experimental
method and examination of differences. Int. Arch. Occup.
Environ. Hlth., 47, 93-118.

Sinn, W. (1981). Relationship between lead concentrations in the
air and blood lead levels of people living and working in the
centre of a city (Frankfurt blood lead survey)- II. Correlations
and conclusions. Int. Arch. Environ. Hlth., 48, 1-23.

Smart, G.A., Warrington, M. and Evans, W.H. (1981).
Contribution of lead in water to dietary lead intakes. J. Sci.
Food. Agric., 32, 129-133.

Solgaard, P., Aarkrog, A., Fenger, J., Flyger, H. and Graabaek,
A.M. (1978). Decrease in content of lead in Danish cereals.
Nature, 272, 346-347.

Spittler, T.M. and Feder, N.A. (1979). A study of soil
contamination and plant lead uptake in Boston urban gardens.
Commun. in Soil Science and Plant Anal., 10, 1195-1210.

Stark, A.D.. Quah, R.F., Meigs, J.W. and De Louise, E.R.
(1982). The relationship of environmental lead to blood lead
levels in children. Environ. Res., 27, 372-383.

Taylor, E. (1983). Measurement issues and approaches. In
Rutter, M. (ed) Developmental neuropsychiatry. New York:
Guilford Press (in press).

Ter Haar, G. (1970). Air as a source of lead in edible crops.
Environ Sci. Tech., 4, 226-229.

Ter Haar, G. and Aronow, R. (1974). New information on lead in
dirt and dust as related to the childhood lead problem.
Environ. Hlth. persp., 7, 83-89.

Thatcher, R.W., Lester, M.L., McAlaster, R., Horst, R. and
Ignasias, S.W. (1982). Intelligence and lead toxins in rural
children. J. Learn. Dis. (in press).

Thomas, H.M. and Blackfan, A.D. (1914). Recurrent meningitis,
lead, in a child of five yuears. J. Dis. Child., 8, 337-380.

Thomas, L. (1979). On meddling. In The Medusa and the Snail:
More notes of a Biology Watcher. new York: Viking Press, Pp.
110-111.

Tolan, A. and Elton, G.A.H. (1973). Lead intake from food. In
Proc. Internat. Symp. on Environmental Health Aspects of
Lead, Amsterdam, October 1972. Luxembourg: Commission of
N. European Communities, pp. 77-84.

U.S. Committee on Lead in the Human Environment (1980). Lead in
the Human Environment. National Research Council, National
Academy Press.

U.S. Environmental Protection Agency (1977). Air Quality Criteria
for Lead. EPA-600/8-77-017. Washington, DC: US Government
Printing Office.

U.S. Environmental Protection Agency (1982).   Quarterly avarages
    of lead from National Air Filter Network.   Research Triangle
    Park, N.C.:   U.S. EPA.
U.S. Food and Drug Administration (1975).   Compliance Program
    Evaluatiion FY-1974. Health Metals in Food Survey.   Washington,
    D.C.:   Bureau of Foods.
Vahter, M. (ed) (1982).   Assessment of Human Exposure to Lead
    and   Cadmium   Through   Biological   Monitoring.   Stockholm:
    National   Swedish   Institute   of   Environmental   Medicine   and
    Department of Environmental Hygiene, Karolinska Institute.
Vostal, J., Taves, E. and Sayre, J.W. (1974).   Lead analysis of
    house dust.   Method for the detection of another source of lead
    exposure   in   inner   city   children.   Environ.   Hlth.   persp.,
    7,91-97.
Walter, S.D., Yankel, A.J. and von Lindern, I.H. (1980).
    Age-specific risk factors for lead absorption in children.   Arch.
    Env. Health., 35, 53-58.
Woods, B.T. (1980).   The restricted effects of right hemisphere
    lesions after age 1: Wechsler test data.   Neuropsychologia, 18,
    65-70.
Wynn, M. and Wynn, A. (1982).   Lead and human reproduction.
    London: CLEAR.
Yankel, A.J., von Lindern, I., Walter, S.D. (1977).   The Silver
    Valley lead study: the relationship between childhood blood lead
    levels   and   environmental   exposure.   J.   Air   pollut.   Control
    Assoc., 27, 763-767.
Yule, W. and Rutter, M. (1983).   Effects of lead on intellectual
    development of children: Critical evaluation of methodology and
    results of studies.   In: Mahaffey, K.R. (ed) Health Implications
    of Typical Levels of Lead Exposure: Dietary and environmental
    sources. Amsterdam: Elsevier (in press).
Zimdahl, R.L. (1976).   Entry and movement in vegetation of lead
    derived from air and soil sources.   J.   Air   Pollut.   Control
    Assoc., 26, 655-660.

CONTRIBUTORS TO THE SYMPOSIUM

Below are listed details of those who contributed to the symposium on "Low Level Lead Exposure and its Effects on Human Beings" which took place in London at the Institute of British Architects from May 10-12, 1982.

Conference Chairman was Michael Rutter, MD, FRCP, FRCPsych, DPM, Professor of Child Psychiatry, Institute of Psychiatry, London.

The following acted as Session Chairmen:

James S. Bevan, MRCGP, D(Obst)RCOG, General Practitioner, London.

John H. Edwards, FRCP, FRS, Professor of Genetics, Oxford University.

Thomas E. Oppe, MB, BS, FRCP, DCH, Professor of Paediatrics, St. Mary's Hospital Medical School.

Robin Russel Jones, MA, MRCP, Deputy Chairman of CLEAR, London.

Robert Stephens, PhD, DSc, Reader in Chemistry, University of Birmingham.

The following delivered papers at the symposium:

Fraser Alexander,   MD, FRCP, DCH, Consultant Paediatrician and Honorary Lecturer, Newcastle General Hospital.

Augustinos Anagnostopoulos,   PhD, Professor of Inorganic Chemistry, Aristotlian University of Thessaloniki, Greece.

Joseph L. Annest,   PhD, Geneticist and Statistician, National Center for Health Statistics, U.S.A.

Irwin H. Billick,   PhD, Program Manager, Lead Poisoning Research, Environmental Research Group, Dept of Housing and Urban Development, Washington DC.

Oliver David,   MD, Associate Professor in Psychiatry, State University of New York.

371

Philip Day,   MA, PhD, FRSC, Lecturer in Chemistry, University of Manchester.

Philippe Grandjean,   MD, Director, Department of Occupational Medicine, Danish National Institute of Occupational Health, Denmark.

Richard Lansdown,   MA, PhD, Chief Psychologist, Hospital for Sick Children, London.

Michael Moore,   BSc, PhD, Senior Lecturer in Medicine, University of Glasgow.

Herbert L. Needleman,   MD, Associate Professor of Child Psychiatry and Pediatrics, Children's Hospital of Pittsburgh, U.S.A.

Clair C. Patterson,   PhD, Geochemist, Division of Geological and Planetary Sciences, California Institute of Technology, Pasadena, California.

Ellen K. Silbergeld,   PhD, Chief Toxics Scientist, Environmental Defense Fund, Washington DC.

Gerhard Winneke,   PhD, Head of the Department of Psychophysiology, Medical Institute of Environmental Hygiene, Dusseldorf, Germany.

William Yule,   MA, PhD, Reader in Applied Child Psychology, Institute of Psychiatry, London.

The following contributed to the discussions:

M. Bailey.   Institute for Construction and Planning Research.

P.S.I. Barry.   Associated Octel Company.

D. Bryce-Smith.   Department of Chemistry, University of Reading.

P. Burney.   Department of Community Medicine, St. Thomas' Hospital Medical School.

R. Carson.	Assistant Director of Environmental Health, Newport Borough Council.
S. Davies.	Private Practitioner, East Grinstead.
H.T. Delves.	Trace Metal Unit, Southampton General Hospital/University of Southampton.
B.W. Duck.	Institute of Petroleum, London.
M.J. Duggan.	Scientific Branch, Greater London Council.
J. Gallacher.	Medical Research Council - Epidemiology Unit.
C.L. Goodacre.	Retired Consultant - FIAT Spa.
R. Hartley.	St. Thomas' Hospital Medical School.
G. Holmes.	Environmental Health Department, Reading Borough Council.
N. Jackson.	Department of the Environment.
D. Laxen.	Department of Geology, University of Edinburgh.
I.B. Millar.	District Community Physician, Bexley Health Authority.
S. Murgraff.	City and Hackney Community Health Council.
S. Pocock.	Royal Free Hospital Medical School, Department of Clinical Epidemiology.
G.M. Raab,	Medical Computing and Statistics Unit, Edinburgh University.
R. Ranson.	Chief Environmental Health Officer, London Borough of Lambeth.
D. Turner.	Associated Octel Company Limited.
N. Walden.	Manchester North Community Health Council.
R.B. Walker.	Environmental Health Department, Luton Borough Council.
N. Ward.	Department of Chemistry, University of Reading.